The Essential Dr. Faith

USING SCIENCE TO BOOST YOUR

• BRAIN • INTIMACY &

• BODY • BOUNDARIES

Dr. Faith G. Harper

Microcosm Publishing
Portland, OR Cleveland, OH

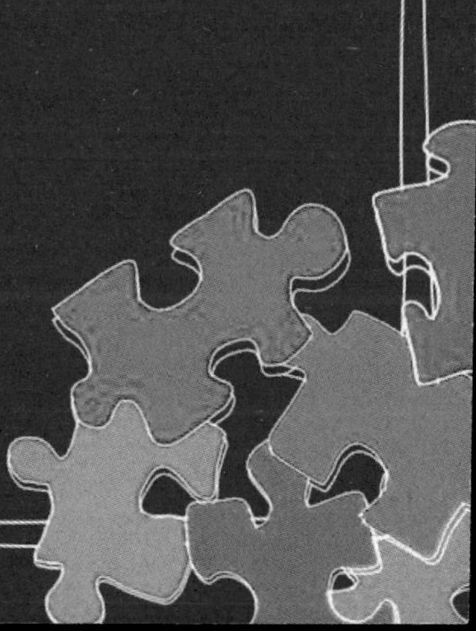

The Essential Dr. Faith: Using Science to Boost Your Brain, Body, Intimacy & Boundaries

First edition - 3,000 copies - November 12, 2024

ISBN 9781648414022

This is Microcosm #835

Previously published as *Unfuck Your Brain* (2017), *Unfuck Your Body* (2021), *Unfuck Your Intimacy* (2019), and *Unfuck Your Boundaries* (2020).

Edited by Olivia Rollins

Book Design by Joe Biel

Cover by Lindsey Cleworth

For a catalog, write or visit:

Microcosm Publishing

2752 N Williams Ave.

Portland, OR 97227

Library of Congress Cataloging-in-Publication Data

Library of Congress control number 2024023017

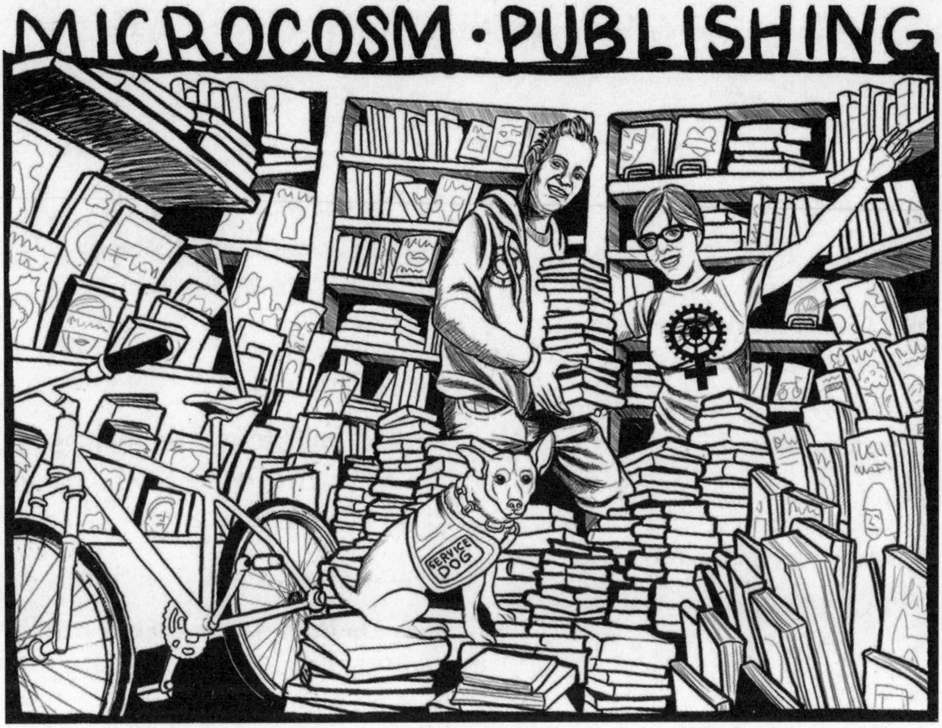

MICROCOSM PUBLISHING is Portland's most diversified publishing house and distributor, with a focus on the colorful, authentic, and empowering. Our books and zines have put your power in your hands since 1996, equipping readers to make positive changes in their lives and in the world around them. Microcosm emphasizes skill-building, showing hidden histories, and fostering creativity through challenging conventional publishing wisdom with books and bookettes about DIY skills, food, bicycling, gender, self-care, and social justice. What was once a distro and record label started by Joe Biel in a drafty bedroom was determined to be *Publishers Weekly*'s fastest-growing publisher of 2022 and #3 in 2023, and is now among the oldest independent publishing houses in Portland, OR, and Cleveland, OH. Biel is also the winner of PubWest's Innovator Award in 2024. We are a politically moderate, centrist publisher in a world that has inched to the right for the past 80 years.

CONTENTS

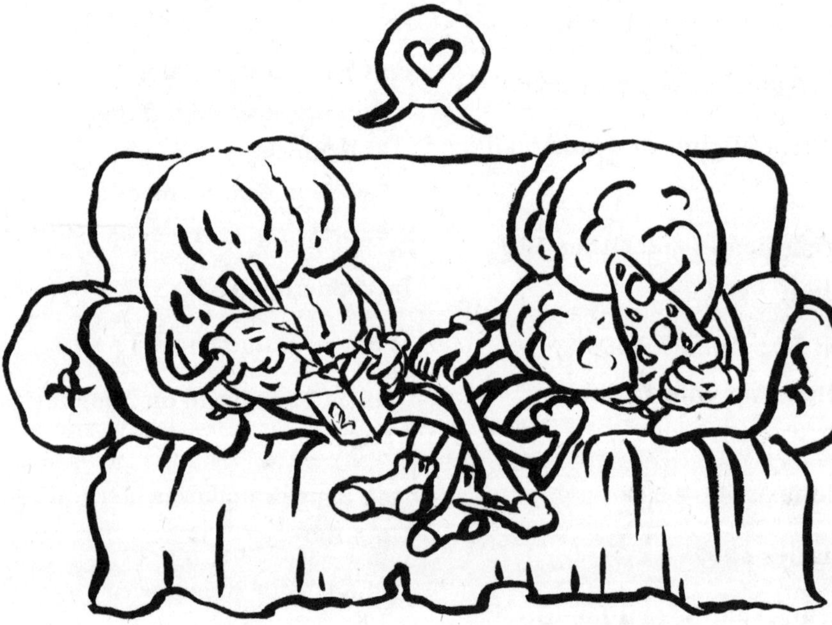

INTRODUCTION TO *THE ESSENTIAL DR. FAITH*

I've written an awful lot of books, zines, and articles around mental health topics. All my books, which are about issues that affect our mental and emotional health, focus strongly on the influence of trauma on our ability to lead the fulfilling, meaningful and sometimes even (whispers) happy lives we keep working our asses off to achieve. And while I hope they all have some level of appeal for readers, there are four that have done especially well in that regard.

So we combined those four into this omnibus edition, collecting them all in one place. TBH, it kinda feels like I'm dropping my first greatest hits album, so I'm bummed to not have woken up this morning with amazing Stevie Nicks hair in a suite at Chateau Marmont. But the fact that these books have resonated with enough people that reorganizing them into an updated volume is already so far beyond my expectations as an author . . . I'll take it.

If you are new to my books, this one is an excellent starter pack to my work. It is also designed to be an easier way to haul around the materials that clinicians and coaches say they use the most. So if you work in mental health and you are running groups and stuff? Carrying one book instead of four is so much easier. So are the roller suitcases. Trust a former hospital activity therapist!

A Note on Edits

Because many topics around mental health have common themes, these four books all had some overlapping content. We made some edits to keep things from getting redundant and to prevent this edition from being a total doorstop. You don't need to read about the markers of trauma four different times, right? Wherever we made those edits, we included a note about where in the book you can find more information on that particular topic.

And for ease of flipping back and forth, we've grouped the recommended resources and references for all four books together at the very end of this tome. So if you're interested in digging deeper into all the research, you know where to go.

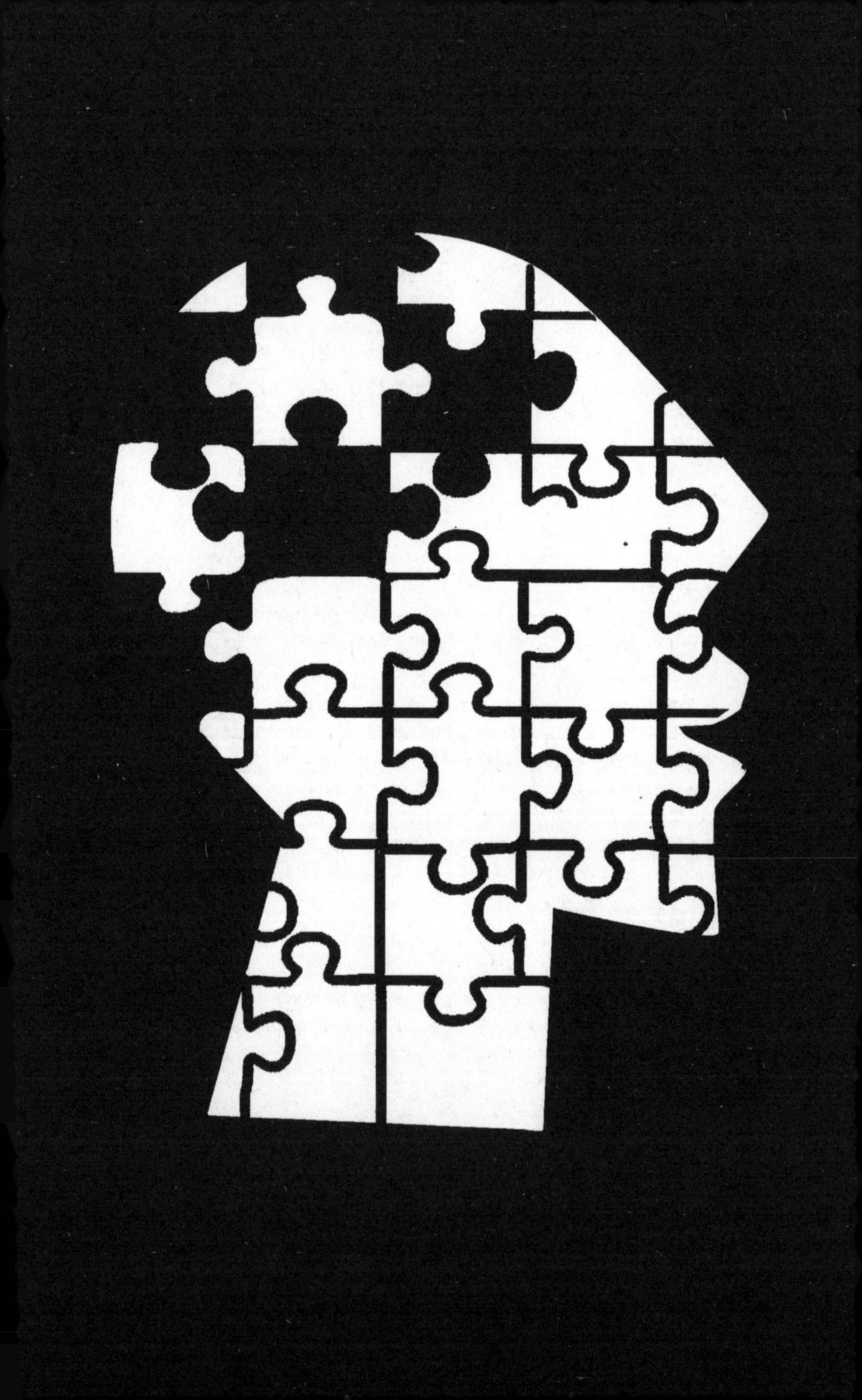

Unfuck Your Brain: Using Science to Get Over Anxiety, Depression, Anger, Freak-outs, and Triggers

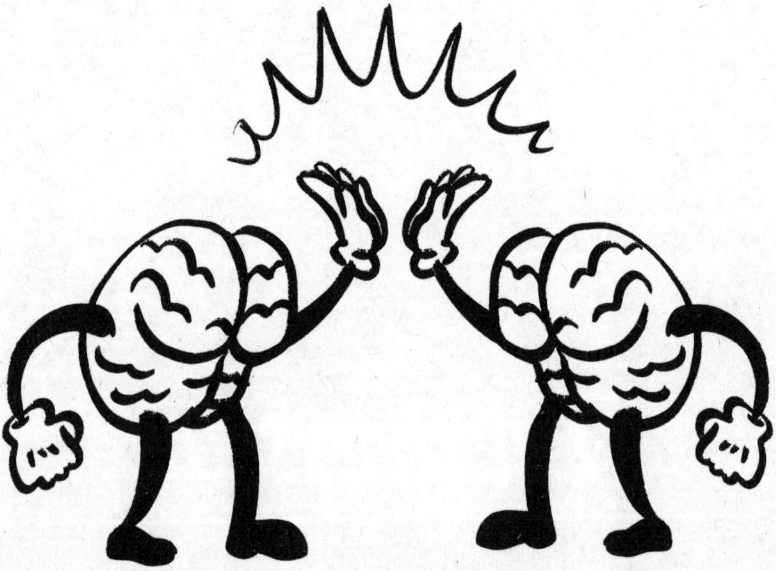

INTRODUCTION

How do our brains get fucked up? Let us count the ways. Anger, depression, anxiety, stress, traumatic grief, substance use, crazy-ass behavioral patterns, dumb-ass relationship choices.

Or as someone said to me recently . . . "Yeah, that's just a typical Tuesday."

So much of what we call mental illness is really a case of brain chemicals gone batshit. And most of this comes from the stressful and traumatic life events we cope with.

We used to hold our poor genes accountable for all the different ways we responded to an environment of stress and trauma. But recent research shows that only two to five percent of the diagnoses people struggle with come from a singular, faulty gene. So we know that the cause of trouble is waaaaaaaay more likely to be our environment and how we cope with it.

These things—anger, depression, the rest of it—are adaptive strategies. If you don't believe anything else I have to say, I hope you believe this part. These feelings are normal. We're wired for self-protection and survival, and that's exactly what your brain is doing when it's acting all fucked up.

Our behaviors are responses to the bullshit we have to deal with day in and day out. Our brains may be responding to big, life altering traumatic experiences . . . but not always. The trouble may also lie in our day to day toxic relationships and interactions . . . the small ways people push our buttons, violate our boundaries, and disrespect our need for safety. And for most people? It's a hot mess combination of the two.

And then feeling fucked up becomes a vicious cycle. We feel weird and crazy for feeling weird and crazy. We feel like we are weak. Or broken. Or fundamentally flawed. And that is the most helpless feeling in the world. Fundamentally flawed means un-fixable. So why bother trying?

But what if you could understand where all of those thoughts and feelings are coming from? And how all the shit going on in your head came to be? What if it were actually entirely understandable? That means it might actually be FIXABLE.

This is important shit. We are way more likely to get better if we know why we are having a certain problem rather than just focusing on the symptoms. If we treat stress, anxiety, or depression, for example, without looking at some of the causes of the stress, anxiety, or depression, then we aren't doing everything we can to make things ACTUALLY BETTER.

It's like if you get a rash (bear with me, gross analogy, I know). You can treat the rash and maybe even make it go away, but if you don't figure out what you were allergic to? Continued issues with rashes are pretty likely.

Same with the brain. If you can understand better why you are doing the things you are doing, the getting better part gets way easier. And it doesn't have to be explained in a super-complicated fancy-pants way to make sense and be useful.

I spent many years as a therapist. A licensed counselor with additional certifications in sexology, integrated life coaching, and clinical nutrition. I still work directly with clients, as a coach (to accommodate working with clients in other states)

My work is trauma-informed, which means I do treat the trauma along with the rest. This does two things:

1. It means I'm actively avoided at parties.
2. My clients are far less frustrated with their progress because they understand the journey we are on and the reasons we are working in certain directions.

I'm not being all self-congratulatory here. My clients do all the fucking work, I'm just the coach. I hold up the huge banner that says "Run this way, Forrest!" at the proper end zone.

I've been in the mental health field for enough decades now for you to say "Damn, you're old," and I can tell you that our current understanding of trauma is fairly new. Several years ago I worked for a program that was the first in town to run trauma recovery groups. In those groups, I saw that focusing on working through trauma histories, rather than on the labels we attached to their effects (depression, anxiety, addiction, etc.) helped people get better. Since that time I've trained in several more trauma treatment modalities, and helped several agencies and programs move into using a trauma informed treatment model.

I'm currently working in a coaching practice and even when the focus is on relationships and intimacy, guess what the biggest issue I run into is? Trauma history. It rears its ugly head everywhere. I found that when I explained everything that was going on in a way that was simple, my clients would say "Oh, shit! That makes sense!" This book exists because nobody else has smushed all that stuff together in a way that is simple and practical. And I have seen how learning the simple and practical part helps people figure out the getting better part way more quickly.

This may be bad for business, but I don't think everyone needs therapy. I hope everyone includes some kind of wellness work in their lives, but we each have to find the route that makes the most sense for us. Some people meditate, some people exercise, some people have a life coach, and some people see a therapist. Some people do something entirely different. It's all good.

Because, hey . . . you do you. But I really believe that everything works better if you understand the why part. And the end-goal of doing things differently, whatever those things may be.

Who is this Book For?

This book is for the people who ask "But, WHY?" all the time. The people who annoyed the crap out of the adults around them when they were little kids by asking questions about how the world worked so they could understand their place in it. Because the why is REALLY NEEDFUL INFORMATION.

This book is for all the people who fucking HATE being told what to do by other people. Who just want the tools and the information that they need to figure out what to do for themselves. You may be figuring this shit out by yourself or with a rock-star therapist who knows better than to boss you around. Either way, you know you are in charge of your own fucking life when it comes down to it, because you are sure as hell responsible for all the consequences.

This book is for the people who are fucking tired of hearing or thinking that they are just crazy. Or stupid. Or lazy. Or "too sensitive." Or just need to "get over" themselves. Who are tired of feeling bad, but even more tired of other people thinking they enjoy feeling bad. Like anyone would choose misery. Like if you could figure out why you were miserable you wouldn't DO something about it. Of course you would. So this book is about why you are miserable so you can do something about it.

What is Going to Happen in this Book?

So, ok. You're thinking: That's all well and good, fancy doctor lady. How is this book going to help? What makes this book all kinds of special and different from the eleventy-billion other self-help books toppling off my bookshelves already? I'm skeptical as fuck right now.

Word. You should be. My bookshelves are crammed full, too. I've probably read most everything you've read.

This book is different, for serious.

First up? I'm gonna lay some science on you. Not complex, dry, boring-as-a-box-of-rocks science, but "Holy shit, that makes sense, how come no one ever explained it to me like that before???" science. I found in my private practice that it DOESN'T take twelve years of college and two hundred thousand dollars of student loan debt to understand this shit. I can generally explain what you need to know about what's going on with the brain in about five to ten minutes (or an equal number of written pages, as the case may be).

Second? I'm not gonna lay all this brain science shit on you and then say "Yeah, that's fucked up . . . sucks to be you" and walk away. I'm going to go through a lot of advice that is actually practical and doable for getting better.

Not everyone has time for an Eat, Pray, Love type of retreat (and clearly, I'm not at all jealous or anything). Most of us have to get up every day, deal with real life, and try to figure out the getting better part during that process. Getting better doesn't mean you don't have to keep doing your own laundry. So we are going to DIY this shit like rock stars. Because you know what? The situation isn't hopeless. YOU aren't hopeless. GETTING BETTER HAPPENS. If you were a client at my office, we would be wrestling these demons back into submission together. This is the next best thing. And it's the shit that works.

Third? I'm going to go through a lot of the treatment options out there. I'm not against medication and Western care . . . BUT I do believe they belong in their proper place among many treatment options. Holistic care means the whole fucking person. And we have to build a plan that works for us. For example, my best line of defense is eating healthy, being forced to exercise now and then, taking herbal supplements, and embracing acupuncture, meditation, massage, and pedicures as part of my wellness regime. And I will fight anyone to the pain (yes, Princess Bride reference) over my belief that pedicures are therapeutic. For my son, it's football, weightlifting, grounding exercises, meditation, a highly structured school environment, neurofeedback, and a combo of both supplements and Western meds. We all have unique needs. Pedicures, strangely, are not on his list. So I will throw in a lot of options you maybe haven't heard about in order to help you create your own plan of attack.

And throughout the book there will be mini-exercises that will help you process the work that you are doing. It's not homework, you don't have to pass a final exam. But having ways to process all the stuff that may come up for you is important. I'm not about to have you carrying my book around with your entrails hanging out because it eviscerated you, FFS. Don't use it if you don't need it. But it's there if you do.

Take Action: Taking Your Own Temperature

How often in life have you genuinely been given permission to feel what you feel? Rarely to fucking never is my bet.

This book is all about working through the types of shit that get in the way of us having the lives we want and the sense of purpose and peace that we crave. The type of bullshit we call traumatic events. It's also for people with huge stress responses, anxiety, grief, anger, depression, and/or addictive behaviors—all the coping skills we develop to get through life without trying to end it.

And that makes for stressful reading. Some paragraphs in here may end up sucker punching your ass because it hits a fundamental truth about your life and experience. And your brain isn't gonna be happy with those feels. Your brain may be all "Fuck this noise and toss that book."

Because we are generally told not to feel negative emotions. They are bad and to be avoided. And we're going to go further into why that is complete bullshit.

But in the meantime, it can be really helpful to tap into what you're feeling. Take your own temperature, so to speak. And have an action plan for if it gets too high. You are going to learn more exercises that you can incorporate later on in this book. But let's start with the simplest first.

Shut your eyes right now and notice:

- What's going on in your body?
- What are you thinking? (It may not be actual thoughts but flashes of memory tapes playing.)
- What are you feeling in response to that? Name those emotions. Rate the severity of them.
- Now what do you notice is going on in your body? Anything different?
- And, seriously, what other shit are you dealing with in your everyday life that's either helping you cope or making it worse?

This exercise might be really hard for you. Lots of people have no fucking clue how they feel. And that's OK, too. You've been trained to be disconnected from that. Told what you felt was wrong. That you weren't allowed.

So if you don't know . . . acknowledge that, too. You may find that as you do this particular exercise over time, you will start connecting to what you feel again. Not knowing does NOT make you a self-help book drop-out. It's just more vital information about where you are right now.

All this exercise does is give you back your power to own what is going on inside you.

You have permission to feel what you feel.

Learning to reconnect with the reality of your experience will help you gather the resources you need to move forward. Because you deserve to. We should honor the past, we should remember it, and we should respect what it has taught us. But we don't have to keep living there. That house is crumbling and toxic and far too small to contain you. It doesn't support our present experience and it sure as fuck doesn't fit into your future goals.

Section One: This is Your Brain on Trauma

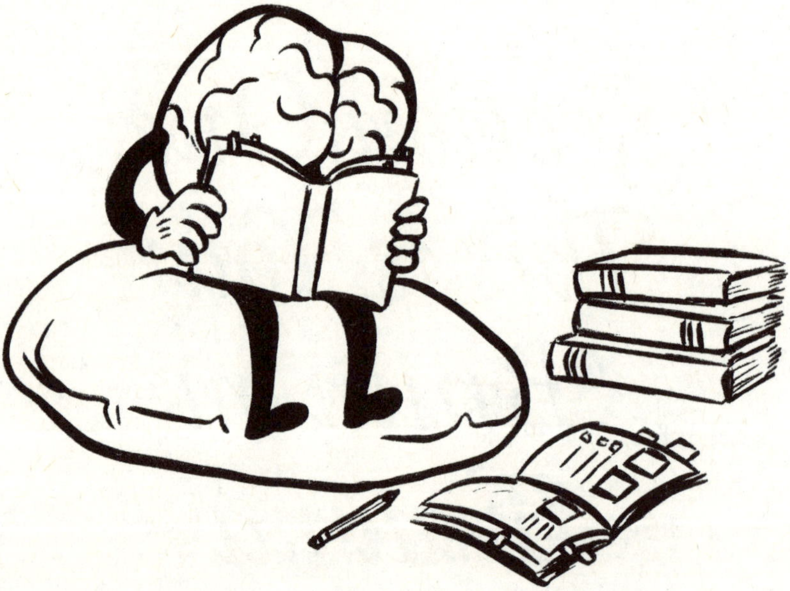

CHAPTER ONE: HOW OUR BRAINS GET FUCKED

Short answer? Trauma.

This book is essentially all about trauma and our traumatic responses. It's also about how we create coping strategies to deal with this trauma—strategies that fancy doctor people call anxiety, depression, addiction, anger, etc.

These strategies are essentially part of the whole complicated process of your brain responding after shit goes down in your life. The brain is really just trying to do its job by protecting you the best way it knows how. But the brain often ends up being a not-particularly-helpful asshole instead. It's like your friend that offers to beat the shit out of anyone who upsets you. Gratifying, but not helpful in the long run.

This book is also about general life bullshittery and other-people's dickitude. The shit that might not be traumatic but gets in the way of us kicking ass at life. The ways we manage stuff that isn't full blown trauma . . . but sure as fuck isn't kittens, rainbows, and teddy bears. Like with trauma, the coping skills we create for THESE situations tend to be less and less useful over time and also downright exhausting.

The good news is, no matter how long you've been stuck in this quicksand, you CAN rewire your response and unfuck your brain.

Why Is My Brain a Big, Hot Mess?

We have a tendency to separate mental health from physical health. As if they don't affect each other in a continuous fucking feedback loop, or something.

Stuff we learn about the brain itself generally falls under the "physical health" category. Thoughts, feelings, and behaviors fall under the "mental health" category.

So where does this thinking and feeling fit in our body? Our mind seems to be this helium balloon floating over our heads at all times. We are holding on to the string, maybe, but it isn't really part of us (though we are still held accountable for all of it).

That image of a disembodied brain isn't helpful. It doesn't make one bit of sense.

And what we actually know about the brain is this: it at least somewhat lives in our gut. Unique microorganisms reside there that communicate so consistently with our actual brains (through the gut-brain axis . . . an actual real thing) to the point that they are referred to as a second brain. One that plays a huge role in guiding our emotions. Ever had a gut reaction? Yeah, that's a real thing.

Which is to say, instead of being a thing that's barely tethered to us and gets us in trouble all the time, our mind actually lies deep in the middle of our body, acting as a control center, taking in tons of information, and making decisions before we are even aware that a decision needs to be made.

Our thoughts, feelings, and behaviors come from HERE. They are rooted deep in our physical bodies, in how our brains perceive the world around us, based on past experiences and current information. So it might be the understatement of the decade to say that knowing what's going on in your brain and how all that shit works is HUGE. And when we totally get all that, we see that how we interact with the world around us is a completely normal response when we take into account brain functioning and our past experiences. If all is bopping along and the landing is smooth, we don't notice any problems. But when we have a rough landing? When brain-traffic control doesn't manage its shit properly, we see the effects:

- Freaking the fuck out
- Avoiding important shit we need to take care of
- Feeling pissed off all the time
- Being a dick to people we care about
- Putting shit in our bodies that we know isn't good for us
- Doing shit we know is dumb or pointless or destructive

None of these things are fucking helpful. But they all make sense.

As we navigate the world, nasty shit happens. The brain stores info about the nasty shit to try to avoid it in the future. Your brain has adapted to the circumstances in your life and started doing things to protect you, bless it. Sometimes these responses are helpful. Sometimes the responses become a bigger problem than the actual problem was. Your brain isn't TRYING to fuck you over (even though sometimes it totally does).

And even if you aren't dealing with a specific trauma? Adaptive coping strategies, bad habits, and funky behaviors all wire in similar ways. And research is showing that these issues are actually some of the easier ones to treat in therapy . . . if we address what's really going on, rather than just the symptoms.

I have found that one of the most helpful things I did as a therapist and do as a coach is explain what is going on inside the brain and how the work we are doing in therapy is designed to rewire our responses to certain situations.

The strategies we work on in therapy (and the strategies and skills people figure out for themselves) are designed to wire the brain back to processing information without triggering some kind of crazy overreaction. This overreaction is our brain's way of adapting and protecting us whenever it perceives a situation as a threat . . . so we are prepared to do whatever we need to do to stay alive. Battle brain ACTIVATE. Even if the "enemy" is just some rando next to you at the bookstore who has no idea they just triggered you.

If we can regain control, then we can respond to these perceived threats in the safest, most rational way possible.

Lemme explain what I mean by that.

Brain 101

So if any part of the book is complicated, it's this part. Because brains are pretty fucking complicated. But this part will only get as complicated as absolutely necessary to explain the shit you are wanting to know about what's going on. So hang with me, we got this.

The prefrontal cortex (we'll call it the PFC), essentially the front part of your brain, is the part that is in charge of executive functioning, which includes problem-solving, goal-oriented behaviors, and managing social interactions according to expectations of what is "appropriate." Essentially, executive function is just straight up thinking.

It's sort of behind your forehead (which makes sense with the name, right?). This is the part of the brain that evolved the most recently, and it's the part that makes us the most different from other species. The PFC is in charge of receiving information from the world and managing our thoughts and actions accordingly.

The prefrontal cortex is also the part that takes the longest to develop as we grow up. It isn't at full capacity until we are in our mid-20s. That doesn't mean that it doesn't exist in children, adolescents, and young adults. And it sure as hell doesn't mean you have a free pass on doing stupid shit if you are younger. But it does mean all our brain wiring creates new and more complex communication networks—new pathways for communication—as we get older and wiser. And if it all goes well, the PFC continues to work better and better—a definite benefit of aging.

Hold on to that if it all goes well part for me, though.

So the prefrontal cortex is the part that is theoretically in charge.

And the prefrontal cortex is, understandably, highly connected to the rest of the brain. The ventral portion (which is just, you know, the backside of the PFC . . . the PFC booty, so to speak) is directly linked to an entirely different area of the brain . . . the part that stores emotions (more on that mess inna second). Additionally, the entire PFC receives feedback from the brainstem arousal systems (don't worry, more on that later, too).

So whatever information is being sent to the PFC from these other parts of the brain impacts that whole thinking thing. There is a region of the PFC called the anterior cingulate cortex (ACC). The job of this region is to manage the dialogue between the PFC (think-y brain) and the limbic system (feely-y brain). The ACC manages the convo in the brain between what we know and what we feel . . . and then makes suggestions on what we should do about the whole mess.

And our wiring in that area is fucking WEIRD. The brain cells here are called spindle neurons . . . they are long, leggy supermodels instead of short and bushy like they are everywhere else. These fuckers can haul some serious ass, to boot. They send signals way faster than the rest of the neurons, so you are hit up with an emotional response fast.

Why those and why there? Only humans and great apes have spindle neurons. A lot of scientists think that they are part of our evolution to higher cognition.

In order to think more, we have to feel more. And then take both into account when making decisions. Emotions are just as important for our survival as thoughts. And you are totally seeing where I am going with this already.

The Asshole Amygdala

So that middle-ish part of the brain that I mentioned? The part doing the tango with the PFC booty? That's the limbic system. This portion is buried a bit in the folds of the brain, behind the PFC. If the PFC does the thinking part, the limbic system does the emotions part. And a lot of that emotions part has to do with how we store memories.

The amygdala and the hippocampus are two key parts of the limbic system. Most of what we now know about how trauma affects the brain is tied into research about the amygdala. The amygdala's job is to relate memories to emotions. True dat. But, to be more specific, the amygdala has been found to only store a specific kind of memory, not all of them. The amygdala doesn't give a shit where you left your car keys. The amygdala's function is to manage episodic-autobiographical memory (EAM). Essentially this is the storage of event-based knowledge. Times, locations, people. Not your great-aunt's banana pudding recipe. Your stories about the world and how it works. The shit that happens to you.

So why the fuck is this important? Episodic memories get stored in the hippocampus as our story about the shit that happens . . . our interpretation of events with our emotional response attached to them. These are memories that are tied to serious emotional reactions. If something happened in your life that was really significant to you, the emotions tied to that memory become attached to it like cat hair or static cling. So when we have an emotional response in the future, the amygdala immediately pulls this EAM file in order to decide how to respond.

What fires together, wires together.

Say you got flowers. Flowers are excellent, right? Sure . . . if your past memories of getting flowers were happy ones. Maybe your partner gave you flowers once and then proposed. So when you're getting flowers in the future, seeing flowers, driving by a flower delivery truck? Nice feelings.

But say you got flowers when a loved one died . . . terribly and suddenly. Some nice person knew you were hurting and sent you flowers. But now even the smell of flowers may make you queasy.

The amygdala has turned the memory of flowers into an actual mnemonic for certain emotions. A mnemonic like ROY G BIV to remember the colors of the rainbow or "Every Good Boy Does Fine" to remember the note breakdown on a musical scale. Shit I've not been able to unlearn from grade school.

The amygdala's job is to make sure you don't forget things that are very important. Remembering important-good is awesome. Nobody bitches about nice memories. Remembering important-bad can sucketh muchly.

It sucks because the amygdala doesn't really discriminate super well, especially when it's trying to protect you. It ROY G BIVs your ass into equating flowers with death. And then you're walking down the street on a spring day and smell the flowers blooming in your neighbor's garden. And suddenly you feel like you've lost your fucking mind, because even though your body is still in your neighbor's garden, your brain is back at your loved one's funeral.

Fight, Flight or Freeze . . . it's the Brainstem!

And that brings us to the last part of our brain convo, where we talk about one final part of the brain . . . the brainstem.

The brainstem is the very base of the brain (makes sense, right?). It is the first part of the brain to evolve into being, and the part that attaches to the vertebrae in our neck and back. You've seen how the brain looks like a bunched up mass of overcooked pasta, right? This is the part of the brain that is starting to untangle itself from the rest of the noodles, straighten out a bit, and transition into being your spinal cord.

The brainstem is our fundamental survival tool. While cardiac muscles regulate basic needs like the breathing in and out and the heart going pump pump pump all day long, the brainstem controls the rate, speed, and intensity. So it will ramp up for a panic attack, for example. Because PAYATTENTIONWEMIGHTBEDYINGFFS. You know, the important stuff.

Being alert, being conscious, being aware of our surroundings? Brainstem tasks.

So when the brainstem is saying "OW OW OW MOTHERFUCKER" or "Danger Will Robinson!" it is actually flooding the prefrontal cortex with a bunch of neurochemicals that change how the PFC operates.

The brainstem may be a basic bitch, but it is sure as hell in charge of a lot.

When the brainstem senses danger, the behavioral actions of the prefrontal cortex become FIGHT, FLIGHT, or FREEZE.

Fight is BEAT THEIR ASS BEFORE YOUR ASS GETS BEAT.

Flight is GET THE FUCK UP OUT OF HERE THIS ISN'T SAFE.

And Freeze is IF YOU PLAY POSSUM AND DON'T RESPOND AT ALL MAYBE ALL THIS WILL GO AWAY.

Don't get me wrong . . . these are essential survival tasks when something dangerous is going on. They are crazy important to our survival. This whole process is our emergency broadcast system, replete with electronic beeping in the background.

The prefrontal cortex takes in some outside information. The amygdala says I REMEMBER THAT! LAST TIME THAT SHIT HAPPENED, IT HURT! HURT SUCKS! And the brainstem tells the prefrontal cortex GET THE FUCK UP OUT OF THERE! WE DON'T LIKE TO HURT!

So we say "Peace out, threatening situation, gotta jet!" Or we fight back. Or we freeze up and play dead and hope the situation passes us over. All kinds of things can feel threatening . . . like a final exam or a bullshit work deadline. But those don't need a HOLY SHITBALLS IMMA GONNA BE A DINOSAUR SNACK response. Except the brainstem evolved to avoid being a dinosaur snack and NOT to deal with bullshit traffic and people who hit the heels of our feet with their shopping carts at the grocery store (though, you could totally argue the point that they are bigger shitheads than hungry dinosaurs).

Squish It All Together? We Got Storytelling Brains

We all understand this to a certain extent, I think. The idea that human beings are storytellers, that is. But only to a certain extent. Because we don't really talk about the fact that this is an actual, evolutionary function. Partially because this is pretty new research, and also because it's kinda weird, when you think about it.

We don't just tell stories because we want to . . . we HAVE to. It's a biological human drive. In fact, we are so wired to tell stories that we even do it in our sleep. This is why we dream.

The brain has a default mode. Everything essentially has a default mode, right? Some sort of resting state. A light switch turned off is in default mode. When you turn on the light, you activate it.

When the brain is activated, it's to concentrate on some kind of outside input. A problem to solve, someone to attend to, something that needs to be done that requires focused, conscious concentration. The rest of the time, the brain is in default mode. Awake and aware, but generally resting.

Researchers have been able to map the brain in default mode . . . and here is where it gets really fucking interesting. The brain in default mode is the storytelling brain.

When our brain is in resting state is when we story-tell. You've totally caught yourself doing this. You're driving home. Nothing you need to attend to, you know this route so well, you aren't really engaged. Storytelling mode ACTIVATE. You're telling yourself a story about what you are going to cook for dinner, or watch on TV, or the errands you have to run. These conversations aren't bullet pointed reminder lists . . . you actually walk through a story of your plan.

A storytelling brain is an excellent fucking thing most of the time.

- Stories are often rehearsals for life events, which makes them really fucking useful if we are getting ready to field test a new skill.
- Stories allow us to hold larger chunks of information than we could otherwise. The PFC is designed to hold about seven pieces of information (plus or minus two). We try to juggle more than that, we start dropping things off the list. Stories, however, help us hold tons more information because they create pathways for remembering far more than we could otherwise.
- Stories are our primary mode of communication with others. According to Lewis Mehl-Madrona, MD, PhD (a well known researcher and treatment professional who incorporates both

Western medicine practices as well as the Lakota, Cherokee, and Cree ancestors and teachers), they are the neural pathways of our collective, cultural brain. It isn't just how we hold information inside, it is how we share it outside.

But clearly the storytelling brain has the capacity to be a serious fucking problem, too. We start telling ourselves (and believing) certain stories about ourselves and the world around us. Our brains are wired to crave certainty. We WANT to see patterns in what happens so we can make better decisions about the world and how we are supposed to keep ourselves safe in it. Brains are stubborn motherfuckers that already have a story they've put together about what is real and true about the world.

You've seen that right? No matter what evidence to the contrary someone sees, they are determined as fuck to stay on course with their decision. It's why elections can be so fucking crazy. Or people lose a fortune in a casino. The emotional brain makes a decision for us and the thinking brain has to scramble to come up with a reason why.

Brains will rationalize the hell out of anything.

Yes, You Can Retrain Your Brain

Brains are adaptable little assholes, and you sure-as-fuck can retrain them. Don't believe me? Well, first of all you should. I'm a fancy doctor. But if you are one of those "Fuck your degree, I want proof!" people, go to YouTube and search for "Lumiere Brothers Arrival of a Train." It's only a 45 second clip. I'll wait here.

So picture this: Paris. 1895. These bros were photography pioneers who presented the first "moving picture" to the public at an art exhibition. They were totes excited about their project . . . but didn't get the expected response. Instead, the moviegoers flipped their shit, and all screamed in terror and hid under the seats. Like, every single one.

The brain's way of perceiving information was telling them all "TRAIN ABOUT TO HIT YOUR STUPID ASS, GET OFF THE TRACKS!"

Because, yeah. Trains were dangerous and moving images of trains did not exist until that point. Their brains perceived the train as a reality instead of a movie.

When you watched this, did your brain freak out? Duh, no. You know what a movie is. Your neural mechanisms have been trained to understand representational train versus literal train.

And now your brain needs to learn real danger versus perceived danger. Remember that everybody's brain has issues with differentiation, especially when it comes to survival. Like the toddler who calls all animals doggies until they learn that there are also horsies, and kitties, and llamas, and great white sharks. The brain is going around yelling DOGGIE DOGGIE DOGGIE all the fucking time.

That is, your brain is presuming danger until it can be convinced otherwise. The amygdala is not trusting the PFC's interpretation at the moment. The minute the PFC is thinking "hmmm, animal?" the amygdala grabs the control stick away from the PFC while screaming DOOOOOOGGIEEEEEE.

That's a lot of mixed metaphors. Sorry about that. Simple version? We have to get the PFC back in charge. Give it a chance to decide if it's an actual doggie or something else. We have to convince the PFC and the amygdala to hug it out and do their respective jobs, which means working the fuck TOGETHER.

It's Official. You Are Not Crazy. A Doctor Just Said So.

Yeah, that was a lot of shit to read about the brain, but it's important shit. Because it means that what we are doing, what we are thinking, and how we are feeling make fucking sense.

Whether you find yourself defensive and combative as fuck, freaking out hardcore, or completely shut off and disassociated, it's your survival mode that is responding. The problem is when this happens during situations that aren't actually life threatening emergencies. The amygdala has hijacked your ability to manage the situation in a rational way using the prefrontal cortex.

It is not a "Hey, let's investigate this situation, have rational conversations, and then determine how we want to respond based on what will best benefit us in the long run" kind of thinking. Your amygdala screamed "DUCK AND COVER!" and all rational responses went out the window.

Duck and cover thinking isn't a bad thing at all. It's the kind of thinking we need when we hear gunshots or tornado sirens. We want to override our executive functioning if we accidentally touch a hot stove. If we didn't, that would mean that while our hand is burning, we are going through an intellectual deconstruction of the experience while our amygdala and brainstem are screaming bloody murder in the background. This is not a postmodern piece of experimental cinema. This is LIFE. We want a brain whose job is to keep us alive, right? Not just remember our locker combination from 6th grade and all the lyrics to Taylor Swift's "Shake It Off," FFS.

But in the process, it also protects us from everything it PERCEIVES as danger, not just ACTUAL danger. Our ability to discriminate between real danger and perceived danger is an imperfect system. The brain is going to err on the side of caution, even if that means you shut down when you don't actually need to.

Say you are just trying to pick up some groceries, but walking through the floral department your brain goes "FLOWERS! ROY G BIV! ABORT MISSION!" And you are in a full blown panic attack, running out of the store before you pass out. And you still don't have any fucking groceries for dinner.

You are all "Damn, Self, that was just the floral department. Just some carnations and roses. No one died, and now I'm stuck eating ramen noodles again." Or maybe you are not even sure why you lost your shit and are thinking "Damn, Self, do you have to be all 50 shades of batshit crazy?"

That rational part? The "just carnations and roses, simmer the fuck down" part? That requires stimulus discrimination.

You know. The ability to decide if something is actually a problem or not.

Stimulus discrimination is a thinking thing, not an emotions thing. Which means it happens in the prefrontal cortex, and once the brainstem gets into freak-out mode, it's really hard to get the prefrontal cortex up and running again. But we can do it. And we are going to talk about how we retrain our brain to respond in ways that better suit life as it is now instead of life as it was in the past.

Our stimulus discrimination response is based on all of our past experiences and habits, and that response is even more ingrained if those experiences were traumatic ones. If a stimulus is attached to a strong memory, the body starts shooting off hormones and neurotransmitters to prepare itself for response. Brains don't really have new thoughts so much as different configurations and mash-ups of old thoughts.

This is why a military vet may freak out at seeing garbage by the side of the road, after being in Iraq and driving through areas replete with improvised explosive devices.

This is why an individual who was abused may freak out over smelling a certain scent they associate with their abuser.

The brain knows its history. It has been trained to do whatever it can to remain safe. It's creating stories about your current experience or possible future experiences based on its past information. It doesn't realize or doesn't trust that you actually ARE safe.

Take Action: Trigger is Not Just the Lone Ranger's Horse

We throw around the word trigger on the internetz like it's fucking confetti or something. But a trigger, in this context, just means the cause part of a cause-and-effect type situation thingy going on.

Sometimes we know straight up what our triggers are gonna be. For example, anxiety may be the motherfucking gremlin on your back. You may know a first date, or a public speaking engagement, or a meeting with your boss is going to send your anxiety through the roof. Or a road trip where you can't find a clean rest stop with a non-sketch bathroom is gonna cause a freak out (And why is there NOT an app for that??? The struggle is REAL).

But sometimes? Not a fucking clue. Like all other mental health issues, we may have a genetic predisposition to certain responses and/or it may be a product of the environment we grew up in or live in now. And that can make figuring out our specific triggers difficult.

Next time you start feeling yourself getting into Eject mode, ask yourself these questions. And later, when you've cooled off, write the answers down:

- What specific emotion were you feeling?
- On a 0–100% scale how would you rate that emotion?
- What were the specific symptoms you felt (your emotional response)?
- What else was going on when it hit? Just write down everything that was going on, no matter how mundane. Because, patterns over time are how we figure out our triggers.

Another method is to keep a mood tracking diary (either an app or old school paper one). This feels like a lot of work, but can really help with figuring out your triggers until you get the hang of doing it mentally throughout your day. Here is a simple format you can copy and use. You can download a printable copy from FaithGHarper.com:

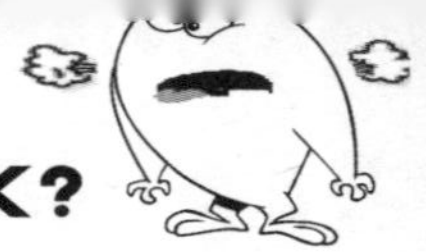

WEEKLY MOOD TRACKER

	MOOD	SITUATION	MAGNITUDE (0-100)	SYMPTOMS
SUNDAY				
MONDAY				
TUESDAY				
WEDNESDAY				
THURSDAY				
FRIDAY				
SATURDAY				

CHAPTER TWO: HOW TRAUMA REWIRES THE BRAIN

Ok, Lady, What the Fuck Do You Mean by Trauma?

A trauma is an event that happens outside our understanding of how the world is supposed to work. A traumatic response is when our ability to cope with what happened goes to shit and it's affecting other areas of our life.

There are lots of things that can operate as a trauma. To be honest, there are plenty of things that are deeply traumatic for many people that aren't really considered by our diagnostic manuals. It's one of the things that burns my ass, because it then leads to people feeling ashamed that their trauma wasn't traumatic enough to warrant attention. And that's some bullshit right there. Because fancy terms and definitions aside? A trauma is a "What the fuck was THAT?" situation.

A trauma can be an accident, an injury, a serious illness, a loss . . . or any kind of life event that kicks your ass.

But in the end? We all experience trauma differently, and are impacted by too many things to list. Creating a list that touches only on the big "diagnosable" categories dismisses other experiences that shouldn't be dismissed.

By one estimate, approximately half of all people in the US will experience a diagnosable trauma although more recent studies have it at about 75%. And about 7 or 8 out of every 100 people will have PTSD at some point in their lives. And that's only diagnosed traumas. The official "rules" for diagnosing a trauma reaction are pretty limited, which means I consider the number way higher than 8%.

Having suffered abuse as a child is a trauma we all recognize, for example. But having dealt with horrific bullying isn't necessarily a recognized trauma . . . even though many people have taken their own lives because they were bullied. So it's not on the list. Because trauma doesn't operate by checking the right box in the right category. Instead? Please believe me when I say your experiences and reactions are valid and real and you are worthy of care and the opportunity to heal.

Because we don't know why some things are worse than others for some people. I know that it is a weird fucking idea, but everyone is different. Everyone's lives, histories, and experiences are different AND our genetic predispositions are different.

And then, get this: We now even know that trauma can actually create genetic changes that can be passed down through generations. If you have a great-grandparent, grandparent, or parent with a serious trauma history, you are wired for a different response than someone who had family members without a lot of life drama. So not only do our genes influence our trauma reactions, our trauma reactions influence our genes.

Seriously, human brain? Could you go fuck yourself on this one?

On a physical level, traumatic response = Amygdala Hijack.

And there are different levels of intensity within that amygdala response. Sometimes we aren't in full-blown trauma mode, but we keep noticing some weird patterns and habits in our thinking and behavior. Maybe you're not in full force freak-the-fuck-out mode but HOLY SHITBALLS, managing yourself is taking away more energy than it should. Ain't nobody got time to spend on the concentrated effort of keeping their shit together for months and years on end.

Short version? We all have our fragile places and we are all susceptible. But for some reason, sometimes we hang in there and sometimes we lose our shit. What's up with that?

How Our Brains Handle Trauma

You know the biggest things that happen to us? The things that we think are the most horrific? These terrible events may not always cause a long-term traumatic response.

About two-thirds of the time, when we experience a trauma, our brains actually don't go into asshole mode. That means that most of the time we are eventually able to find a way to make sense of the trauma and recover from it without having enormous long-term consequences. This doesn't mean you didn't deal with something epically craptastic. It just means you were able to find your way through the experience without a long term amygdala hijack.

In a perfect world, bad shit wouldn't happen. Heh, yeah. Good luck to all of us on that one. Second-best scenario is that when bad shit happens, we duck and cover then come out unscathed. And honestly, we do most of the time. Look back on all the fucked up things that you had to handle in your life that didn't create epic crazy-brain in the long term. Not that it was an immediate and flawless recovery, though, right?

Most of the time, it takes about three months to reestablish equilibrium after a trauma. That is, after about 90 days, our emotional sensors are no longer operating at hyper warp speed mode, and return to normal.

Using the word normal is total bullshit, of course. Of course, it's not really normal, no matter how well you recover. Traumas change us forever. So this so-called normal is more of a new normal, in that regard. We find a way to live and cope with the situation that happened, the loss of what the world had been, and an acceptance of what it is now. We still experience feelings surrounding whatever happened—feelings that may never completely go away. But our amygdala isn't super haywire over the situation after a few months. Hijack mode, deactivated.

But approximately a third of the time, after a trauma, we don't recover to a new normal. We have a trauma response instead. And we develop PTSD—Post-Traumatic Stress Disorder.

What is PTSD? The Oxford dictionary defines post-traumatic stress disorder as:

"A condition of persistent mental and emotional stress occurring as a result of injury or severe psychological shock, typically involving disturbance of sleep and constant vivid recall of the experience, with dulled responses to others and to the outside world."

Good definition. Fancy one. But the unfancy version? PTSD is failure to recover from a traumatic event. And PTSD is a fucking DEMON.

The National Center for PTSD (VA.gov) has collected research in this regard. What makes you more likely to experience PTSD? A lot of the indicators they found make a ton of sense:

- Being directly exposed as a victim or an in-person witness
- Experiencing something that was very severe, or the person was hurt badly as a result of the incident
- Traumas that were long-lasting
- Believing you were in danger or someone you loved was and feeling helpless to protect them or yourself
- Having had a severe physical or emotional response during the traumatic situation

Our backgrounds can make us more susceptible to a trauma response, as well:

- Having had other traumas at a young age
- Having other mental health problems or having family members with mental health problems.
- Having little support from family or friends, either by not having many people in your life or being surrounded by individuals who don't understand your experience.

- Having recently had stressful life changes, or having recently lost a loved one.
- Being female or in a minority cultural group (because you are statistically more likely to experience a trauma to begin with)
- Already using mind-altering substances like drugs or alcohol
- Being younger
- Having less education
- Coming from a cultural group or family system where you are less likely to talk about problems.

No surprises there, I don't think. But the last item on that list is HUGE. Go read that again. When we talk about things, they get better.

But why? Why some people and not others? What's the brain science behind all of this?

It's not about the nature of the trauma so much. Or the severity of it. Or even totally a function of our wiring and our experiences. Those things have an impact on our ability to heal, for damn sure. But if it was that easy we could create an anticipatory flow chart to help us nail down who is going to develop PTSD and who isn't. But we can't, because how we heal is as much about our present and near future as it is our past.

Research shows that when we can't get to a new normal, it's because the brain's ability to process the experience is disrupted during the first 30 days after the trauma happened. This is why PTSD cannot be diagnosed in the first month. We don't know yet if we're going to get our shit back together or not.

Those first 30 days are critical. We need time and space to recover, to process what happened, to find ways to make sense of how we want the world to work and our experience of how life actually unfolds. In this time, we need relational supports. Our brains are hardwired to connect, and we get better in connection to other people. We'll dig into this in Chapter 3.

Not having this time and these connections is a damn likely indicator that we are heading into trauma response territory.

And not having this time, or these people, happens for a lot of really good reasons.

See, generally speaking, traumas are not stand-alone experiences. Trauma is often complex and continuous. For example, people who are in abusive relationships well know that one-time offenses rarely happen. The violence is cyclical and ongoing. If you serve in the military or work in a high risk profession, you experience terrible things regularly and know that they can occur at any minute of any day. Trauma puts us in survival mode for those first 30 days. And traumas may be coming so fast and furious that we don't have a moment to stop and breathe. So our brains shut down the trauma-processing experience so we can continue to survive.

The brain is actually being a protective motherfucker when it says "We are still in the foxhole and can't deal with this shit right now!"

Sometimes it isn't a matter of continued trauma, but the demands of our everyday lives that cause this shutdown. Sometimes we don't have the time and space to heal from our grief experience. Because we have to keep getting up in the morning, getting to work, feeding the dog, finding our kid's missing left shoe. There is only so much work our overtaxed brain can handle. Taking care of OURSELVES often becomes a luxury we can't afford, rather than a necessity we can't ignore.

And sometimes our brains just have no mechanism to make sense of the trauma. No matter how much time and space we give ourselves for healing, we can't find a place for the traumatic experience that gives it the meaning we need to move on. That's the storytelling brain again, stuck in telling the same story that just doesn't work.

Whatever the reason, the brain can shut down the healing process at a moment's notice and our "new normal" becomes a trauma-informed experience rather than a healing one. We start avoiding any reminders of our trauma because compartmentalizing is the only way we feel safe.

And human beings are some seriously adaptive motherfuckers. Avoidance techniques can work really well for a really long time.

What Trauma Looks Like on an Ordinary Day

How do you know you're dealing with trauma?

Once you start operating from a trauma-informed experience (whether full blown PTSD or not), you can see signs of the following in your life as the brain's way of managing your trauma with adaptive strategies. Which is just a grad school word way of saying we create great ways to avoid our trauma responses so we don't have to deal with them. But it's a foundation that was built on unsteady ground. Cracks start to develop.

- Arousal – The amygdala is always wearing its crazy pants and you find yourself freaked out when you shouldn't be or don't want to be. You may or may not know why. But your brain may process something it considers a threat that you aren't even cognizant of and all of a sudden you are falling apart in the middle of the grocery store.

- Avoidance – You find yourself avoiding things that trigger arousal. Grocery store was bad? I can order my groceries online. Really don't need to leave the house for groceries, right?
- Intrusion – Thoughts, images, memories related to the trauma experience start shoving their way up. The things that your brain was protecting you from don't actually go away. And they start bubbling to the surface without your consent or willingness. This isn't the same as rumination, where you worry over a bad memory intentionally; it's when stuff shows up when least expected. And you can't manage everything that is bubbling up.
- Negative Thoughts and Feelings – With all this other stuff going on is it any wonder that you never just feel good? Or even just OK?

These are the essential four horsemen of the PTSD apocalypse. It's how we diagnose full-blown PTSD. When they're present, it means that at some level you are reliving your trauma in your head at any given moment.

But not everyone having a trauma response has full-blown PTSD. A PTSD diagnosis is a checklist, in the end. Someone who is evaluating you for this diagnosis will be looking to see if you have a given number of these symptoms or more. So some people meet some of the criteria for PTSD, but not enough to warrant a diagnosis.

But not meeting criteria for PTSD does not put you in the all-clear or make you magically feel any better, right? You are clearly not OK now and there is a pretty damn good chance that it is gonna get worse.

The VA figured this out when studying 9/11 first responders. Of the people who had some symptoms of a trauma response but not full blown PTSD, 20% showed a symptom increase that qualified them for a PTSD diagnosis two years later when they were reassessed. Go fucking figure that if you keep reliving your trauma, those connections keep reinforcing in your brain.

Thoughts, feelings, and behaviors that are driven by our trauma response can be really difficult things to understand. Not just for the people around us, but even for ourselves. Have you ever had a moment like that? When you were thinking "What the actual FUCK, brain?" We feel clueless and the people who love us feel helpless.

But let's give our dick-for-skittles brain a break here. It's the brain trying to make sense of shit. Shit that may not actually make sense in reality. So it goes all over-reactive in how it demands you respond to certain events. It reminds you of your stories. And those certain memories trigger negative emotions. And the brain reacts in a protective way without you even realizing what's going on.

Ok, then. What kinds of symptoms do we need to watch out for? Good question, smart cookie! The list is a pretty long one.

Reliving the Trauma Symptoms:

- Feeling like you are reliving the trauma even though it's behind you and you are physically safe.
- Dreaming like you are back in the traumatic event (or maybe a similar event).
- Having a huge emotional response when something or someone reminds you about the trauma. Like freaking the fuck out, even though you are currently safe and/or lots of physical symptoms (sweating, heart racing, fainting, breathing problems, headaches, etc.)

Avoiding the Memories of the Trauma Symptoms:

- Doing things to distract yourself from thoughts or feelings about the trauma, and/or avoiding talking about it when it comes up.
- Avoiding things associated with the trauma like people, places, and activities. And a lot of times these areas of avoidance get bigger and bigger. Like avoiding a certain street that an accident happened on. Then the whole neighborhood, then driving at all.
- Needing to feel in control in all circumstances, like sitting in places that feel safest in public spaces, not having close physical proximity with other people, avoiding crowds. (If you work in a field where safety training is a big thing, this may be automatic and not necessarily mean PTSD.)
- Having a hard time remembering important aspects of the trauma (blocking shit out).
- Feeling totally numbed out or detached from everything or just about everything.
- Not being interested in regular activities and fun stuff. Not being able to enjoy shit, even if it should be enjoyable shit.
- Not being connected to your feelings and moods in general. Feeling just . . . blank.
- Not seeing a future for yourself, like just more of the same versus things getting better.

Other Medical or Emotional Symptoms:

- Stomach upset, trouble eating, only craving foods that are sugary (therefore more comforting to a stressed out body)
- Trouble falling asleep or staying asleep. Or sleeping a lot but for shit. Either way, feeling fucking exhausted all the time.
- Not having enough fucks in your pocket to take care of yourself in important ways (exercising, eating healthy foods, getting regular health care, safer sex with chosen partners).
- Soothing symptoms away with substances (e.g., drugs, alcohol, nicotine use, food) or behaviors (e.g., gambling, shopping, or dumb endorphin-producing shit like playing chicken with trains).
- Getting sick more frequently, or noticing that chronic physical health issues are getting worse.
- Anxiety, depression, guilt, edginess, irritability and/or anger. (A HUGE number of mental health diagnoses are really just a trauma response that is not being properly treated, sadly.)

Is it any wonder that we get all confused about what is a trauma response versus some other diagnosis? So the easy diagnosis is PTSD. But trauma responses, like I mentioned above, can wear a Halloween mask of other stuff. Depression and anxiety are two big ones. Sometimes trauma responses can even hide themselves as bipolar disorder and schizophrenia. I have worked with more than one person that had a label of a thought disorder like schizophrenia, but when we started discussing the content of their "voices" we realized they were trauma flashbacks. Trauma responses can also disguise themselves as ADHD, anger and irritability, attachment and relationship issues, and a twisted sense of right and wrong.

There is nothing wrong with any of these other diagnoses in and of themselves. Diagnoses can be necessary to get insurance to pay for services. They also serve as a tool among clinicians—a shorthand that is only meant to mean "these symptoms present." And these diagnoses can absolutely exist on their own, without a trauma trigger. But the problem with getting real help is when trauma IS the root cause.

And that is how we set ourselves up for failure. Trauma-related diagnoses are actually more successfully treated than many other mental health issues, if we understand what the symptoms are a response to and handle them in that context.

Brain unfuckening is a completely possible thing.

Ok, So It's Not Really a Trauma. But I Still Have a Fucked Brain. What's Up With That?

Ok, so you picked up this book because you figured you have some unfuckening to do. But the trauma stuff doesn't really ring a bell for you. That's not your thing. But you don't like some of the stuff going on in your head, and want to do something about it.

Maybe you have a habit of reacting that's less intense than a trauma response, but works essentially the same way. Even if your amygdala isn't in terrorist hijack mode, your memories and emotions are still wired together, right? Your amygdala has its groove going in a bad habit that is making life harder for you in dumb ass ways.

What is a habit? A settled or regular tendency or practice, especially one that is hard to give up. We did something and it worked. We continued to do it and it continued to work. At some point maybe it stopped working as well, if at all, but our asshole brain is still grooving along with the story that it works, because it hasn't figured out a better option. So it's still going to trigger an amygdala response, tying memory to emotion. It may not be a hugely overactive trauma-informed response, but it is there nonetheless.

This is why addictions are so hard to treat. Learning to STOP doing something is really hard, once we have wired a particular response. Hence the "Addictions" chapter of this book. Even if you are all, "Yeah, not a heroin addict, doesn't apply," consider reading it anyway. Pretty much great info for everybody.

And yes, behaviors and thinking patterns can TOTALLY have addictive qualities.

For example, maybe you grew up in a house where no one talked about their feelings. It wasn't encouraged and everyone else became uncomfortable if you tried. You learned pretty quickly that talking about your feelings was clearly against the rules. You weren't abused, you weren't traumatized. But, at the dinner table, if you said, "My best friend and I had a fight today and I'm really sad and angry," it would elicit a response of "That happens sometimes, dear, please pass the potatoes."

So if you tried talking about your feelings and were continuously shut down, you probably wired a connection in your brain that having these discussions made other people uncomfortable. This maybe made you feel anxious, or guilty, or frustrated.

Cue 20 years in the future. Your Boo wants you to talk about your feelings. You go into this weird-ass emotional fog whenever you try. Anxious, guilty, frustrated. Boo is all "WTH?" and you have no idea.

The good news is that the info in Chapter 4 will work for you, too. And it will work faster, because the story doesn't have the far deeper groove that a trauma creates. Your work will be more about pattern recognition and clarity rather than a deeper rewiring response. You'll rock that shit out in no time.

I Love Someone With a Serious Trauma History

This is seriously tough, isn't it? You have someone that you care about so much that is really struggling with their trauma recovery. You want to HELP. And feeling unable to do so is the worst feeling in the world. You're at risk of serious burnout and secondary traumatization. Because yeah, watching someone live out their trauma can be a traumatic experience in and of itself.

Two things to remember, here:

- This is not your battle.
- . . . but people do get better in supportive relationships.

This is not your battle. You don't get to design the parameters, you don't get to determine what makes something better, what makes something worse. No matter how well you know someone, you don't know their inner processes. They may not even know their inner processes. If you know someone well, you may know a lot. But you aren't the one operating that life.

Telling someone what they should be doing, feeling, or thinking, won't help. Even if you are right. Even if they do what you say . . . you have just taken away their power to do the work they need to do to take charge of their life. There are limits to how much better they can really be if they are continually rescued by you.

. . . but people do get better in supportive relationships. The best thing to do is to ask your loved one how to best support them when they are struggling. This is the type of action plan you can create with a therapist (if either or both of you are seeing one) or ask them in a private conversation.

Ask them. Ask if they want help grounding when they are triggered, if they need time alone, a hot bath, a mug of tea. Ask what you can do and do those things, if they are healthy things to provide.

It may be helpful for them to have a formal safety plan for themselves (there are resources for sample safety plans at the end of this book), with what your specific role will be. This will help boundary your role, and keep you from setting up scenarios where you rescue or enable dangerous and/or self-sabotaging behavior.

You may need to set hard limits. You may need to protect yourself. This isn't just for your well-being, but will also help you model the importance of doing so to your loved one.

Love the entirety of them. Remind them that their trauma doesn't define them. Allow them consequences of their behavior and celebrate the successes of newer, healthier ways of being. Be the relationship that helps the healing journey.

Take Action: Name that Bastard

Give your negative reactions an actual persona to inhabit. Name it after a heinous ex, a shitty grade school teacher, or Kim Jong-un. Create a whole character for that fucker.

Emotions feel so huge and so nebulous that transforming them into an actual, defined entity that you can battle really helps. Then you can have convos with Donald Trump's Epic Hair Swirl (or whomever, but personally I think all things negative should be named after that hair) whenever it comes calling.

Now you can focus on that entity the way you would on an actual person that was threatening you in a real-world situation. You can negotiate, you can yell back, you can lock it in a box. It's now at a manageable size of your choosing, with the appropriate amount of ridiculousness in its presentation so you can laugh at it while you kick its ass.

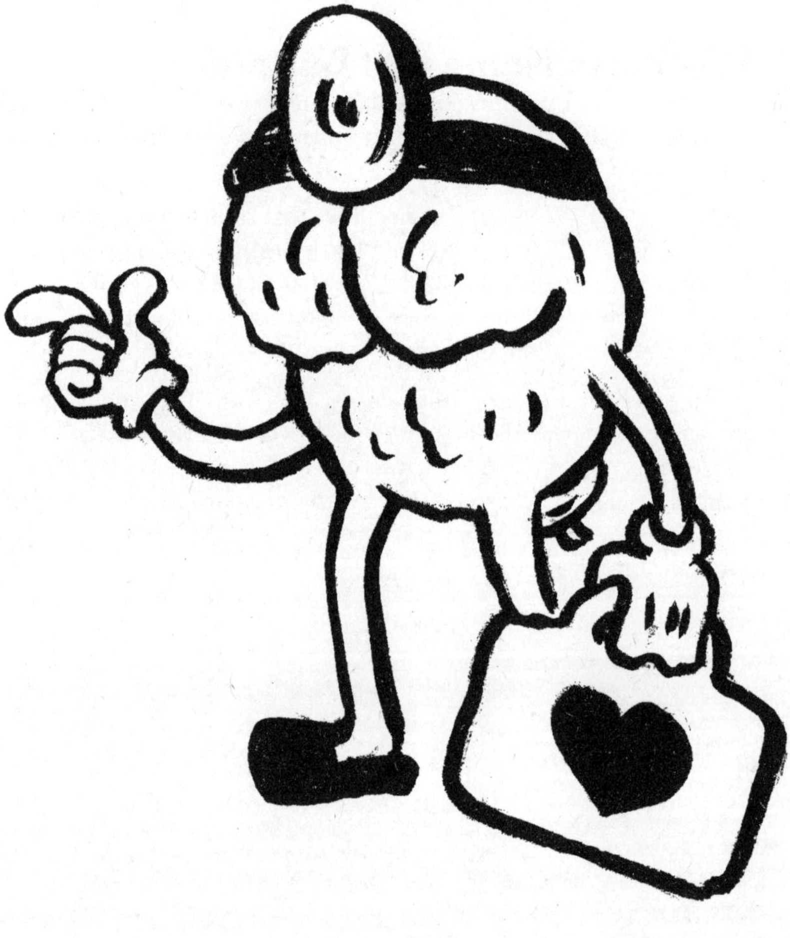

CHAPTER 3: UNFUCK YOUR BRAIN

If we called the first two chapters of this book "This Is Your Brain," the rest of this book would be called "This Is Your Brain on Therapy."

I've worked with children, youth, and adults in recovery from trauma throughout my career. I've found that the following analogy works well for most everyone. Kids like the grossness of it, adults like the symbolic understanding that they get.

Trauma is like a wound that has crusted over but hasn't fully healed. It looks closed, but the infection is still burrowed in under the skin. It festers even when we don't realize it is there, or when we find ways to ignore it. But what happens if we don't clean out that wound?

Kids like this part.

"It gushes out EVERYWHERE! Blood and pus and it HURTS and it's SUPER GROSS!"

Totally.

We have to clean it out for it to heal.

But what about the scar it leaves behind?

Adults like this part.

Scars are badges. They are a reminder that we healed.

We create new ways to feel safe that don't cause us more harm in the long run. We process our experiences with people who are safe and trustworthy and care about us. We retrain our brains to THINK rather than REACT. Those wounds? We treat them.

The Fancy Science of Unfucking

Because our emotions are tied so closely in the brain to our memory, it makes sense that memories of past events coupled with current experiences can elicit a really strong response.

But our brains aren't actually wired to hold on to certain emotions for long periods of time. Emotions are designed as part of our information feedback circuit.

WE LIKE THAT! MORE OF THAT!

~or~

THAT SUCKS! MAKE IT STOP!

Our emotions influence our thoughts and behaviors. They are meant to be a physiological signal to the rest of the brain. Once they have done their jobs, they are then meant to dissipate.

Do you know how long an emotion is actually meant to last?

90 seconds. Seriously, just one and a half minutes for an emotion to run its course.

But you are calling "bullshit" right now, I know. Because if that were really the case, why do our emotions last hours, days, or years? 90 seconds? Not so much.

Emotions last longer than 90 seconds because we continue to fuel them with our thoughts. We do this by telling ourselves the same stories about the triggering situation over and over.

We also continue to fuel them with our behaviors. My favorite definition of crazy is doing the same thing over and over and expecting different results. So when we are reactive instead of proactive, we keep reinforcing the pattern.

Say you got in a terrible car accident driving down First Street. It makes total sense that driving down First Street would send your brain into a shit-fit panic. So you avoid First Street. Eventually avoiding First Street is your modus operandi to the point that anything that involves being in the vicinity of First Street doesn't happen. You don't WANT to have a meltdown over the thought of driving down First Street. You want your life back, FFS! But as long as you continue to avoid driving down First Street, you are deepening the groove of that behavior and the feelings of panic that you associate with remembering the accident.

Thinking about the accident becomes something you can't control. Rumination is a form of unwelcome, obsessive attention to our own thought patterns. It's a stuck point. An error in the coding. You ruminate about the accident to the point of thinking you are losing your mind, because it feels like the rumination has taken control.

Basically, we continue to feed that particular emotional response (anxiety, fear) and those particular thoughts (accidents happen on First Street) by continuing with the same adaptive behavior we originally used to keep ourselves safe (don't drive down First Street, bad things happen there!). So we keep the feedback circuit in a perpetual cycle.

Ok, yeah, maybe. But what about all those non-rumination memories? The feelings we will go to the end of the earth to avoid. Instead, maybe you refuse to give ANY attention at all to the idea of driving down First Street.

Ruminate? Not fucking LIKELY.

Fucking brain wiring again. Avoiding a certain emotion makes you hold on to it just as much as ruminating over it does. Remember the infection analogy? It's just festering in there.

Both ruminating and avoiding work exactly the same way . . . a Mobius strip of nothing really ever changes and we aren't going to get anywhere. Rumination is a way of insisting on making sense of an experience, but doing it in a nonsensical way. And avoiding is just refusing to acknowledge it at all, at a conscious level. Rumination and avoidance are ways of trying to control our experience, rather than taking it as the information that it is meant to be and finding ways to process through our responses.

When we hit upon a situation where control is taken away from us, even the memory of that event is SERIOUSLY the most uncomfortable situation in the history of EVER. It's a reminder that we have far less control over the external world than we would like to have. And that is deeply scary shit. Both rumination and avoidance are ways our brain reacts in an attempt to get control back. If I fixate on it, I can figure out a way to keep it from happening again. If I avoid it, I can erase it from existence in the past, present, and future. It feels way safer than remembering something, recognizing it for the event that it was, and then letting it go.

To get to a place where we just feel what we feel? To sit with it for that 90 seconds? To remember that it's just information from our body, part of our feedback circuit? That it doesn't define us? Change anything about the essence of who we are? That it may not even be ACCURATE information about the situation? REALLY FUCKING HARD.

Being triggered means being on shaky ground. We just want the earth to stop moving. We want a sense of control back. If we get a sense that what we thought was solid beneath us was never really solid at all, that means we have to live with constant ambiguity. And ambiguity is completely counterintuitive to the things our brain is trying to do and continuing to tell us in order to help us stay safe. Ambiguity pushes the button: Threat Alert Level Red.

Remember all that fancy brain stuff from the first chapter? Because our brains are hardwired to keep us alive, the instinctual part of our brain takes over when we feel threatened. But unlike the other species we share this planet with, when the threat is over, we aren't good at discharging that threat feeling, getting all those hormones and neurotransmitters out of our system, and going back to our everyday lives.

And the prefrontal cortex cannot control our instinctual responses; it can only elaborate on them. It can offer different information and different ways of responding. It can test new scenarios. The PFC provides feedback. It can negotiate. But it is NOT in charge in times of high stress. You are not crazy for wondering if your thinking brain has been hijacked by your animal brain. You feel that way BECAUSE IT HAS.

And quite frankly, your animal brain is irritated as fuck at all your epic ingratitude at how hard it is working to keep you alive.

It's not a sign of weakness that it keeps happening. It's a hard-wired survival instinct. You can't forcibly take control back through sheer willpower. Animal brain will win every time and smack you down with a "Hell, naw" when you try.

Healing trauma means working through our shit, rather than trying to overpower it. Instead of full-frontal, Braveheart-style attack, we create ways of having new convos that are safe and supported. We don't push out of our comfort zone, we create a larger bubble of comfort zone that helps us roll along until we realize we don't need it anymore.

Getting Unfucked Immediately After a Traumatic Event

Ok, remember when I was yammering on about all that first 30 days stuff? That this is a really critical time for trauma recovery? Yeah. Because, holy shit. If we are given the time and space to process a huge, horrible thing that happened to us? That makes all the difference in the world.

If you have experience with the military, or with first responders (firefighters, police, EMS) you've heard terms like "after-action report" or "incident debriefing." In a similar way, if you have ever been through the kind of traumatic incident where professionals (police, doctors, etc.) got involved, at some point you had to tell your story.

Talking about what happened is a good first step for most people. The problem with that is if we only get to process at a Dragnet level. You know, "just the facts." It has the potential to separate us even further from the emotional content of our experience by focusing on a recitation of events, rather than a processing out of emotionally-laden memories.

When any event happens, it transforms in that instant from an occurrence to a memory. If we are given the space and support, we are empowered to process that memory on the emotional level it was stored at. "Just the facts" is only meant to be the beginning of the healing process, because it is not nearly as helpful as "all the feels."

So if someone has handed you this book after a very recent trauma event? They are saying they are there and they want to help.

Or maybe you picked it up yourself because the little voice in the back of your head said you should. Either way? This is the time to take care of yourself, tough stuff. You need the space to heal.

I haven't really found a huge difference between the things that help you heal when a trauma is fresh versus what to do when it is older. But I have found that healing is way easier when we dig into it right away and don't give our brains the opportunity to start mapping out bullshit signals that fuck us up. I also found that if you're able to do the work now, you are far less likely to struggle with chronic mental illness as a result of your trauma, or at least it will be less severe/more manageable.

And I also know you are worth the time it takes to focus on yourself and your healing. No matter how silly it feels, or how busy you are, or how much everyone around you is dismissive or uncomfortable with the process.

You deserve every opportunity to heal.

Unfucking Way Later

Then there are us unlucky motherfuckers who didn't get a chance to really unpack our trauma during that 90-day re-stabilization window. That means we have more months, years, or decades of brain fuckery to untangle. This is not a hopeless situation at fucking all. Because if this is you? You are a SURVIVOR. Your brain figured out ways to keep you going when everything around you was crazy. And it WORKED.

The problem is, it isn't working well anymore. Instead of being a solution, it's become a problem. So your brain has to be put back on its leash and retrained.

You need to teach your brain to use the prefrontal cortex to discriminate between real threats and perceived threats again. When the feedback system works the way it's intended to, the amygdala doesn't go nuts and send every message to the brainstem to activate freak-out mode.

A lot of the work I do in my private practice is guiding people through processing their stories while helping them stay grounded in the present. This helps us remember that we are in control of our experience at this point in our lives, even if we weren't in the past. It is amazing to realize you can feel something and not have it overwhelm you. That right there? That is what taking your power back really means.

If someone has a partner or supportive friend or family member available, I show them how to help with the process as well. We figure out exactly what their role will be so they have a way of being supportive, rather than freaking out and making the situation worse. (Some of the dumbest stuff is done with the best intentions, right?)

Many people do this work in therapy, but not everyone. Even if you are working with a therapist, a good therapist is going to operate as your sideline coach, giving suggestions and feedback from the outside perspective. If you are working through any of these issues, you are the one doing the hard part, whether your supports are friends, family, or helping professionals, or just your own damn determined will to get better.

Whether you have help or are going it on your own, I've found that knowing why these techniques work makes them work that much faster. Knowing how the brain is wired to work helps us feel less frustrated, stupid, and guilty. Because one of the biggest barriers to getting better? Shame. Shame from ourselves and shame from others that we aren't already better. Or that we had an issue to begin with.

And fuck that.

Remember what I said about you being a survivor? If you have crawled through all these years, months, decades of muck, fighting with a haywire brain, YOU DESERVE TO FEEL BETTER. You deserve your life back. You are not fundamentally, unfixably broken.

Let's do the thing.

Take Action: Ride the Wave

Emotions last 90 seconds. They are a signal in the brain that something needs your attention. They are meant to only last long enough to actually get your attention, and they dissipate after you decide on your course of action.

The problem is we tend to do one of two things instead of paying attention. We either perseverate (without action) or go straight-up avoidance mode. Both make brain fuckery worse.

Try setting aside five minutes to sit with the anxiety you're feeling instead of fighting back. All this means is being mindful of your present emotional experience. You can free-write as you are processing. You can practice your breathing. You can do anything other than avoid or distract from the feeling. The point is to retrain yourself that it won't last forever. You may be this feeling's bitch for a few minutes, but this is not a permanent state of being. I swear on my Roomba it won't last forever . . . and I love my Roomba, it's employee of the month every month!

If you attend to what you are feeling, you get over it way more quickly than if you avoid it. I've noticed I'm bored with myself about 3 minutes into committing to sitting with my feeling for 5. I'm ready to go make a cup of coffee, read a book, find the cookies I hid from myself, or do anything other than perseverate.

Take Action: Put It On Ice

A lot of therapists used to encourage clients to wear a rubber band and snap it on their wrist if they felt an urge to self-harm, or were having spinning thoughts, or considering an impulsive behavior. But, um, snap a rubber band on yourself enough times and you will tear the fuck out of your skin. So we're not doing that anymore.

But the point of the rubber band was legit. We were trying to help people disrupt the current focus of the brain by encouraging it to attend to another pain point. Ice works much better without causing lasting damage. Seriously, try it. Grab an ice cube and squeeze. Your brain is gonna be all "OW! WTF you doing that for??" and it disrupts the signal. If you have an impulse to self-injure to manage anxiety, you can actually place the ice on the part of the body you typically hurt instead of doing the other harm behavior.

The cool thing too, is carrying ice with you isn't obvious. You can bop around in your day, and grab an ice cube out of your cup without people going "What the hell is that about?" I have worked in group programs where everyone carried water, so handing someone a cup full of ice to use if they got triggered didn't make them feel singled out to their peers.

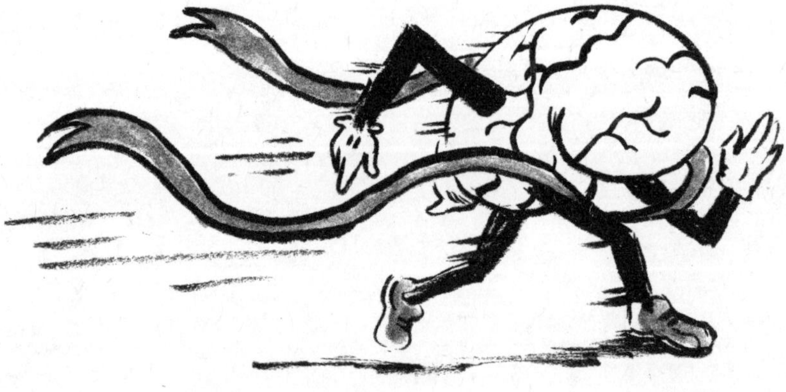

CHAPTER 4: GETTING BETTER: RETRAIN YOUR BRAIN

A Framework for Getting Better

So this is the general section of the book. Here is how we retrain the brain bullshittery that's going on. Of course, not everyone has the same responses to situations. If they did, fixing shit would be easy and I wouldn't have a job. So topics related to some of the specific things that happen to people are coming up in later chapters. You know . . . depression, anxiety, anger, addiction, grief responses, and stress. All parts of the human condition at some point in every life.

But first I want to lay a stage-wise model on you . . . an idea of sequence for how trauma happens that helps us understand how to better fix that shit. I am WAY aware that no one ever fits into a fancy model in which we complete certain steps and then VOILA, ALL BETTER . . . and let's add some fucking jazz hands to the mix while we're at it.

Life does what it does, and half the time we are just hanging on for dear life. So what other people call stages, I call a framework. It's good to have an idea of where you are in the process, at any particular moment. So you can focus on what will work best at that moment. And if later on today (or next week, or next year) you are five steps forward or two steps back? That's where we go in. No biggie.

Ok, you are squinting at me now with suspicion that we are gonna go all traditional self-help workbook bullshit with a helping of Dr. Phil hollering "How's THAT workin' for ya?" Maybe a tiny bit. But only the shit that works best, nothing extraneous. It's all about the brain science behind it. And F bombs. Because I have a fancy PhD and can say fuck as much as I want. So stick with me, and let's figure out what works for you.

Back to frameworks. One of the best frameworks for understanding how the brain heals from trauma comes from Judith Herman's book Trauma and Recovery. Her grown-person labels (and my less traditional examples) are listed below:

1. Safety and Stabilization

Holy Shit! That's over, right? I can sit down for a second without someone kicking my ass now? Would that be possible, Universe?

If trauma means that our sense of safety in the world has been violated, regaining that sense of safety feels almost impossible. That event became a seriously strong memory which continuously triggers our "fight, flight, freeze" response. Safety and stabilization is the process of understanding everything that is going on with your brain and of taking control back over your body when this happens. It's the brain reboot when all this shit gets triggered for you. Herman's book focuses on this stage, and so does mine. Because it's the hardest part to get going . . . and nothing else happens without it.

2. Remembrance and Mourning

What the FUCK was that? What happened? Shit ain't supposed to go down like that! That kicked my ass HARD.

This is the part we call a trauma narrative. It's the space to be allowed to process your story when you have the skills to do so without being triggered to all shit. It's about owning your story and not letting your story own you. It's about the trauma as you remember it, and the thoughts and feelings that are bundled up with the event memories. If we think of trauma as emotions trapped in the body, this is how we metabolize them out. This can be done in all kinds of safe ways: with a therapist, with an awesome loved one, in a support group, or even by yourself in a journal.

3. Reconnection

So, maybe, just maybe, the whole world isn't complete bullshit and I can still generally be OK again. Not to say that wasn't some fucked-up shit. But not everything is fucked-up shit and not everyone is a total fucking asshole.

This is a fancy way of saying, "taking your life back." It means finding a way to have the trauma fit into its rightful place within the entirety that is your life, rather than taking over and controlling every aspect of it. It's about finding meaning in your experience. This can be so hard to wrap your head around, I know. This doesn't mean that the situation wasn't horrible and fucked up, but it does mean that you can use it to make yourself stronger, to support others, to not let it own you. It means having positive relationships that are defined by everything you are instead of just your trauma. It can also be about reconnecting to your spirituality, if that has been an important part of your identity. It means knowing that no matter what else happens . . . you have YOU in your corner. A fucking survivor anyone would be lucky to have on their side.

I admit this is all easier to explain than to do, but let's talk about how to get started.

First Things First: Safety and Stabilization

The following section is full of activities that engage the prefrontal cortex and override the brainstem take-over that puts you into fight, flight, or freeze response. Teaching the PFC to focus on something else disrupts the whole asshole brain hostile takeover response.

Bruce Lipton, in his book The Biology of Belief, compares trying to stop an amygdala hijack to screaming at a tape player because you don't like the song that's on. It's just playing the tape, yanno? It doesn't have the capacity to realize you want to stop the tape, rewind the tape, or fast forward. It's firing the danger signals and has no more capacity to stop rolling as a tape player has to stop playing a song once the Play button has been pushed. Even if it's Nickelback, FFS.

You CANNOT have a logical conversation directly with the amygdala. ANYTHING you want to do has to be a negotiation with the amygdala by the PFC. Because the amygdala is in protection mode (or terrorist mode, depending on your patience with its bullshit at the moment) and is the one in charge. This is where we re-stabilize ourselves and reestablish our sense of safety. By getting our PFC to sneak in and pause the tape, we can negotiate with the amygdala to chill the fuck out, sit the fuck down, and let the grown-ups get back to work.

Yes, you can actually do something else and think of something else. But you do have to train yourself how.

This trauma response didn't creep up on you overnight, right? You didn't go to bed one night feeling all fine and dandy and wake up the next morning all kinds of hot mess. Your brain created its response network based on the information it was receiving over time, so learning to be un-fucked is also going to take time.

Some days are going to be better than others. You may do awesomely well then get hit like a ton of bricks with all kinds of what-the-SHITSTORM-just-happened???!!!???

Those days are balls, aren't they?

None of that shit makes you a failure, it means you are still growing. I tell my clients "It really is going to be OK in the end. If it's not OK yet, that means we aren't at the end."

And bits of OK now and then give us the breathing room and resting space to store energy for our next battle against that anxiety-trying-to-eat-our-face-off thingy. Ok, that's not the technical term, but it should be.

The biggest component to making this shit work is to practice these techniques when your brain is not in asshole mode rather than trying to learn them when you are already completely stressed. Trying new soothing and coping techniques when you are feeling your best self will help you figure out which ones work for you.

Because as you well know, taking back control of your brain when it's been hijacked is really difficult.

There is an expression: Amateurs practice until they get it right, experts practice until they can't get it wrong. I'm not trying to go all inscrutable Zen koan on you here . . . the idea is that the way to Carnegie Hall is practice, practice, practice. Proving you can do something once is easy, getting so good at it that it becomes second nature is way harder.

But that's what rewires a trauma reaction. Do it so often it just becomes what you do. On Tuesdays we wear pink. And when we are triggered, we use our fucking coping skills.

Trying good coping skills out while you are NOT in freak-out mode will make it easier to access them when you are. Having people around you that feel safe to you and that can help prompt you to use your positive coping skills can be invaluable.

Of course, it probably seems that panic comes on at the worst possible time, when you are on the freeway and alone in the car, for example. So having a set of simple coping skills as well as the more complicated ones is invaluable. It might be a literal talisman (a stone you carry), a mantra you say, or the coping cards from the exercise below. Yes, they seem cheesy as fuck. But they WORK so damn well, I gotta throw the idea out there.

Take Action: Create Coping Cards

The problem with all the coping mechanisms below is that chances are you can't fucking remember them in the heat of the moment, at least at first. So when you find a mantra, a grounding exercise, a fact about anxiety, or another statement or image or action that helps you, put it on an index card. Hole punch your cards, put them on a snap-shut key ring, and you have a set of coping cards you can flip through when panic hits.

It sounds epically nerdy, I know. But I have had so many clients end up loving the shit out of their cards and using them all the time. They're a way to remind the PFC to be in charge of the control stick and ground itself in reality. It's cheese with extra cheese sauce, but that's what works when we are actively rewiring brain bullshittery.

Grounding Techniques

I get asked a lot to teach just one skill to people. New counselors, new foster parents, and first responders who aren't counselors but end up helping people manage a mental health crisis all ask, "What's the one universal thing that anyone can do to help someone having a rough time?" and the best answer I have is to help people ground themselves back in their bodies and in the present.

When triggered, the brain is reliving a past event instead of responding to the present moment. Grounding activities help you get back in your body and the present moment rather than reliving your memories. Grounding is one of the best ways to manage emotional pain, because it helps you remain in the present and remember that the pain itself is based in memory, and doesn't have the power to hurt you in this moment. I hear all the time from people that they use the shit out of this skill.

Some people don't want to unpack their story and process their trauma. And that's OK. But everyone wants a way to manage all the shit that comes up when they are experiencing a trauma reaction. Grounding helps a lot. Seriously. It's the best way of saying "Hey, amygdala? Slow your roll, FFS."

Mental Grounding

Mental grounding techniques are intended to keep you in the present moment by focusing on your current situation and surroundings. You are gonna use mantras or make lists. And yes, you can say these out loud. To yourself, to someone else. If you're on the city bus and don't want to draw attention, you can go through your list mentally or mutter under your breath. Whatever works. (. . . and if you put in headphones, people will think you are singing to yourself and not responding to internal stimuli.)

For example, you might describe all the colors in the room, or an object you are holding.

It may be repeating a safe phrase to yourself over and over. One of my favorites that I've heard is "FUCK YOU, AMYGDALA!" It apparently works beautifully for that individual!

Some people like to play a kind of categories game, where they name all their favorite movies, or books, or something that requires a different kind of concentration.

Some people will go over their schedule, either in their mind or out loud, or the steps needed to complete an activity.

All of these mental grounding activities are a way to remind your brain of where you are in the moment and that you have more control than you realize over what is going on inside you when your panic button has been tripped.

Physical Grounding

As young children, we are in our bodies and in our experiences all the time. It isn't until we get older that we realize our bodies can be in one place while our mind goes somewhere else. This is great when your body is in math class but your brain is on the playground. But it becomes more problematic as we get older. Have you ever found yourself arriving at home without remembering anything about the trip it took to get there? Physical grounding techniques are ways of reminding us that we are in our bodies and that we have ownership of that experience.

Physical grounding can include being mindful of our breathing. Simply notice your breathing, in and out. When you catch yourself wandering, remind yourself to focus back on the breath.

You may try walking and noticing each step you take. If you find that you walk and still ruminate, try carrying a teaspoon of water while you walk, and focus on trying not to spill drops of it.

Touch objects around you.

Sometimes specific sensory objects are especially soothing. These are usually suggested for people who respond differently neurologically (you know who you are, my neurospicy folks) but they can help everyone. Things like: A cotton ball with lavender oil on it kept in an airtight container that can be opened and sniffed to trigger a calming response. Something to chew on (gum, beef jerky). Play-doh that can be squished, glitter bottles that can be shaken, a talisman in your pocket like a polished stone or something of spiritual significance. A ring that you can spin on your finger.

Jump up and down.

Make sure your feet are touching the floor. Try taking off your shoes and feeling the ground beneath you.

Eat something slowly and be mindful of all the flavors and textures. Grapes or raisins work well for this. Interestingly? People who don't even like raisins (and I raise my hand here) are not bothered by them when using them for this exercise. (Check out Unfuck Your Body for more detailed instructions on this one.)

If you feel safe to be touched, have someone you trust put their hands on your shoulders and remind you gently to remain in your body.

If touch isn't going to make things worse? Give someone a hug. Go get a massage. Cuddle with your boo. Touching and being touched releases oxytocin. Touch is also good for the heart and the immune system. So get on that.

Soothing Grounding

Soothing grounding is essentially self-compassion and self-care in a difficult situation.

Think of things that make you feel better. Visualize things you enjoy, such as the beach or a sunset. A sunset on the beach? I'm down with that.

Remember a safe place and picture yourself surrounded by that safety.

Plan an activity or treat you can look forward to in the near future, like a cupcake from your favorite bakery, a hot bath, a movie you've seen 100 times and still adore, a baseball game and a bowl of popcorn, or a hike in your favorite park.

Carry pictures of people and places you care about and focus on these images.

• • •

You can play with all of these different forms of grounding, and develop ones that work best for you when you are feeling most distressed. If you are intrigued by the idea of doing more work in this area, you may want to check out some of the recommended reading at the end of this book as well.

But above all else? You totally got this shit. Your brain has done its job in keeping you safe, and now you are ready to take the reins back and move forward in your life. And that's excellent, isn't it?

Getting Help with Grounding

If you have someone who is supporting this work, share this with them and ask them to prompt you through your re-grounding process.

If you are reading this to help someone who is struggling to try new coping techniques, this is something you can offer gently or even model, without saying, "Hey, I'm going to help you with your fucked brain right now." For instance, I might drop some essential oils on the lightbulbs in my office and talk about focusing on the scent. I'm already usually barefoot, so I will talk about how I like to feel my feet directly against the ground. I may gently discuss the colors on the walls, the textures on the blankets in the room, the sensory materials we have for kids that all of us adults love too.

If I notice panic coming up in a friend or family member I know well enough to touch even when they are triggered, I may put my hands on their shoulders and press down very slightly while talking to them about what I notice going on.

Many counselors are now using sensory tools that our occupational therapy cousins have been talking about for decades. Small weighted blankets with just enough size and weight to place across your lap, feet, or around your neck can also be really helpful.

Mindfulness Meditation

Ok, first of all let's start by getting all definition-y. We tend to use mindfulness and meditation as interchangeable terms. Or in a non-interchangeable but still confusing-as-fuck way. They aren't really meant to be interchangeable, but they aren't really meant to be confusing-as-fuck either.

Meditation is when you intentionally set aside time to do something that's good for you. There are all kinds of meditations (prayer, exercise, art, etc.).

Mindfulness is both a general awareness of the world (noticing your existence and the existence of everything else around you) AND formal meditation practice. It's two things, not one.

So you can meditate without being particularly mindful and you can be mindful without meditating. But meditation and mindfulness overlap when we do mindfulness meditation, which means that we are setting aside time for that intentional focus on our awareness of the world . . . which includes the workings of our own mind.

Unfuck Your Body includes a lot more content on mindfulness and meditation, including info on how they operate in the brain and the body and how you can practice them in a trauma-sensitive way, along with a handful of specific meditations you can try. I've included some of my favorite books on the subject in the recommended resources section for that book, because there are people who are way smarter than me about this shit. But for now, here's the basic guideline to get you started.

Sit upright. If you can do this without back support, like on the floor on a cushion then good on you. If you need a straight back chair, do that. If you can't sit at all, that's OK, too. Get yourself in whatever position is most comfortable. The reason sitting is better than laying down is that the point is to fall awake, not fall asleep. But the point is also to not be in screaming fucking pain, so don't stress it.

Soft-focus your eyes so they aren't closed but they are seeing without actually seeing. You know what I mean. Be visually spaced out because what you are really going to be paying attention to is inside you.

And now you are going to breathe in and out. And focus on your breath. If you have never done this before it's going to be weird and hard. But for the record, if you have done this a zillion times chances are still good that it will be weird and hard.

If you catch yourself being distracted, just label it "thinking" and go back to focusing on your breath. Thinking isn't a failure in the least. It's gonna happen. And noticing it and bringing the mind back to the present moment is the point. So it's a total win.

A lot of people feel awful during meditation, thinking they suck at it because they are continuously distracted by chatting thoughts. That's OK. Your brain is desperately seeking to story-tell. All kinds of distracting stuff is going to come up. You are going to think about what you need to cook for dinner. Or a conversation you had at work. Or whether or not you should buy new sneakers or go to a movie this weekend.

Because the default network of the brain is storytelling mode, remember? And you aren't distracted by external events, so the default mode has all kinds of stories to tell you. But here is the thing about mindfulness meditation . . . research shows that it disrupts the storytelling process of the default network. When we used to think the only way to do that was a distraction by outside events and stimulus.

And I'm not even going to pretend that this shit is easy to do when you are spun up. But it's important to at least try. Because part of a panic attack is the stories our brain starts telling us about the attack itself. And it's generally not a pretty story. Because the chemicals released during an anxiety or panic attack are designed to get your breathing ramped up and your heart racing. So your brain is insisting that you are going to have a heart attack or stop breathing. That's not actually going to happen. When you catch that thinking, remind yourself that's a biochemical response, but not reality.

Keep breathing. The continued, conscious effort to breathe and untense will slow your heart rate back down and help you get more oxygen flowing. It's a literal chemical counterbalance. Meditation releases every chemical that counteracts brain fuckening: dopamine, serotonin, oxytocin, AND endorphins. And it's cheaper than Crossfit. Six thousand years of Buddhist practice has something going for it, yeah?

Treat your bodily reactions like any other random thought. Itching is common. If you catch yourself itching, label it thinking three times before succumbing to the urge to scratch. You may be surprised at how often your brain is creating things for you to focus on. As an early meditator, my nose would start to run. My meditation instructor got wise to my epically awesome self-distraction skill and started keeping tissues by her cushion for me. I wasn't allowed to get up. I used a tissue and went back to my breathing. Of course, if you have real pain, don't ever ignore that. Rearrange yourself for comfort and don't be a hero.

If you have someone helping you through this, they can prompt your mindfulness by saying something like, "Hey, what are you noticing going through your head right now?" or progressive relaxation by saying, "Ok, let's start with your hands. They're really clenched up, can you spread out your fingers instead of balling your hands up?" Sometimes meditation feels more doable if you have someone meditating with you—it helps you feel supported and kept on track.

Prayer

So we just defined mindfulness meditation, right? Meditation is no more than listening to. Meditation is the process of quieting ourselves down enough to hear what's going on inside us. Our minds are brilliant at creating endless amounts of chatter that we often talk back to without listening first. Meditation is the willingness to hear yourself before you speak.

What does prayer have to do with it? You may be rolling your eyes up in your head at me over this one, I know. Prayer? I don't do religion. But what we have, as a culture, agreed to call prayer is just talking to. Speaking to ourselves or something bigger than ourselves about our wants, needs, desires, and intentions. Remember the storytelling brain? Prayer is a natural mechanism of the storytelling brain. Talking through our situation in this manner can be far more powerful than talking to a friend, family member, or therapist. It's a grounding experience that helps us be more aware of our thoughts, feelings, and behaviors. This is what is going on. This is what I want. This is the help that I need.

Music

Because who doesn't like music, right? Only the same people who hate the smell of home baked bread and don't understand how adorable fluffy baby sloths are.

Do you know how much of our day we spend listening to music? Like FOUR fucking HOURS. Music is primal. MIT scientists recently figured out ways to prove that we have specific neurons in the brain that pay attention only to music, ignoring all other audial noises. Brains have music rooms. And, just maybe, music existed before speech did. And that's why speech developed at all . . . to go with our music. And look at how much of our early architecture was designed around our need for music. Across cultures, places of worship were designed around our need to create music in communion.

Music is both primal and communal.

And we all use music in different ways. Some people want music that is soothing when they are distressed. Others want to hear things that are loud and thrashy and match what is going on inside. Still others want things that are upbeat and danceable so they can have their own personal dance party.

I grew up listening to old blues albums on vinyl while the other, less weird kids were watching Sesame Street. So guess what is most soothing for me? Old blues albums on vinyl. Or when I need a pick-me-up, I like to pull up the music I work out to. It has a cadence that I connect to physical movement. I may use it to dance around to while cleaning the house, or even while driving to prepare myself for the event I'm driving to.

What works for you?

Having music that helps your brain connect to either a relaxed state, or an energized but not panicked state can be really beneficial. Especially now when everyone, including those baby sloths, have smart phones that they can queue up a playlist on. So create a couple of playlists. Think about what your songs are. What's your fight song? Your personal anthem? The songs that reflect your best self? The songs that remind you that life is worth living? Have them ready when you need them.

Self-Compassion Exercises

Self-compassion is the total polar opposite of self-esteem. Self-esteem comes from the outside. Do great on a test? Great for self-esteem. Fuck it up royally? Self-esteem is shot to shit.

Self-compassion means being as kind to yourself as you would your best friend. It is an intentional honoring of our imperfections as humans. It doesn't mean we let ourselves off the hook for things we fuck up, and it's not an excuse to be a dick. In fact, people who are self-compassionate are also more driven to be better human beings because they think they are worth the effort.

Treat yourself with kindness, understanding, and self-respect. Ask yourself, what would you say if this was happening to your best friend? What would the Buddha say to you right now?

Amazing things have happened when I have taught people the self-compassion skills suggested by Kristen Neff and Christopher Germer (see the recommended reading section for their work). The first time it happened, I was teaching a roomful of therapists working on their research PhDs. One of these people also happened to already be an MD.

So, you know. Strong, focused, high achievers like whoa. I asked them to put their hands over their hearts and remind themselves that they experience suffering. That this suffering is part of the human condition. And to give themselves permission to be kind to themselves and forgive themselves their imperfections.

The aforementioned MD/PhD/SuperFancyPants therapist? She did the exercise and tears started to roll down her face. This person, who I looked up to as amazing, had never slowed down long enough to give herself the same level of compassion she showed to the individuals she worked with.

Try it yourself.

Put your hand over your heart and voice your experience of suffering. Remind yourself that suffering is part of humaning. Tell yourself that you are allowed kindness and forgiveness, and that starts as an inside job.

Mantras/Positive Self-Talk Strategies

Does this make you feel like Stuart Smalley? I always felt cheesy when I tried positive self-talk but I also found that it WORKED. Think of it as talking over that bullshit tape the amygdala is playing.

Yes, I know you are freaking out right now. It will pass and you will feel better. Keep breathing.

You've got this. It may not feel like you do. But your success rate for getting through serious bullshit is 100%. You aren't about to break your winning streak.

You know what sucks? This right now. You know what helps? This isn't permanent. And you've totally earned a cookie for dealing with this today.

Your self-talk strategies can be put on your coping cards if you are using them. And this is absolutely something you can ask for help with. Let people know which mantras you are using and have them remind you of them when you are struggling.

Exercise

I know, I know. Fuck Crossfit and fuck spinach smoothies. But exercise releases endorphins. Short version of that? Endorphins have mad ninja skills . . . they block our perception of pain and enhance positive feelings . . . both of which counterbalance the stress response. Which means those superfit people who say they get a runner's high? Totally aren't lying. Freaks of nature, maybe. But totally telling the truth.

You are totally allowed to choose a form of exercise you can tolerate. I am not a fan of sweating and physical exertion in the name of health. But my doctor keeps telling me that reaching for a cookie does not count as a sit-up, so I gotta do SOMETHING. I do enjoy swimming, walking, and hiking . . . they are way more relaxing and meditative for me than competitive team sports (but if that's your thing . . . go on with your weird-ass self!). Even better is when I go hiking with my bestie. We get exercise and get to talk shit about everyone we know in the process.

Find something that doesn't suck. It can be as intense or gentle as you want, but try stuff. Most places will offer a free class or free week so check shit out. I had a client who fell in love with boxing by trying out a free class. It was great exercise AND made her feel more empowered and in control of her experiences.

Get Yourself Outside

Sometimes the doing of anything feels like way more than can be handled. Remaining vertical is difficult enough, there certainly isn't going to be any meditation or exercise or any other woo-woo shit.

If you can't do anything else, try to get yourself out in some sunshine. Even if it's just to sit on a bench while drinking your afternoon coffee or something. Sunlight increases vitamin D production and serotonin. Both of which will give you a little chemical boost without having to pop a pill. It's hard to sit in the sun and feel like ass at the same time. And trust me, I've tried. I usually perk up despite myself.

If you live in a gray and gloomy place, you may want to invest in a personal sunlight lamp that you keep in your workspace. When my brother left Texas to go to school on the East Coast, he found himself battling seasonal affective disorder (SAD). He just wasn't getting enough sunlight to battle low-level blues. The lamp made a huge difference.

When You're Ready: Remembrance and Mourning

Once you have a number of skills down that help you manage the responses that have been managing you, you may be thinking about working through your story.

The good coping skills part is really fucking important. So many people feel forced to talk about what is going on with them without a way to feel safe in the process. It's triggering as hell and ends up retraumatizing them.

So these techniques are things you only do when you are ready, when and if telling your story is something that is going to help you move on, and with someone who can be with you in that experience.

Writing or Journaling

Writing or journaling exercises, especially when taking the time to be slow and deliberate and put pen to paper, can be a good start for sharing your story. Things may come out that you didn't realize were there, or that you needed to say. Some ideas to get you started may include:

- Using a workbook that includes specific writing prompts related to your situation. For example, many individuals who have dealt with childhood sexual trauma have found the writing exercises in The Courage To Heal by Ellen Bass and Laura Davis to be very useful. I have clients that complete the exercises between sessions and we review what they wrote together.
- Write letters to other people. Not letters you will actually send, but what you would want to tell these people if you could. They

may be the people who hurt you. Or it may be the people who you love but who don't understand what you are struggling with. Figuring out what you want them to know might be a good starting point for understanding your own process. And maybe starting a new conversation with them, if possible.

- Write a letter to your future self. Write about everything you went through to get to the healthiest place you are working toward in your future. List all the things you went through and how you got through them . . . as if you already have. What you come up with may surprise you.

Telling Your Story

This simply means talking about your trauma and other things that have impacted your life, as you remember and perceive them. This isn't about literal truth, but the story you have been carrying with you that has affected your wiring for so long.

We talked about the brain being a storytelling brain. Creating a new story means first understanding the one we are now carrying around. Sometimes the story ends up surprising us. We don't even realize all the hateful shit we are telling ourselves until it happens in our out-loud voice.

Preparing people to do this part is a big part of trauma therapy. But many people are able to do it with the help of friends, family, or other loved ones. While group therapy can be really beneficial, this probably won't be the place where you tell all the details of your story, as it can be a triggering experience for other group members. In my years of group work, we would create a title for the event (e.g., "when the rape happened"), when processing issues surrounding the event, but wouldn't discuss details of the event itself during group.

The actual work of sharing the story usually starts with a trained therapist . . . because we have the skill set to hold space for you and are able to sit with all the strong feelings that are coming up for you without judgment, correction, or our own experiences being triggered.

If you do want to have this conversation with a friend, family member, or other loved one instead, keep in mind that the person may be going through their own shit. Hearing your shit may not be something they can handle, and that's totally fair. They may think they can, but then realize they are getting triggered. Before you start, give them permission to stop at any point. Many times people share their stories with a therapist first and then invite the loved one in and share the story again to that person, with the therapist present to help the process.

Reframing Your Story

Telling our story in a coherent way can often help us figure out the parts of the story that don't make sense, or to see other perspectives. We may find that there was more going on than is on the tape we have been playing over and over in our heads. It doesn't make horrible experiences less horrible, but it can help us find meaning and work towards forgiveness.

Remember all that brain science stuff about how we have an emotional response and then we create a story to back up that response? One of the best things you can do to challenge that is to think about how you are thinking.

Here's the magic. Brains are changing all the time . . . and we can shape that journey. Yes, trauma changes our genetic structure but we can change it back. Life experiences reshape our DNA moment by moment. The Dr. Faith guide to epigenetics would be a whole other book, but what you need to know is that we are not destined to a prison of our past experiences.

1) Think about the story you tell yourself and others. Review the story that you shared from the exercise above. What aspects might be missing? What else needs to be included?

2) How is this a story of your survival?

3) Who are the other good guys? The caretakers and the helpers? What did they do and how did they do it?

4) What about the things you did that you aren't proud of? In what ways were they the best decisions you were able to make for yourself at the time? What did you learn from them that you can use moving forward?

Getting Back Out There: Reconnection

Reconnection means reconnecting to ourselves and to the world around us. It is how we re-engage, make peace with our brains, and live the life we want again. This part can be a struggle, because we are so often pushed to do this before we are ready . . . before we feel safe. And clearly it doesn't work that way. When your "reconnection" is forced by the will of others, it becomes another form of trauma . . . because your power was taken away from you. Again.

You do this when YOU are ready. And yes, you may need to push yourself a bit. But now you have the grounding and coping skills to remind yourself that you are safe.

You got this.

Using Your Story to Create Meaning

The healthiest people are the ones who find meaning in chaos. The ones who can find the pony in a pile of shit every time.

It doesn't make the awful things that happen any less awful with bullshit like "Oh, that was God's will, there was a lesson to be learned in that." Because if God wanted me to learn something, there were far easier ways of making that happen, I'm pretty sure.

But we can learn skills of resilience and strength through the terrible things that happen. They can make us better, stronger, more compassionate, more engaged human beings.

1) Learn from your past. Your past is your learning experience, not the well-worn rut your brain keeps trying to live in. What have you learned that you want to carry forward? What have you learned about yourself and your capacity to survive and heal? What can you let go of so you can move on?
2) Learn from your future. You know where you want to go, what kind of person you want to be. Ask that person what you need to do now to get there. Ask them to share their secrets of success.
3) Use both in your present. Continue being aware of what and how you think. What from your past are you carrying? What from your future? What do you have to offer others as a benefit of what you have gone through? What empathy and support can you share? How can you help others not be alone? How can you advocate for change in your community?

Finding Forgiveness

Forgiveness is serious, deep, and powerful magic. So many people think that forgiveness means forgiving those who have hurt them. And there is truth to that. But more so, I have found people really are working to forgive THEMSELVES. The person they are angriest at and ashamed of is THEMSELVES. And they have been carrying the weight of that around for years.

Reminding yourself that you were doing the best you could with the information and skills you had at the time is hugely important. And remembering that the people who have hurt us are also broken and fucked up is almost as important.

Thich Nhat Hanh is a well-known Vietnamese Zen monk and teacher. He is the man Martin Luther King Jr. called "an apostle of peace and nonviolence" when nominating him for the Nobel Peace Prize.

He is also a man who had a very abusive father growing up. He talks about picturing his father as a three-year-old boy, before the world reshaped him into the angry man he became. And he states that he pictures himself as a three-year-old boy, standing in front of his father. His three-year-old self smiles at his three-year-old father, who then smiles back.

He doesn't call it a forgiveness practice, but it absolutely is. Remember self-compassion from above? Compassion is integral to forgiveness. First ourselves, then others.

Building Relationships With Safe Boundaries

Nobody sets out to have shitty relationships. But we do have a habit of picking people to be with who allow us to keep playing the same tapes over and over. When you have ownership of your story, you can figure out how to stop the tape and get back in charge of your brain, and you will be amazed at the amount of bullshit you were putting up with around you.

You will be able to articulate clear boundaries for yourself and unfuck your relationships in the process. You may start letting people out of your life, when you realize they can't deal with your new backbone. That can be a really difficult thing to process. Make sure you have healthier people around you that support your boundary work while you make this transition.

If your boundaries have been violated in the past, you may not know how to create boundaries that aren't too rigid or too permeable. Start by asking yourself the following questions:

1) Is this a person who challenges me to be my best self or are they here because I prefer them to being alone?
2) Is being alone the same thing as being lonely? If not, how do I tell the difference and how do I manage them as different situations?
3) Have I (or am I) communicating my boundaries effectively or am I expecting other people to figure out what I want?
4) What are my boundaries? What are deal breakers? What is possibly negotiable? What is not an issue?
5) Have these boundaries changed over time? Do I see them maybe changing in the future?

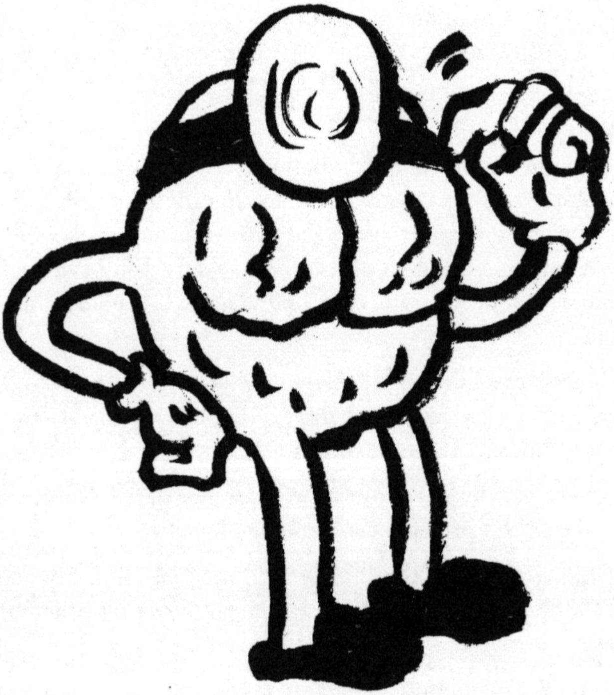

CHAPTER 5: GETTING (PROFESSIONAL) HELP: TREATMENT OPTIONS

There are lots of ways to kick your brain's ass back into shape. And a lot of them will be things you do on your own.

But sometimes on your own isn't enough. If you aren't getting better, or not getting better at the rate you would like to see, it might be useful to get help from someone who has the skills, resources, training, and perspective on your situation that you don't have.

My intent here is to help you consider different ways you can best bring yourself back to wellness. Many of the things I have found to help are things that have not been common in Western medicine practice. I've noticed that this is seriously changing, though. And changing fast.

About 10 years ago I had a client discharge from the local state hospital with melatonin instead of Ambien and I think I actually squeaked out loud, I was so excited. Ambien is a pretty strong sedative, typically prescribed for insomnia. You've probably heard stories of the crazy shit people have done sleepwalking on Ambien. Melatonin on the other hand is a supplement you can purchase over the counter. It's a hormone that we naturally produce that helps us tune into our sleep cycle. Many of the people who use it have found that it not only helps them fall asleep, it helps them stay asleep—without the prescription requirement, side effects, and price tag of Ambien. That particular change was the first step I saw on a shifting focus in medicine. I am seeing more and more Western practitioners (like myself) incorporating complementary, holistic treatment or referring our patients out for it.

Yes, I am one of those people who loves woo-woo. But I believe in evidence based woo-woo. Anything I have ever suggested has mad research behind it that I can show to my clients and the other people involved in their care. I've had some amazing convos with medical doctors in my community when I've touched base about adding neurofeedback instead of Xanax and shown them the research on why. Neurofeedback works much like biofeedback, giving you real time information about your brain waves, which allows you to learn how to control many symptoms that most people use Xanax or other hard core prescription meds for (there will be more on both of these treatments later in this chapter). Neuro is often used in conjunction with talk therapy . . . and I've seen it work when talk therapy has hit a wall.

And I also believe in never, EVER asking anyone to try anything I haven't tried myself. And I share my experiences with them.

You'll read about a lot of kinds of complementary medicine below. It is called that for a reason. It is intended to augment, not necessarily replace. I was trained in traditional talk therapy. And I would NEVER suggest dumping the prescription medications that have helped people stay alive.

So let's review the treatment options out there that may be of benefit to this brain business that is going on with you.

Also, Unfuck Your Intimacy includes more specific guidance on ways to heal from trauma (especially when it's interfering with your intimate relationships), so check that out if you think you'll find it helpful.

Traditional Talk Therapy

So, yeah. This is my jam. My training is as a licensed professional counselor, which is talk therapy. Talk therapy has a great capacity to heal, in support of other treatments or sometimes alone. A good therapist has the benefit of their training and a perspective on your life that you don't have because they aren't living the experiences you are living, at least at this time. They can provide insight, coaching, and interventions to help on your getting-bettering journey.

If you are working through trauma, look for a therapist who has had trauma training and find out which kind of training and what certifications they have. All this should be on their website, and don't be shy in asking if it isn't!

If you know you prefer a certain style of therapy, like cognitive behavioral therapy for example, look for that information. If a certain spiritual background is important to you, seek that out as well!

Allopathic Meds

Allopathic just means mainstream treatment. Western medicine. The shit we already know about. The prescription stuff. Nothing wrong with allopathic treatment, medication saves lives. Allopathic medication eliminated polio, FFS. If I break my arm, I don't want someone to rub herbs on it, I want it reset and cast.

The problem? As a society, we are moving more and more towards medication as the first (and only) line of defense for managing mental illness, rather than focusing on the root causes. Anxious and depressed?

We have medications for that. And rather than using them to help alleviate symptoms while doing other work on the root causes, it becomes a routine of constant medication adjustment with little other support.

This leads to over-medication, tons of side effects, and then more medications to manage the side effects. We are seeing more and more stories of people medicated to the point of toxicity.

And medications don't really work as well as their manufacturers spend advertising billions for us to believe. Most people end up not taking them after a while for just that reason. And the World Health Organization confirmed a long term study which showed that in third world countries where antipsychotic medications are not even available, recovery rates were actually HIGHER. Because if the medications weren't available, they couldn't be the focus of treatment. So the causes were treated. A sense of meaning and community was provided instead. And people got better.

Allopathic medicine doesn't have to be—and often shouldn't be—the endgame of your treatment. But in some cases, it helps the getting-better part happen faster. My friend Aaron is an MD (yes, a REAL doctor who can prescribe meds, unlike me who just talks about shit) uses this analogy:

Imagine you are in a boat in the middle of the ocean and there is a leak in the hull. You might be able to drop a pump down in the bilge and keep enough water out to make it to shore. You might be able to reach down under the water and patch the hole. But, it would probably work a lot better if you used the pump to lower the water level so you can get at the hole better. The medicine is the pump that will keep you afloat while you and the therapist patch the hole together.

Yeah, yeah. Meds help sometimes. But how? If we know that a trauma reaction changes brain chemistry, what are meds doing to help fix it? To unrepentantly jack another Dr. Aaron analogy?

Imagine you are an Air Force base. Everything is fine then all of a sudden all the lights go out and the radar goes dead. You aren't going to assume that just because a second ago everything was fine it still is. You are going to assume an attack. When you have a mood disorder your radar has lost communications to the rest of the base, so it assumes an attack, all the time. We are going to reconnect communications so your threat detector, which we assume is doing its job, is talking with the threat response unit again.

Both of these analogies are brilliant, right? Medication as a tool. Medication as something potentially life-saving. NOT medication as singular cure-all. And it should never be a mechanism for controlling people instead of symptoms, which is happening more and more. Certain populations, like those in prison systems and foster care systems, receive psych meds at way higher rates than their peers. Which is way too fucking Orwellian for my perspective on healing.

There is a growing trend of distrusting allopathic psych meds. But one side effect of this trend is that it is actually INCREASING the stigma and shame about mental illness.

The more we can do to encourage the body's own ability to adapt and heal, the better. Medications can be an integral part of that journey, although they are rarely the only tools we use. Educating yourself and advocating for yourself about prescription medications will greatly increase the likelihood that they are used properly with you. There are good quality informational portals like the Mayo Clinic, WebMD, and FamilyDoctor that can help you read more about the different types of medications for mental health issues so you can make a more informed decision about what you put in your body.

Naturopathic Meds

I know, I know: "Here, chew this bark" seems pretty sketch.

In Unfuck Your Body, I talk a lot more about supplements, including why they can be sketch but don't have to be if you're using quality products (and especially if you're getting guidance from a professional). For our purposes here, I'll just say that I'm a huge fan of using whole food and herbal supplements in support of or instead of prescription medications. It is something worth talking about with your healthcare provider. Lots of Western medicine docs are getting on board, and there are lots of legit holistic practitioners out there, as well.

When it comes to managing stress, anxiety, depression, and other trauma related symptoms, there are certain formulas that have been used with efficacy for centuries. Kava is a good example. As is St John's Wort . . . and perhaps others you have seen on the news. My recommendations are usually dependent on the specifics of my client's presentation and trauma reactions, but that's an entirely different book. And yes, one I promise I'm writing!

It is SERIOUSLY worth seeing an herbalist, Chinese medicine practitioner, or a clinical nutrition practitioner before you start buying out your local health food store. You don't have to purchase fancy and expensive plans to get quality information to get you started.

Other Complementary Therapies

Complementary therapies are not designed to diagnose or treat conditions. They ARE designed to support the body's natural ability to heal. I love the approach of giving my body and mind what it needs to care for itself whenever possible. A lot of treatments have tons of support behind their efficacy. And many of them can be used either alone or with Western practices (like traditional talk therapy or allopathic meds). Some of the most common, with the most research behind them include:

Acupressure/Acupuncture

Acupressure and acupuncture use the same principles, but acupuncture involves using the actual needles in the skin while acupressure involves the tapping of certain points instead of breaking the skin.

However, whether tapping or using needles, it works by stimulating certain points on the body to promote healing and/or reduce pain. What is really interesting is that as we learn more about the vagus nerve system, we are seeing lots of commonality in nerve mapping and 5000-year-old acupuncture charts. We know that trauma reactions are a whole body response when we look at the bullshit the limbic system tries to do to us, right? A lot of this response is communicated in the body through the vagus nerve I just mentioned. So there is something to all that weird fucking needle stuff, after all!

If you are interested in a combo deal of acupressure with talk therapy, there are forms of acupressure that some therapists use . . . most frequently Emotional Freedom Technique (EFT), which combines acupressure and self-talk strategies. The EFT is something you do yourself with guidance from the practitioner, using the same main activation points an acupuncturist uses (bonus if people touching you squicks you out). The self-talk helps you reframe the stories your brain has been telling you while creating new ones in the process. There are a ton of free videos that walk you through the basic process, though a therapist will help you modify the scripts to work through your specific situation.

Massage

Everyone knows what massage is, I don't have to explain it. But people are surprised when I suggest it as healing for emotional issues, not just physical pain. First of all, physical pain can absolutely be a symptom of depression. But even if that isn't going on, massage can be a safe way for people to learn to relax and feel comfortable in their skin. So many times after a trauma we feel disconnected from our bodies. I also realize massage can be very triggering for certain types of trauma. Definitely don't force yourself out of your comfort zone. Some people are way more comfortable with a pedicure and a foot massage than with a full body massage. Some people prefer a hot bath or hot tub soak rather than having someone's hands on their skin. Anything that feels safe for you while helping you reconnect with your physical body can really help you unfuck way faster.

Chiropractic Treatment

What? Chiropractic care for mental health issues? Isn't that for bad backs? Beyond again, the fact that depression can manifest as physical pain, chiropractic is a holistic form of treatment that operates from the idea that adjustments can facilitate nervous system support. Pain and nervous system support? Totally huge parts of a trauma reaction for many people. And sometimes these physical symptoms are far worse than the emotional ones.

Many chiropractors (as well as massage therapists and acupuncturists) also build nutritional assistance into their work, as well.

Energy Healing (Reflexology, Reiki)

Energy healing is one of those things that seemed super weird, even for me, for many years. Then I read more about it and tried it for myself and wow. So, energy healing is based on the idea that our bodies operate on all these frequencies that we can tap into to promote our healing. Weird? Not so much. One study showed energy healing being as effective as physical therapy. UCLA now has a whole fucking LAB that studies electrical activity in the body. And UCLA is a state funded school. Tax money invested in energy healing. That's some serious street cred.

Reflexology focuses on applying pressure to areas of the ears, hands, and feet with the idea that these areas are connected to other points throughout the body (and polyvagal theory bears this out). Reiki (a Japanese term for guided life force energy) is the channeling of energy from a practitioner (or from one's own self) into the person who needs healing in order to activate the body's own healing process. These forms of energy healing (among others) help us find the stuck points in the body where we tend to hold our trauma, in order to better release them.

And BTW? Acupressure (tapping work like the EFT I talked about) is considered a form of energy healing as well as a form of acupuncture.

Biofeedback/Neurofeedback/Alpha Stim Treatment

Biofeedback is the electronic monitoring of bodily functions that help people learn to control responses that were previously automatic. Neurofeedback focuses specifically on the brain signals with the same intent to help individuals learn to manage their brain responses. We have far more control over our body and brain responses than we realize, and both bio and neuro can be great ways to augment or even speed up our unfuckening by giving us immediate feedback when our brain and body starts to get into fight, flight, or freeze mode. You essentially play a video game with your brain. It sounds as Tron as all-fuck, but you are set up with a Pac-Man type game or something similar, which you can only complete when you keep your brain waves in the optimal zone for your wellness. An example? My son did neuro work to help him with self-control and impulse management. Protocols were set in his game that helped him focus on that part of his brain. When winning the game, he actually felt the pressure of the blood rush to that section of his prefrontal cortex. And we could even see changes in his handwriting after just a couple of treatments!

I also include Alpha-Stim treatment in this section, since even though it is a passive treatment, it falls under the same principles. Alpha Stims are devices designed to increase alpha brain waves (which are the great combination of calm+alert that we all crave). It works like neurofeedback, except the machine does the work for you rather than you training that brain state yourself. It helps with sleep, pain, anxiety, and a host of other conditions. I do use an Alpha Stim in my practice, especially when clients are working through a trauma narrative that is important to them but is causing a lot of "tough therapy day" hangovers. I have also had clients use them to have fewer symptoms in their daily lives without other medications. Alpha Stims have to be purchased with a prescription in the US, but any licensed provider can prescribe them, not just a medical doctor.

Nutrition Changes

When we are stressed we crave sugar like whoa. The brain needs glucose to maintain willpower and energy . . . which is why dieting is so hard. You are deprived of the glucose you need for willpower. Typically, the more stressed and busy we are, the worse we eat. So it's a vicious fucking cycle and ridiculously frustrating.

I know there are lots of nutrition wars out there. Figuring out the best plan for you can be exhausting (Paleo? Keto? Vegan? Gluten Free? THE FUCK I'M SUPPOSED TO EAT?). Short answer? Our body works best when we take care of it, eating the whole and healthy foods humans ate for centuries. And any diet you follow is going to make you more mindful of what you are putting in your mouth, for damn sure. So I'm not hell-bent on you choosing one over the other. In fact, everyone has different dietary needs, which is why my cookbook, (The Revolution Will Include Cookies, Say Something Real Press, LLC, 2016) offers variations in each recipe for some of the more common ones.

And seriously, getting help from a clinical nutritionist, Chinese medicine practitioner, or trained naturopath who incorporates nutritional work can be well worth the investment. I do clinical nutrition work in my practice. I have worked with many people only once or twice on diet modifications and supplements and that's all they really needed: some basic assessments and advice to help them through the overwhelming information out there.

I go deeper into nutrition in Unfuck Your Body, but for now, there are certain basics that can help enormously without getting into weird food-cult status.

- If we eat healthy about 85% of the time and enjoy treats about 15% we can maintain good functioning.
- Stay away from industrial foods as much as possible. The most important thing to remember about food labels? Trying to avoid foods that have labels. The more refined and machine-processed a food is, the more likely it is for your body to not recognize it.
- The movement away from gluten is more about the genetic modification of the wheat in the US and less about gluten itself, at least for most people (Celiacs and people with severe allergies aside). While moving to France or Italy would be ideal, the best thing we can do in the US is move away from gluten and grains that have been modified as much as possible. I live in South Texas so we live on corn tortillas anyway. Many individuals that are entirely grain free use coconut or almond flour. If you miss wheat like a physical pain, try the original einkorn wheat flour in your baking instead of the crap from the grocery store shelves.
- Many people who can't tolerate dairy do fine with raw milks. I can, my son can't. But it may be worth trying.
- Chemical sweeteners are total ass to your body. Aspartame, saccharine, sucralose? The ones that tend to come color coded in yellow, pink, and blue? Cutting calories is not doing you any favors in the long run. A good calorie free sweetener option is stevia.
- If you suspect something is making you feel worse, try dumping it out for 21 days. See how you feel. Add it back in. Notice a difference? Your body will totally tell you what it needs.

Peer Supports

There is a huge body of research that shows that peer-to-peer support partners (as the federal agency SAMHSA refers to them) are an enormous part of many people's wellness and recovery processes. This makes sense. Someone who has similar lived experience has a level of empathy, understanding, and compassion that other people don't. There are phenomenally caring treatment providers out there, but we often connect to the people who have also traveled the same path we are on.

There are lots of names for this role in communities, including recovery coach, sponsor, family partner, and systems navigator, to name a few. There are also clinical professionals with lived experience who may share that experience as part of the work they do with people.

If peer supports are available wherever you are seeking treatment, give it a try. Someone who has been in the same hole you are in is sometimes the best person to talk to about finding the way out, doncha know?

Natural Supports

These are the people who love you just because you belong to them. Your family, your friends, teachers, coworkers, etc. that go above and beyond their role in your life to support you getting better. Having people who love us just because they DO is so, so, so important to getting better. Use them! If they ask to help, let them! It takes far more strength to accept help than to reject it. Be strong enough to allow others into your life.

Choosing The Right Provider

This chapter is about a wide range of treatment options, not just your decision to choose the red pill or the blue pill. Along with all these options, it's also important to choose the right provider.

There is no magic way to do this, other than asking for recommendations and feedback from people you know, asking the provider questions about their practice, and finding someone else if the fit isn't good.

Check out a potential provider's web presence as much as possible. Do you get a feel for them and their style? Feel comfortable with the idea of seeing them? Do they share a worldview on healing that matches your own?

Create a list of what is important to you in a treatment provider and your goals for treatment. If the work you are doing doesn't match those lists? Time to move on.

The important thing to remember about treatment is that it is not rent-a-friend. Treatment works when it is designed to help you process, heal, and move forward. If your time with this person becomes a time to perseverate and regurgitate rather than gain insight and release, it is doing more harm than good. Finding providers you like working with because they support you and guide you toward healing is vitally important. A good provider will not have their feelings hurt if you feel you will do better work with someone else. In fact, they should offer referrals and suggestions of who else you could connect with. The point of therapy is getting better . . . not working with a particular person.

This is your care and your life. You don't owe your provider anything except payment for the services they provide.

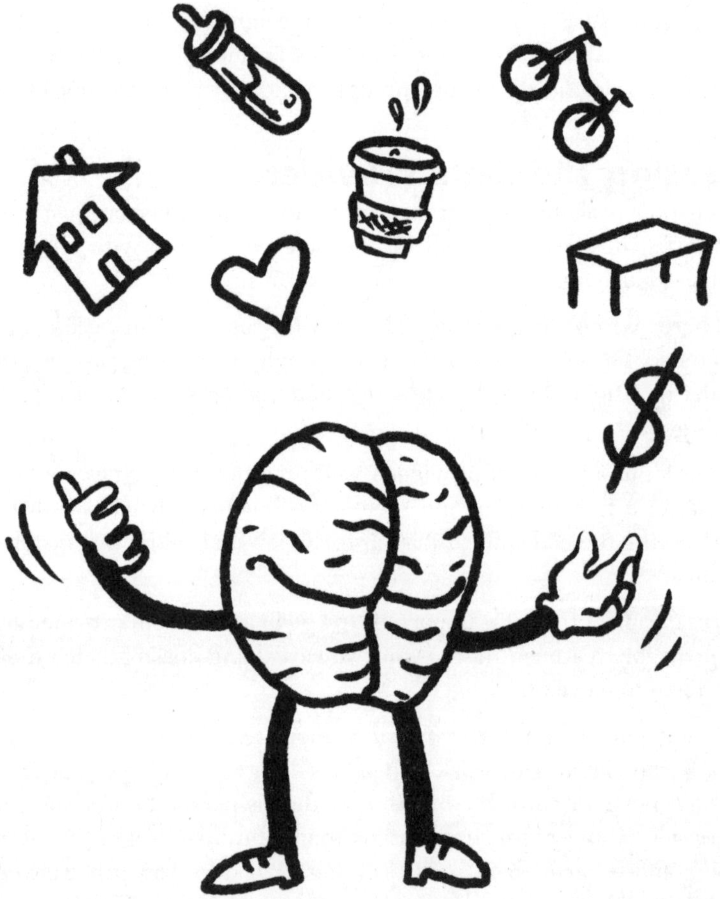

Section Two: This is Your Brain on Life

We are all cursed with living in interesting times. Even when shit is rocking along and our lives are generally positive, they are not curated for a focus on calmness, dullness, and space to think and chill. Remember when vacation was meant to be a time to have fun and adventures? Now it's a time to go away and sit somewhere and be as quiet, non-thinky, and non-doey as possible. I work with so many people who just need more time in their lives to chill. They aren't crazy, they are just fucking exhausted.

And this is an actual, real thing. We have a lot of physical illnesses, like Fibromyalgia, that might be better explained as adrenal fatigue. We may be getting a bit into woo-woo territory here, but it makes hella sense when you look at what's going on with the body during our stress response. Our adrenals secrete the hormones that help us react to stress in the longer term. If these hormones end up in chronic demand because we are under chronic stress, it makes sense that hormonal production would start to taper off. While full-fledged adrenal insufficiency will show up in blood work, smaller declines in adrenal functioning won't.

But they may be showing up in other ways such as exhaustion, body aches, weird skin discolorations, loss of hair, lightheadedness with low blood pressure, etc. It's like the body becomes Miss Clavel from the Madeline books, announcing, "Something is not right."

There's tons more on all this in Unfuck Your Body. For our purposes here, yes, it is also quite-fucking-likely that our continued stress response (whether trauma-induced or not) is responsible for a shit-load of mental health diagnoses. Depression and other mood disorders, anxiety, anger, and addictions all have clear ties to the body's continued worn groove of a physical stress response.

Um, what? Keep your shit straight, lady. You just said stress hormones were secreted through the adrenals. So what the fuck does that have to do with mental and emotional health?

Excellent question, smarty pants! True story about the adrenals . . .

BUT the adrenals (and all other glands) don't secrete anything until the pituitary gland (in the brain) says so. The adrenals (among others) may play the heavy, but they're under complete control of the pituitary. They may give the pounding but they didn't give the order for the pounding.

And who does the pituitary take orders from? Boom, back to square one.

The brain (specifically, the hypothalamus) is the actual master gland, the head coach. The head coach coordinates with the starting quarterback, the pituitary gland, which then calls the plays for the whole rest of the team (hey, there body). The hypothalamus and the pituitary gland control the hormonal system AND the nervous system through their constant convos. All physical body regulation starts back in the brain.

So what's the magic answer, then? I wish I were the badass bitch with the magic answer. But as you well know, the real magic answer would be less stress. And that would be an utterly dick answer to give you . . . because that's not remotely possible most days, is it? So instead, we have to focus on better stress coping so we can manage our business without losing our minds and trashing our bodies.

This half of the book is the part of our mission (should you choose to accept) where we start looking at the specific ways our bodies and minds express stress. The great fuckening, if you will. Hang with me while I nerd out. I promise a lot of what you've been thinking, feeling, and doing is going to make epic amounts of sense.

CHAPTER 6: ANXIETY

Don't you just love dictionary definitions? Anxiety is . . . the state of being anxious.

Well, no shit.

Interestingly enough, the word "anxiety" (and its definition of "being anxious") isn't one bit modern. In fact the word "anxious" was used MORE in the early 19th century than it has been in the early 21st.

You know what that means? Anxiety is a classic human condition that we have been grappling with for centuries. Modern living is sure as hell stressful. But modern life is not the source of human anxiety. Humanity in and of itself is an anxiety-provoking experience for so many people.

As a nerd is wont to do, I looked up the root of the word "anxious." It's from the Latin anxius, which is from the Ancient Greek anko, which means "to choke." Fucking word, they got that right.

Anxiety covers a lot of ground: It can be the experience of unease at its most chill. Distress at medium heat. Straight up panic at a full boil. And as those ancient Italians well knew, it's a hugely somatic experience. That is, it's something you feel in your body as much as it's something that controls your thoughts.

And it's always the most uncomfortable feeling ever. Your body is intentionally making you feel off balance so you have to attend to shit. There's a fancy term for that: Disequilibrium.

So here is our working definition: Anxiety is a state of full body disequilibrium at a level of intensity that demands immediate attention and corrective action on your part. It can be in the face of a real or perceived threat, either present or anticipated.

That right there is why anxiety is so hard to ignore. The whole point of the body producing that feeling is to demand your full attention like a naked, raging toddler running through the street in a snowstorm with a fistful of gummy bears in one hand and a bloody machete in the other.

Quite a visual right? Sure as hell not something you can readily disregard in the course of your day.

Anxiety demands every ounce of attention we have to give it, no matter how inconvenient the time or how unnecessary the anxiety actually was to begin with. So you can see how this relates to trauma reactions, right? It's really easy for anxiety to be your default setting if you have the kind of history that tells you to constantly be on guard.

Symptoms of Anxiety

Thoughts and Feelings Symptoms

- Excessive worry
- Rumination (hamster wheel thinking patterns)
- Irritability/Anger (Weird, right? Anger is the culturally allowed emotion so we substitute that one a lot for what we are really feeling. Check out the anger chapter of this book!)
- Irrational fears/specific phobias
- Stage fright/social phobias
- Hyper self-awareness/self-consciousness
- Feelings of fear
- A sense of helplessness
- Flashbacks
- Obsessive behaviors, pickiness, perfectionism
- Compulsive behaviors
- Self doubt
- A sense that you are "losing it" or "going crazy"

Physical Body Symptoms[1]

- Trouble falling asleep or staying asleep
- Inability to rest
- Muscle tension
- Neck tension
- Chronic indigestion
- Stomach pain and/or nausea
- Racing heart
- Pulsing in the ear (feeling your heartbeat)
- Numbness or tingling in toes, feet, hands, or fingers
- Sweating
- Weakness

1 You are totally reading the physical body checklist and thinking . . . this is the same list for everything from anxiety to Ebola. Which is why so many people end up in emergency rooms thinking they are having a heart attack when they are having an anxiety attack. It's also the same reason many people have missed the fact that they were having a heart attack because they were also having an anxiety attack. In Mental Health First Aid training, we suggest that if you see someone with potential anxiety attack symptoms, you ask them if they know what is going on and has it happened before. If they say "no" then treat it like the potential emergency situation it may be and call 911.

- Shortness of breath
- Dizziness
- Chest pain
- Stomach pain
- Feeling hot and cold (feeling like having chills and fever without running a temperature)
- Shooting pains/feeling like you have had an electric shock

Of course there are tons more symptoms. These are the more common ones and a complete list of all the things you may experience with anxiety would be an entire pamphlet of list-ness. You can find lots of great lists all over the interwebz, including ones that break down all the different categories of anxiety symptoms.

A lot of other things we do are adaptive to managing anxiety as well. Obsessive-Compulsive Disorder is totally an anxiety response. Cutting and other self-injury behavior may not stem from anxiety in all people, but does for many. So many diagnoses out there stem from just a few core issues. Anxiety is totally one of them.

But yeah. Anxiety symptoms. There is a lot of nasty shit our bodies do to us to get our attention and make us correct course.

Any of those hit home? You probably aren't reading this if the answer to begin with was "nah, I'm always chill."

Do I Have Anxiety or Am I Just Anxious Sometimes?

You ask the most awesome questions! Like any other mental health issue, the answer lies in whether or not anxiety is controlling your life, rather than being a legit way of your body telling you to get off your ass and do something.

Clinically speaking, if you say it's a problem, I will agree that it's a problem. You know you the best.

Some people want a more formal way of self-check. There are a lot of anxiety assessment scales out there. The one you see quite often is the OASIS (which stands for Overall Anxiety Severity and Impairment Scale). It's well backed up by research and it's free to use, since it was developed by the National Institutes of Health (NIH).

OASIS doesn't have a magic cut-off number (as in: below this you are fine, above this you are batshit anxious). But it can be a good starting point for opening a conversation with a treatment provider or even just to reflect on your experiences.

The OASIS questions ask for you to reflect on your experiences over the past week and rate them on a scale of 0–4, with 0 being no probs, 1 being infrequent, 2 being occasional, 3 being pretty frequent, and 4 being constant fucking companion, thanks for the reminder.

Yeah, I'm translating a bit there. You can see the entire scale with the exact wording online, download it and print it if you want. (tinyurl.com/jnubjvx)

The exact questions themselves are as follows:

- In the past week, how often have you felt anxious?
- In the past week, when you have felt anxious, how intense or severe was your anxiety?
- In the past week, how often did you avoid situations, places, objects, or activities because of anxiety or fear?
- In the past week, how much did your anxiety interfere with your ability to do the things you needed to do at work, at school, or at home?
- In the past week, how much has anxiety interfered with your social life and relationships?

Having a "holy shit that's me!" moment? You are so not alone. The Kim Foundation notes that about 40 million American adults ages 18 and older (18.1% of people) in a given year meet the criteria for an anxiety disorder and 75% of individuals with an anxiety disorder had their first episode before age 21.

Anxiety Really Does Sound a Lot Like Stress

Yup, totally. And anxiety often comes from chronic stress. The big difference? Stress has external triggers. I know, I know, so does anxiety, but hang with me.

Stress can produce anxiety, but it can also produce a ton of other emotional responses (depression is probably the biggest). Anxiety is an internal response to stressors.

Think of it as a workflow process. If stress, then anxiety. Or any other number of uncomfortable emotional states. It all happens so fast it ends up mashed together in our brain. But there is definitely a cause and effect thing going on between the two.

A good book if you are interested in learning more about this is Why Zebras Don't Get Ulcers by Robert Sapolsky.

So Where Does this Anxiety Shit Come From?

Generally speaking, the human body works hard to maintain its chill point. So why is the body intentionally making you all bonkers-batshit with this anxiety thing? That makes as much sense as cheerfully banging your head into a brick wall, dunnit?

And once again, it all comes back to brain wiring. I am clearly a one trick pony in that regard.

Short version: We are wired to have strong emotional responses because those responses keep us alive. Feeling anxious is absolutely an important survival skill.

Longer version: If something triggers an anxiety response, your body gets flooded with norepinephrine and cortisol. Here's what those do:

Norepinephrine is released through your central nervous system (Hah! Nervous!) in order to prepare your body (which includes your brain) for action. It increases your focus and attention as well as your blood flow, blood pressure, and heart rate.

Cortisol is the classic stress hormone. It increases blood sugar and suppresses the immune system. Many people with chronic stress also gain weight, specifically as "belly fat," due to the constant cortisol production. The important thing to know here is that when cortisol is released with its partner in crime, norepinephrine, it creates strong memory associations with certain moods, to create warning signals of what you should avoid in the future.

The interesting thing here about anxiety as a stress response? The good thing? Anxiety means the body is still fighting back. This is fundamentally different from depression, which is essentially a wired response of learned helplessness (this is Robert Sapolsky stuff again).

Anxiety symptoms are active coping skills in the face of threat. The problem is only when the brain has decided that most everything, most everywhere is a threat. And, boom. That right there is a trauma response.

Even once you've figured out your triggers, anxiety isn't something you can willpower your way out of. As you saw, we have the asshole twin chemical combo going on. So in the here-and-now moment of anxiety or a straight up panic attack, you gotta do something to metabolize those chemicals. When anxiety hits, you have to face it head-on.

Any of the exercises at the ends of these chapters or in Chapter 4 can be used to help manage anxiety in the moment. Give your anxiety a goofy name or persona. Carry ice to hold as a reminder. Do some deep breathing exercises.

When you aren't feeling anxious, you can work on longer-term self-training to rewire your brain.

Self-Training for Learned Optimism

Like all other brain retraining, there are certain things that can really help combat chronic anxiety. It isn't a magic bullet, better-immediately type cure, but the idea of training yourself to be optimistic has some merit behind it. There is a guy named Martin Seligman who is a legit big deal in my field. He was studying learned helplessness when he noticed that there are certain qualities that those obnoxiously, cheerful Susie-Sunshine optimistic people generally have:

Permanence: Optimistic people don't dwell on bad events, and approach them as temporary setbacks. If they get neg'd on, they bounce back more quickly. They also believe that good things happen for reasons that are permanent. Essentially, the world is fundamentally in their favor.

Pervasiveness: People who are happy monkeys tend to keep failure in its proper place. They recognize failure in one area as only belonging in THAT area, rather than meaning they are a failure at ALL THE THINGS ALL THE TIME. They also tend to let the things they are good at inform the rest of their lives, rather than keeping that in its own space. Sucking at basketball doesn't mean you will now make a shitty risotto. And if your risotto rocks, it is an indicator that YOU rock. And that you should cook more often. And invite me for dinner, I love risotto.

Personalization: Our cheerful buds blame bad events on bad circumstances rather than bad selfhood, but take credit for good circumstances as indicating that they are good people. So basically failures are events, not people. But successes are people, not events. If you dig me?

Understanding what makes an optimist gave Seligman an idea. If we can learn helplessness and pessimism, then why can't we learn optimism and a positive outlook? Especially if we know the three big indicators we are shooting for? Interested in figuring out which way you wire?

Take Action: Challenge Your Neg Gremlins

Seligman created an ABCDE model designed to help you reframe your thinking as optimistic. And yes, it looks a ton like Albert Ellis's Rational Emotive Behavior Therapy (REBT) and Aaron Beck's Cognitive Behavior Therapy (CBT). We all borrow from each other's shit all the time. Therapists and researchers are assholes like that.

Think about the last time you felt anxious and write down some notes for each of these five letters:

In Seligman's model the A stands for Adversity. What bullshit is going down that generally triggers your anxiety response?

B stands for Belief. What are your beliefs about this event? Be honest, if your anxiety is triggered a lot, you are probably running a thought pattern in the direction of "THIS IS FUCKED!"

C stands for Consequences, though really it should stand for Cookie. Seligman didn't agree with me that once you think that shit's fucked you should go have a cookie. Instead, he wants you to look at how you reacted to the situation and to your beliefs.

D stands for Disputation. This is where you literally argue with the neg-gremlins your brain is throwing down and focus your attention on a new way of coping. Remember the storytelling brain? Create a new story to use instead.

And finally, E stands for Energization. What was the outcome of focusing your attention on a different way of reacting? Even if you were still pretty anxious, did you handle the situation better than you may have in the past? Over time, with doing this, do you notice that your anxiety is starting to fizzle out FINALLY?

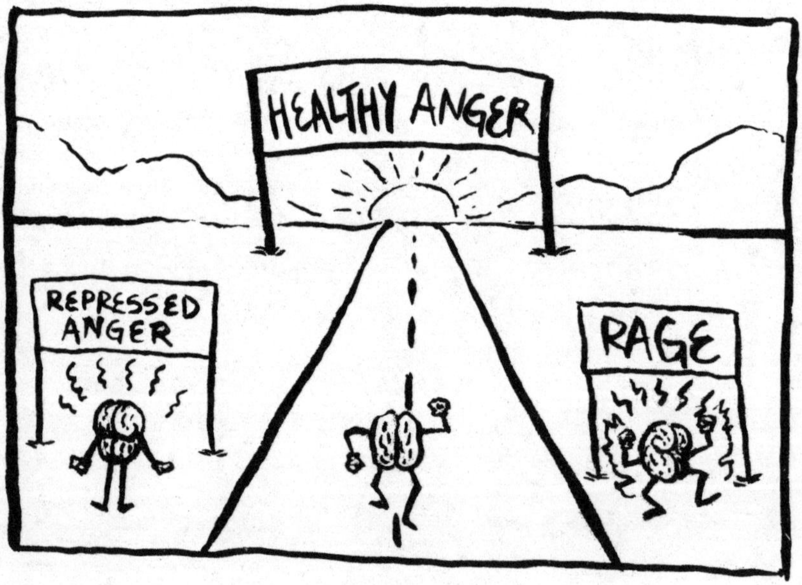
HEALTHY ANGER
REPRESSED ANGER
RAGE

CHAPTER 7: ANGER

If you have ever looked up a definition of anger, it tends to be not very helpful . . . usually a synonym rather than a definition. You read shit like that and you are thinking "No, no . . . I know what irritation is, antagonism is, rage is. They are all forms of anger. But what the fuck is anger actually made of?"

So anger is an emotion. Yeah, no shit. But bear with me. The word emotion derives from the Latin emovere, which means "out-move."

OK. NOW we are getting somewhere.

So, first off? General reminder:

Emotions are instinctive responses that are triggered by outside events and inside memories of past events. They function in the middle part of the brain, separate from the reasoning and cognitive processes in our prefrontal cortex.

So anger is an out-movement instinctive response. That makes sense, right? At its core, anger is an instinctive response designed to protect us from harm by pushing us into concerted action.

Boom. There we go. An operational definition of anger that is actually helpful.

Anger (and anger induced aggression) are activated in the same way that other emotions are. For anger, the specific activation triad is the amygdala, hypothalamus, and periaqueductal gray neural systems. Each type of threat activates these areas in different ways. Which is excellently geeky, but not so important to this convo.

The important thing to remember is that if we think we are at risk? Being threatened? We are going into brainstem fight club mode. Anger is how we prepare for that fight. The interesting part is that anger gets a lot of input from the PFC. All emotions do, obviously . . . but anger is pretty interesting in that the expression of it varies wildly in different cultures. Which means a lot of anger responses are taught, therefore PFC-negotiated. What's up with that?

A Culture of Anger

Why is everyone so fucking pissed off all the fucking time?

You don't have to look for a video on YouTube to see someone losing their shit. Just hang out at a grocery store, church parking lot, or mall food court for a little while and you will see someone flip the fuck out over something pretty damn minor in the grand scheme of things.

Maybe this person has been you at some point. Or someone you love. Or someone you barely tolerate but have to put up with.

There are a lot of theories about why we have all this anger, and they all make a lot of sense.

We are:

- Overdistracted
- Overstimulated
- Overcrowded, and
- Overinundated in everyday life.

Wouldn't anyone lose their shit?

But in plenty of other countries that are just as over-everything'd, you don't see nearly the same amount of anger responses as we do in the US and Europe. One Swedish researcher was fascinated by the cultural differences and compiled a review of studies about anger, comparing anger in the US, Japan, and Sweden and her findings were fascinating. She demonstrated that in Japan, for example, individuals are explicitly taught that there is an enormous difference between what you feel inside and how you present that to the world. It isn't something that Japanese citizens just pick up from those around them, but from the actual school curriculum.

In Japan, you are taught how to handle negative emotions.

But in contrast, when Americans are asked to explain uncomfortable emotions, they really have a hard time doing so. They often describe emotions as internal, not things that have consequences in behavior. But there is one interesting exception: Anger.

Anger, for some Americans, is considered a positive force of change that helps us overcome obstacles, cope with fear, and become more independent. One study found that 40% of individuals in the US considered their anger to have positive consequences over the long term.

That means that in the US, anger is not only acceptable at some level, it's often seen as a GOOD thing.

And our cultural rules and values about anger are getting us in some serious fucking trouble.

- "I reached my boiling point!"
- "I was blowing off steam!"
- "I blew my stack!"
- "I was berserk!"
- "I went nuts!"

- "I unleashed my anger."

The underlying message in these symbolic explanations is that anger is in control of us, we are not in control of anger. Maybe that's why we love those movies where Liam Neeson kills everybody.

We speak of anger in a way that leads us to believe that anger is valid, it is in charge, and it must be acted upon. Our expectation is that anger requires retribution . . . and we see that our job, then, is to ensure a corrective response. From the time we are children, that anger is not only permissible, it's a positive means of addressing situations.

This isn't to say that anger is always bad, or always a negative force. No one has ever gained equal rights in this country by asking politely for them and having them handed over. And the energy that anger gives us can help us respond appropriately in certain situations.

If my children are in danger, my anger response will drive me to protect them. But my anger at the cashier for going on break after I finally get to the front of the line I've been waiting in? Probably not productive for anyone involved.

What is Anger?

Anger, like all emotions, isn't good or bad or right or wrong.

It just is.

Emotions are information, designed to help us make decisions that will protect us and keep us safe. They are triggered in the middle part of our brain, in our amygdala, based on the information we are processing and our memories of past situations.

Positive emotions are a type of "carry on" feedback. Our brains telling us "Yes! Yes all cookies! Yes hiking with friends! Yes funny movies! These things feel nice, let's do all these things!"

Negative emotions are the polar opposite. They are the cat scrunched up in the corner, ears flattened and growling. "No! Do not want! Does not feel good or safe or nice at all! Make it stop!"

Anger triggers the fight/flight/freeze response I was yammering on about back in Chapter 1.

Feeling some serious fucking anger is a normal part of being a human being. Losing your shit is not.

As I tell my clients . . . you are allowed to BE crazy, but you aren't allowed to ACT crazy.

Being irritated as fuck because someone jacked the parking spot you were waiting for?

Totally legit.

Going postal over it? Not so helpful.

Not so helpful to everyone around you, not so helpful to greater society, and . . . for purely selfish reasons . . . not so helpful to you.

When we lose our fucking minds on a regular basis, we are wiring our brains into a constantly heightened state that eventually fries our circuits (and pushes away everyone we love in the process). We program ourselves to always be on the alert. So we react with far greater speed than we used to, and perceive more situations as being dangerous, hostile, or threatening. We are constantly jumping at shadows.

Our brains never get to rest and recharge and we start struggling with many other conditions associated with this wiring change. Added up, those conditions are known as autonomic nervous system dysfunction. Many common health problems (heart disease, high blood pressure, food allergies) as well as many common mental health issues (depression, anxiety, PTSD) are related to a continued heightened response.

And back to anger right here, because anger is the worst offender in this regard.

To borrow a famous Buddhist expression, anger is like holding onto a hot coal and expecting the person we are angry at to get burned.

Anger is a Secondary Emotion

And you know what is really fucked up about anger? This emotion that we culturally believe is driving us to success? It isn't even a primary emotion.

I know, you are now asking: And what the fuck is that supposed to mean, fancy PhD lady?

It means that while anger may be the first emotion we recognize at some level in ourselves, and the emotion we act (or react) upon, I guarantee you it actually isn't the first thing you feel in any given situation. Anger is a secondary emotion.

The best model I have seen to explain anger uses the acronym AHEN.

AHEN is as simple a conceptualization as you can get.

- Anger is triggered by
- Hurt
- Expectations not met
- Needs not met

Of course, it is a little more complicated than that in that we aren't usually limited to just one of these triggers but a big glob-ball of all of the above.

Here's how to use AHEN. Next time you are pissed as all get-out, ask yourself the following questions:

1) Am I hurt? Did something happen here that made me feel insecure? Unsafe? Unvalued? Unworthy? Unappreciated? Just plain old sad as fuck? Of all the things that have kicked me in the nuts over the years, why is this situation particularly nasty? Was it the person who I perceive as doing the hurting? Is it a particular situation that bothers me more than others? Has this been a problem for me in the past? Is this one of those fucking TRIGGERS people yammer on about?

Break this shit down . . . why the hurt?

2) Did I have expectations that were not met? Was my little brain bopping along expecting a certain thing to happen and it didn't happen? Was that a realistic expectation? (Be honest here, aiight????) If it was realistic, is it some life changing shit when it didn't happen? Someone took the parking spot you got to first. Dick move. Reasonable expectation that they would follow civilized parking lot protocol? Fuck yeah. Otherwise we are 3 inches away from complete social chaos . . . people need to follow some fucking rules, FFS. But is it life changing? Not so much. You find another parking spot (eventually) and get parked (eventually). Then, hopefully, you move on. So break this shit down next. Was it a reasonable expectation to begin with? Did the world fucking end because it wasn't met? Some shit is for-real serious, some isn't. Tell yourself the truth here. Is this an expectation worth getting all hurt over?

3) Did I have needs that were not met? This is a tough one. Because how do you define what a need really is? If you are Buddhist, you may not think they exist at all, right? On an existential level you are all kinds of right. But on a physiological level, the brain is wired to keep you alive. If something threatens the brain's sense of equilibrium, you are gonna get flooded with fight back chemicals, straight to the amygdala.

Certain things are going to trigger this fight response more than others. Imminent danger is a duh. We need to feel safe. We need to perceive our loved ones as safe. If your brain perceives a threat to you, your sweetie, your kids, your pooch? It's on. Protect what's important to you! Get mad!

There are other kinds of safety needs we can't discount. Human beings are hardwired for relationships. We need the stability of relationships in order to be well. Our brains know this, even when society tells us "You don't need no one but your own damn self, playa'!" That's some bullshit. We live communally not because we are overcrowded but because we have to do it to survive. So with that need comes the need for emotional safety. We need to feel secure and supported in our relationships with other people. We need to have a good idea of what to expect. We need to feel loved. This is more than some dickwad jacking our parking space. This is about our fundamental human need to feel supported by others in the world. We need to know that we are safe with the people we love, that they love us back, and that they are not going to hurt us, at least not intentionally.

We need to get out of dark alleys at 2AM. We need to get away from the erratic driver swerving next to us on the freeway. But we also need a community of people who love us silly and make us feel secure.

The anger that kicks us in the ass for the longest is when that contract gets broken. When the person with whom we most needed to be safe did something that made us question that safety.

You can see why I have stuck with this model of understanding anger for years now, I'm sure. It helps make sense of so many of the situations we have to navigate on a daily basis.

Knowing where anger comes from is way more than half the battle. It's like 90% of it.

How many times have you had an "Oh!" moment when you realized why you felt a certain way and then the feeling just . . . melted?

And then there is the other 10% of the time.

Shit be real and managing it is hella hard.

But like we talked about above, dealing with anger is like dealing with any other piece of information that we need to take into account to resolve a situation. It isn't a good or bad thing and it doesn't have to be the driving force of our decisions.

Take Action: Where Does Your Anger Come From?

When was the last time you were angry? When you aren't in actual imminent danger or under actual threat, and after you've used the AHEN model to break some shit down, evaluate the following questions:

1) What are the underlying roots of your anger? Once you figured them out, were they legit or were they more about you and your history than about the present situation? If you aren't sure, reflect on when you first noticed that you were angry. What was going on around you . . . sights, smells, noises, people? What were you doing? What were others doing? What were you thinking about? Any particular memories coming up at that time?

2) If the roots are legit, are they something that needs to be addressed or is it one of those bullshit daily life things that just happens? Speeding ticket, fucked up drive thru order, etc.?

3) If it needs to be addressed, what is the best way to do so? How do you correct the situation with as little disruption as possible? What can you do to keep from getting further hurt in the process (physically, emotionally, and mentally)? Can you keep the hurt to others minimal (physically, emotionally, and mentally)? Does it need to be addressed immediately, or can it wait until you are calmer and feel safer? Is there anyone else you can talk to that is going to have a healthy, supportive perspective . . . a counselor, friend, mentor, family member? Someone who knows you, loves you, and will totally call you out on your shit if need be?

4) After you act (instead of react), then evaluate the results. Did it work? Is this a strategy that you can use again? Are you still angry or are you feeling better and safer now?

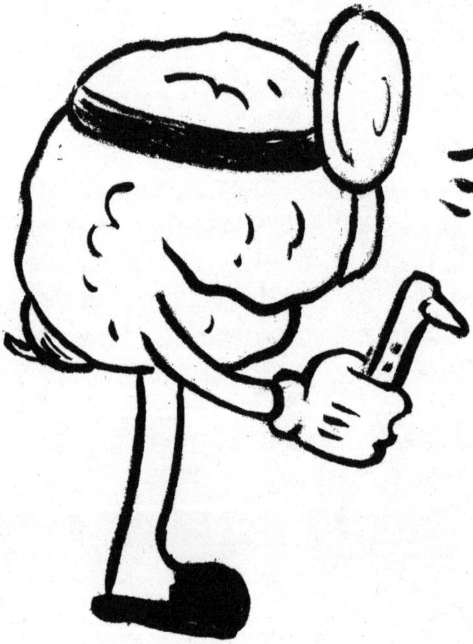

CHAPTER 8: ADDICTION

Let's start with one universal truth right off the bat.

Practically everyone is addicted to something, at some point in their lives.

Yep, quite possibly you. Definitely me. If you picked up this book with the intent of helping someone you care about, one of the first things you can do is recognize your own struggles with some form of addiction.

Yeah, I know that seems a seriously dick thing to say. But bear with me for a second, this is gonna make sense.

The spelling of the word "addict" is unchanged from the first use of it in the mid 16th century. It was used to describe someone who was bound or devoted. Still dead-on now, innit?

Addiction was originally defined by early mental health professionals (Freud and the like) and the first peer recovery group facilitators (AA and the like) based on what they saw, heard, and could measure at the time. Consensus was that addiction is a function of cravings plus compulsive use. It was a simple model, and was our first start in providing addiction treatment. But it really didn't encompass all the complexity of addiction.

While our understanding is by no means complete, we now know that addiction is WAY more than craving plus use. The neurobiology of addiction is epically complicated, though new research is starting to give us different insights than we have had in the past. We know that substance addictions set off the pleasure pathways in the brain like WHOA . . . although at different levels for different people. Which helps explain why some people are more prone to substance addiction while others find that the same substances make them feel fucking awful. We also know that the anticipation of use can set off all kinds of dopamine signals in the brain . . . which totally explains addictive behaviors where a mind altering substance isn't being used at all.

Gabor Maté, in his book In the Realm of Hungry Ghosts, offered this definition of addiction, which I have used ever since I read it, even in my dissertation.

"Addiction is any repeated behavior, substance-related or not, in which a person feels compelled to persist, regardless of its negative impact on his life and the lives of others.

Addiction involves:

1. Compulsive engagement with the behavior, a preoccupation with it
2. Impaired control over the behavior
3. Persistence or relapse despite evidence of harm
4. Dissatisfaction, irritability, or intense craving when the object—whether it be a drug, activity, or other goal—is not immediately available."

Some addictions are clear. The woman with the fresh track marks over years of scars. The man who loses his home and car to gambling debts and now is hiding from dangerous creditors.

Some of what we term addictions are out-of-control behaviors that cause huge problems in our everyday lives, even though we are able to get up and function in some areas every day. This applies to those of us who take out a bag of chips or a tray of muffins after a tough day. Or go shoe shopping for our 8th pair of black sandals that we are never going to wear.

There are addictions that excuse us from society altogether, those that keep us barely afloat within it, and those that become a barrier between us and the rest of the world. It's only a matter of degree, in the end.

How do we define when we cross over into addiction territory? As a relationally-trained former therapist and current mental health coach, my answer is a simple one. When our addiction becomes our primary relationship. Maybe not in our hearts and heads. But in our behaviors, definitely. When we don't have control over our addictions, we are spending time, resources, and energy on the addiction instead of the people we love. And instead of, let's face it . . . ourselves.

Where Addictions Come From

Where do addictions come from? And why the fuck do I say that practically everyone is some kind of addict?

When we engage in an addiction to the point of it taking precedence over our relationships with people, it's a problem. It's a coping mechanism that has moved from soothing us to controlling us completely.

Addiction is the domain of the sensitives. The empaths. The people who notice early on what is dark, hidden, and broken in society. We learn that pointing out these discrepancies is grounds for punishment. We are told that good boys and girls don't notice such things. And if they do, they CERTAINLY don't talk about it. So we start taking on responsibility for all this shit that is dark and broken. We swallow it down and it starts eating us alive. Everything must be our fault. We clearly aren't good people. Relationships aren't safe. The only way to get through is with a mechanism of coping and support.

If you have had a trauma, if you have been hurt so badly in a way that makes you not trust the world, you are far, far, far more likely to be susceptible to addictive behavior.

At some point in most people's lives, we start using something to help us feel better. We are hungry for something that we aren't getting. So we start feeding that need with other stuff. Substances, behaviors, activities. Whatever we choose probably helps for a while. It soothes the raw hunger that we are feeling, and helps us forget about what we really need.

In reality, addictions are just coping skills gone awry.

There is a huge, gray, fuzzy margin between healthy coping and addiction. It's a big, blurry area where we start losing control over our coping skill, be it a substance, an activity, or a behavior, and it starts controlling us and taking over more and more of our lives.

Coping skills are intended to help us stay grounded and get through difficult times. They aren't intended to replace reality, or replace our real relationships. So when we can't entirely be with the people we love . . . When we can't entirely feel safe within ourselves . . . That means whatever we are using to get us through is operating as an addiction.

How We Heal

There are two basic categories for addiction treatments. The traditional model of addiction treatment is abstinence based. That is, you cannot engage in the addiction at all . . . that's the only mechanism of healing. The other is harm-reduction. This method is more of a negotiation with the addiction, finding ways to reduce the harm that is occurring in our use. Let's talk about how some of these treatments might work in practice.

Abstinence Based Treatment

I grew up within the framework of AA: Alcoholics Anonymous. My father was in recovery, so we spent enormous amounts of time at AA meetings, events, conferences, and having our house full of people new in their sobriety. AA was unique when it was created some 80 years ago. The idea is of people with lived experience sharing their support and helping others on the path to finding their own sobriety. It's based on giving yourself over to a higher power, whatever that happens to be for you. Many people who struggle with faith-based services are uncomfortable with this framework. And other prescriptive elements have emerged in some groups that feel exclusionary. For instance, many groups believe that sobriety means no mind-altering substances, even medications for a mental health disorder.

It's a shame because the AA model also can be of great benefit to healing. Higher Power? For some people that may just be the greater community surrounding you. Healthy relationships, attunement to your own authentic voice. It doesn't have to be an omnipotent God of some form. And you shouldn't have to give up the medications that are keeping you sane while letting go of the addictions that sent you on the road to crazy.

And there are plenty of groups that do honor those differences in beliefs, whether it be AA, NA, OA, DDA, or any other twelve-step program. There are meetings available online 24 hours a day, and in most communities throughout the world. There are meetings that focus on special groups of individuals who may not be comfortable in general meetings, such as Lambda AA, which was created for LGBT individuals in recovery, and the Wellbriety movement, which focuses on the specific needs of indigenous individuals.

There are other plans outside the traditional twelve-step model that are also abstinence-based, such as SMART Recovery, Save Our Selves/ Secular Organizations for Sobriety (SOS), and Women for Sobriety. These programs have also been around for some time, but focus on newer research about making sobriety effective. These programs generally also have more of a focus on self-efficacy/internal locus of control rather than relationality/higher power support.

That's a simplification, but my point is that there are sober living options outside of the twelve-step model. And a variety of options means a larger chance of finding something that makes sense for you.

Harm Reduction

There are two times when harm reduction treatment is the best bet:

1) When it is what you HAVE to do.

2) When it is what you WANT to do.

So, here's the thing. Some addictions can be given up entirely and recovery can be achieved through total abstinence. One can live forever without drinking alcohol or purchasing a lottery ticket, after all.

But sometimes we don't have any fucking choice about abstinence. Food addiction? Still gotta eat every day. Most work addicts aren't independently wealthy to where they can just quit their job and instead go meditate at an ashram in support of their recovery.

Sex addiction? While I suppose you could make the argument that abstinence is an appropriate treatment strategy, I haven't yet worked with anyone that would agree that giving up sex was an option. And considering most of them had long-term partners, their partners wouldn't agree either.

What's more, some people do not WANT to let go of the substance or behavior that is the source of their addiction. For example, someone sex positive may want to continue to use porn that is conscious and affirming, without having their use of porn take control of their lives. Or they may want to use substances in a controlled way, rather than in a way that is impacting their lives in a negative manner.

And yeah, I get it. Some addictions are so insanely dangerous that abstinence is likely the only thing that will save your life. Crack cocaine? Not something you want to try to use in moderation.

But most abstinence-style recovery programs do not allow for a harm reduction detox—or the use of less harmful substances to mitigate the effects of not using the harmful ones. For example, there has been enormous debate surrounding the use of methadone (legal) and marijuana (legal in some states) to support recovery from hard drugs.

Some substances require a medical detox (alcohol and heroin being the two big ones) to prevent serious medical complications or even death. Detox is not the same thing as addiction treatment and recovery, of course. It's only meant to get you through the medically dangerous part of getting rid of the poison in your system so you CAN move on to treatment and recovery.

Of course, some substances are just a bitch to detox, even if they don't involve medical risk. Anyone who is a caffeine addict? You know how bad it feels when you don't get your fix. Refried ass is an apt term.

Straight detox (whether inpatient medical detox or chaining yourself to the bed and away from the coffee pot) can be a huge barrier for many people. While there are more and more medical programs that are no-fee, these programs obviously can't make up for lost wages during the stay, provide childcare, etc.

For all these reasons and more, harm reduction is becoming a more frequent treatment option for many people.

There are formal, nation-wide programs like Moderation Management. And there are lots of treatment professionals who use a wide variety of harm reduction strategies in their practice as part of therapy. And yes, I am absolutely one of those treatment professionals.

Instead of thinking that you have to be completely abstinent before digging into the emotional stuff, I believe that addictive behavior is a way people manage their traumas, and that we need to work on the underlying trauma and find other ways to cope with it before we take away that coping skill. Until the addiction becomes the least helpful coping skill that someone has, it's going to be hella hard to treat.

Unfuck Your Addiction

So here is what I ask clients to do.

This is clearly the world according to Dr. Faith. I am no more right or wrong than anyone else, but I have been doing this work for a very long time and have found ways of supporting recovery that work best for the individuals I work with and my own worldview/treatment style.

Now, anyone who says they have the BEST way to treat addiction is a fucking liar. I would never claim such nonsense. So take my suggestions for only what they are—suggestions. Use anything that works for you and dump the rest.

1. Consider addiction's role in your life as a replacement relationship.

Shit ends up in the addiction zone when it starts replacing our authentic relationships with the people around us and with our own self. We end up in service to the substance or behavior that is the point of our addiction. It isn't just something in our life, it becomes the most important thing in our life. Addiction recovery is a recognition of that. Maybe you don't feel that you have any relationships worth saving. Maybe you don't even think that YOU are worth saving. I'd beg to differ, but it's not up to me. I would suggest, gentle reader, that you give space to the possibility that there are good relationships out there to be had. And your current addiction is a nasty, dirty parasite who is never gonna love you back the way you deserve to be loved. When you are hanging out with your addiction, consider what needs are being met and if this is really the ideal way of handling them. Once we become conscious of our engagement with the addiction and remind ourselves we are choosing the addiction over ourselves and over others, it becomes harder and harder to continue to make that choice. Don't step into your usage without being mindful of what you are doing. It gets harder and harder to fuck over yourself and the people you love when you are doing it with intentionality and ownership.

2. You're in charge of yourself. You really are. Even if you feel that you aren't. Even if you feel that you never have been.

Ultimately, your use will change because you want it to. You will change because you want to be better, because you want your relationships to be better. Even if you get remanded by a court into treatment, whether or not you stay sober will ultimately be up to how badly you want to, right? No matter what people tell you to do, whether or not you do it is ultimately up to you. Remind yourself that when you feel yourself bristling against authority. What do YOU want for yourself? Is what you are doing getting you there?

3. It's far easier to START doing something new than STOP doing something old.

A lot of really great clinicians are fearful of working with individuals with addictions because they think the idea is to get someone to stop doing something. I take the opposite approach, focusing on adding healthier behaviors and building healthier relationships rather than focusing on the addiction itself. We may build awareness around some of the history and/or behaviors surrounding use, but we don't generally focus on the use itself. If you build a healthier you, the addiction often becomes less and less needed as a coping skill. I was asked recently "How often does therapy consist of just getting people to get out more?" And the answer is? A helluva lot!!! You don't have to go balls to the walls superhealthypants, but can you add in one small thing that makes you feel better instead of worse every day? And can you pay attention to how you feel when doing THAT thing instead of the addiction thing?

4. Remember that sobriety and recovery are spectrums.

You get to choose the best point for yourself on that spectrum and you get to choose when that changes. Do abstinence if that works for you. Do taper + harm reduction if that works better. Part of your journey is figuring out who you are and who you can be in relation to your addiction. I have worked with people who soon learned that playing a game of poker would spiral into heroin use within a month. Only complete abstinence kept them safe. Then I have worked with other people who tapered hard drug use with marijuana. A few gave up the marijuana too at a later point (it isn't legal in the state I live in, so using had some inherent risk) and some continued to use marijuana instead of other drugs successfully for years with no relapse. As alluded to in mentioning the legality of marijuana in my state? You are, of course, responsible for all the consequences of your behavior. For example, if you are mandated to go in for drug screenings and you pop hot, you can't blame this book.

5. Stop the bullshit.

With yourself, with others. Blowing smoke up people's asses, convincing yourself that you are making good decisions when you know very fucking well that you aren't? Stop that. You may not have had much control over your life up until this point but consider this my permission slip to you to TAKE IT BACK. Accountability through and through. If you engage in your addiction, own it with honesty. Don't blame anyone else. Remind yourself that your engagement in your addiction is a choice you are making. Make it consciously. Instead of telling yourself "my partner broke up with me so it's their fault I'm using, I just can't handle all this," try "My partner broke up with me and that triggered all my struggles with abandonment. I'm choosing to use because it's the coping skill that has worked best for me and trying something new feels overwhelming." You may find it harder to hurt yourself with your addiction when you take a mindful sense of responsibility for it.

6. Figure out your triggers.

If you squeeze your eyes shut, you will continue to bump into shit. If you keep your eyes open to the terrain, you can start putting together a map. When you catch yourself doing the thing, ask yourself to retrace what led to it. The HALT acronym is a big one in addiction treatment . . . am I hungry? Angry? Lonely? Tired? If you pair awareness triggers with accountability for your actions it becomes increasingly hard to stay on the addiction path.

7. Forgive yourself your fuck-ups.

You are a fuck-up. So am I. Yaaay for being human. Have some self-compassion for that fact. Self-compassion is the opposite of self-esteem. It's about your insides rather than your successes and failures on the outside. It means you forgive yourself your failures and your human bumbling. And no, this doesn't mean you get to be a hedonistic fuck-face. In fact, if you are aware of your human frailty, and take care of yourself in the moments where you are your most fragile and off-kilter, research shows you actually take more responsibility and accountability for your actions. Kristen Neff wrote an amazing book called Self-Compassion. Read the thing if you haven't. Changed my life.

8. And forgive the fuck-ups done unto you.

I hear you. Some terrible shit has happened to you. Seriously awful stuff. Awful stuff will continue to happen. Sometimes people are just as balls as they can be. Forgiveness isn't about them, it's about how much bullshit you want to carry around with you. I'm guessing not that fucking much. Forgiveness doesn't mean allowing ongoing dickitude. Instead, it will help you set better boundaries so you know how to better protect yourself in the future. And it will open the door for you to have more real conversations with the people around you, instead of continuing to only converse with your demons.

9. Anticipate your continued imperfect humaning.

Do your best to do your best. But seriously. You're gonna fuck up. You may even relapse. And you know what? We either win or we learn. So take the fuck-ups as new ways of getting good information about yourself. What did you do differently this time? What can you take from this experience and do differently next time? Honoring our fuck-ups with clarity is brave as fuck. And you so have every capacity to be brave.

Take Action: Where Can You Say Yes?

Addiction is often treated like a lack of willpower. Nancy Reagan told us it was simple enough . . . all you have to do is just say NO.

So that becomes our internal dialogue. Why can't we, sometimes? Why can't we just say no? It leads to a shame spiral and blocks our ability to be self-compassionate.

If addictions are replacing other relationships, that's where our first steps in healing should begin.

So sit down and make a list:

What can you say "yes" to?

Not as a replacement for your addiction. Not instead of or a giving up of something else. Life isn't a zero sum game, after all. And being told to give up the thing that has helped you the most in the past isn't fair. I know that's your end goal, of course. But we don't have to start there if you aren't ready.

Just say yes to something new. Something you used to love but don't do anymore. Something you always wanted to try.

Expand the boundaries of your life back out by adding something. What happens? What shifts? What else do you need now? What do you no longer need?

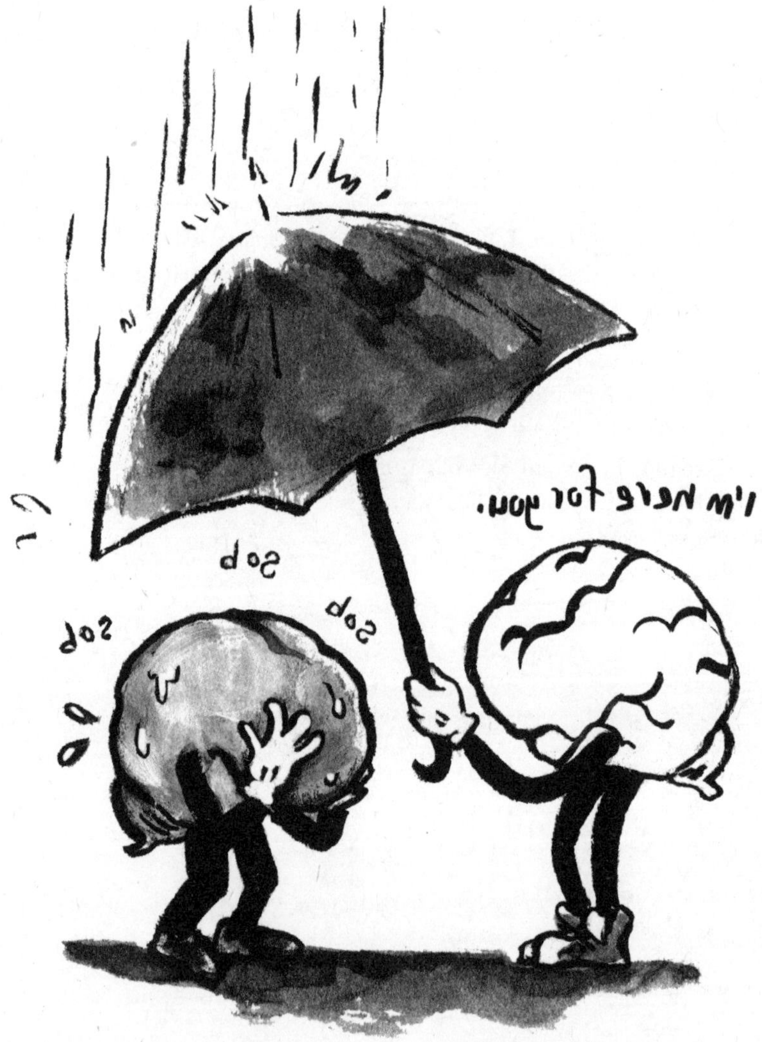
i'm here for you.
sob
sob
sob

CHAPTER 9: DEPRESSION

Depression is one of those words we throw around and use as a label so indiscriminately it's lost its meaning. I've been guilty of it and I bet you have, too. I used the word depressed to express how I felt when Whole Foods stopped carrying my favorite ginger cookies, even though pissed as fuck with a preposterous sense of entitlement would have been a way better description of my state of mind.

Depression is not your team losing in overtime, losing your favorite watch, getting fired, or breaking up with a partner. Granted all of these things have different levels of suckitude, but at their core they are all losses that cause understandable levels of grief (which is the topic of the next chapter). Grief and loss can absolutely be traumatic, and can absolutely lead to depression. But with proper space and time to heal, we heal. Depression is a far more insidious problem. And sometimes it doesn't have anything to do with an identifiable loss.

Just like anxiety, depression is related to the biochemistry of stress.

Anxiety is an over-response to stress hormones. It's the body trying to go into survival mode to protect itself, based on what it thinks to be true. Anxiety is a biochemical over-response to stress.

Depression is the body's way of saying nothing I do is going to help anyway, it all sucks ass no matter what. Depression is a biochemical learned helplessness response to stress.

Depression is the body's way of saying if nothing I do makes any difference, there is no point in enjoying ANYTHING. Robert Sapolsky defines depression as "a genetic-neurochemical disorder requiring a strong environmental trigger whose characteristic manifestation is an inability to appreciate sunsets." I define it as a clinical case of the fuck-its.

In his book Tribe, Sebastian Junger writes about depression in relation to anger in how it is triggered as part of the fight-flight-freeze response. If anger is preparing you to fight, then depression is your brain's way of turtling up . . . to not get noticed, to not be too active, to not do the things that might put you in more danger.

Depression is not the same thing as sadness, grief, coping with trauma, or coping with loss. Depression is the complete shutdown of all the things that make being human a joyful experience. The biggest, most consistent symptom of depression is anhedonia, which is a tongue-twister way of saying an inability to feel pleasure. If you look at that word, you can see it essentially means not-hedonistic. If you struggle with depression, you have all kinds of feels. Guilt, shame, anger, irritability, hopelessness, overwhelming grief. But you rarely have experiences of pleasure, gratitude, connectedness, and joy. And if you do reach out for them, you feel them snatched away more often than not. Depression is the thief of all the wonderful things that make human-ing worth it.

The word depression comes from the Latin word deprimere, which means to press down. Yup, exactly. Depression operates as a literal anchor into the muck. An actual diagnosis of Major Depressive Disorder requires that anhedonia be present every day for at least two weeks. Other symptoms that are also really, really common are:

- Low energy/fatigue
- Low level chronic pain
- Jacked up concentration, difficulty making decisions
- Feeling guilty and/or worthless
- Sleeping a ton or sleeping for shit (whether not sleeping at all, or sleeping badly)
- Feeling either super restless, or really slowed down (like moving underwater or brain wrapped in cotton)
- Intrusive thoughts of death (morbid ideation) or suicide (suicidal ideation)
- Change in eating habits (and five percent or more change in weight either up or down because of it)
- Irritability, anger, low distress tolerance

How Does the Getting Better Part Work, Then?

The bad news is there is no magical path for healing depression. However, that's ALSO the good news. That means you get to find the path that works best for you. And fuck anyone who tells you that you aren't healing correctly. Because there is no magical answer about what treatments you should seek out. The important thing is to be aware of the many options available for you to choose from . . . especially when there are people who are going to try to push their worldview about treatment on you.

Only more recently have mental health professionals started to incorporate trauma-informed care in their work. If depression is predisposition + trigger, then wouldn't it make sense to look at some of the possible triggers? We've already covered all this, I know. But as a general reminder?

Very little of our genetic programming is set in stone. Two to five percent of all diseases TOTAL are related to a single faulty gene. However many, many, MANY diseases are lurking in our DNA and can be turned on by the right conditions. The shiny-human super fancy term for this is epigenetics.

Whoa, wait a fuckin' minute here, Doc. Does this mean that my depression that was turned on could turn back off again?

My pain in the ass therapist answer is: That's a hard maybe.

If you know or at least have a hardcore suspicion that your mood disorder has a big-assed trauma taproot then it might make a fuck-ton of sense to treat the trauma along with the other symptoms.

Whoa, lady, does this mean I may not need to be on meds forever? Maybe I won't pass it down to my kids? Maybe it won't keep getting worse year after year like it has been?

More hard maybe answers there. Blech. I wish I knew the magical equations in that regard. I can tell you that people tend to have a way better handle on their mood disorders if we unpack the trauma fuckery. They manage present and future triggers way better. Sometimes they aren't nearly as impacted. At the very least they know to go "Shit just got real again, I need some Buddha-damn help right about now." If they are on meds, they are often able to at least decrease, or find ways of not having to increase year in year out like they have been.

And yes, I have seen complete remission of symptoms a number of times. It is possible.

People don't need to unconsciously perpetuate the cycles of trauma in their own kids, either. They teach them the healthy coping skills that they have learned. (Great book? Trauma Proofing Your Kids by Peter Levine.) And if their kiddos end up struggling as well, they are the first to advocate for help immediately and early to keep them from struggling through the system. And they aren't going to allow any bullshittery from the school system and the mental health system as they get that help. Because no fucking way are they gonna let their kids suffer the way they did.

This is another one of those tough subjects, I realize. It's hard to be cheerful about an illness that tends to eat people alive. But like everything else, I really believe that understanding the biochemical roots of the problem is enormously helpful in feeling less trapped and crazy. You are not defined by your depression. You are not weak, and you didn't do anything wrong. You didn't deserve this. You are not being punished. You hit the perfect storm of genetics + trigger and you are now dodging and weaving while running your ass off toward getting better.

People struggling with depression (or any mental illness) are ANYTHING but crazy.

They are survivors, fighting back against brain chemistry that is entirely at odds with all the things that make life worth living. Those of you who are living this? Who are saying "Fuck you, Depression, you don't get to win today"?

You are the bravest people I know.

Keep fighting.

Activity: What I Want Back

Depression's fundamental difference from sadness is how much it steals from us when it strikes. It's like a police state where not just behaviors are punished, but crimes of thought as well. Depression takes away our lives and our will for life.

Have you ever been in this place? Are you in this place now?

I would love for this to be the time that you pick up the phone and start asking for help. Help from family and friends, help from professionals. But I know how hard it is to make that call . . . and how hard it is to actually get the help you are begging for. It feels overwhelming.

I also know that if you are reading this book and

have gotten this far, that's where you are headed. You are starting to get a glimmer of a thought of "Fuck this shit, I want my life back."

And if I am right? What do you most want back? Of all the things that make life worth living that depression has robbed you of, what are you missing the most right now? It may not be the biggest thing, and that's OK. In fact, it's great because it may be easier to wrestle it away.

You don't have to do anything about this yet, unless you want to. But the intent of this exercise is to start with the thought crime that depression has forbidden you from having. The thought that you can do better and deserve to do better. The thought that there is a world out there that you have the right to participate in and maybe even enjoy.

Let's start right there. Write those thoughts down. Remember that world. That's the beginning of your new story.

CHAPTER 10: THE IMPORTANCE OF HONORING GRIEF

Remember how we talked about the trauma recovery timeline? While there is no magic number associated with the time we need to heal, researchers have found that ninety days is the basic timeframe for reestablishing equilibrium. And the first thirty days are the most fragile and necessary part of that process. When something disrupts that experience, we are far more likely to experience long-lasting symptoms of trauma, which can look like depression, anxiety, or any number of mental illness labels.

Part of avoiding a trauma response is having the space to grieve. Grieving what hurt you. Grieving what you lost. Grieving the life that you wanted that isn't the same now.

Mental illnesses like depression and anxiety have strong genetic predispositions, but research also shows that they still require a triggering event. Unresolved grief often acts as exactly that trigger. Not having the space to heal can create actual biochemical changes in our brains.

It's also not too late, you know. It doesn't matter if it's been thirty days or thirty years. For many people, healing an established trauma response may include going back and doing the grief work you were never allowed in the first place. Grief scares the fuck out of us, whether it is our own or someone else's. It feels like a freefall that is completely dark and completely bottomless.

When we don't allow or aren't allowed our grief process, this can often lead to an experience of "traumatic grief." That is a level of unresolved grief that turns into mental illness. Let's work to stop that bullshit and focus on honoring grief.

That starts with how we talk about it, how we support others who are grieving, and how we ensure we get the support we need in our own healing processes. Grief is the fundamental process of letting go. In her book How Can I Help? June Cerza Kolf notes the statistic that the number one fear experienced by human beings is the fear of abandonment. C. S. Lewis, in his book A Grief Observed, stated:

"No one ever told me that grief is so much like fear."

Grief is a realization of the certainty of abandonment. It is our worst fear made reality.

It makes sense, then, that we don't really talk much about grief. It scares us shitless. We fear that discussing it will somehow invoke it. While we know at an intellectual level that abandonment is unavoidable throughout our human existence on the planet, it still knocks us sideways when it happens.

When we discuss grief, our first thought is always of death. But grief is the experience of any kind of loss, any type of abandonment in our lives. Grief can come with the loss of a job, the loss of a relationship (through any means, not just death), or the loss of a way of life we have come to know and expect. We can grieve changes even if they are happy ones. Getting married can be an amazing thing, but we may still grieve the loss of our single days. Becoming an adult is something we all looked forward to, until that moment we had to grieve the freedom of childhood and the ability to hand over decisions to someone else.

Our cultural expectation is to possess rather than release. Loss (abandonment) is a forced release for which we have few mechanisms to heal ourselves or support healing in others. We don't talk about the inevitable letting go of that which we think we possess.

What Is Grief?

Grief means, most simply, deep sorrow. The word grief comes from the old French grever, which means "to burden." Grief becomes a literal burden we carry.

Gabor Mate, in his book In the Realm of Hungry Ghosts, discusses how emotional pain lights up the brain the same way physical pain does. When we hurt, we LITERALLY hurt. It is just as much a bodily burden as a broken bone or serious physical illness.

That's a simple definition of grief. But grief has a habit of never actually being simple. There are different kinds of complicated grief:

- Grief can be complex, especially when you experience lots of losses happening close enough to each other to get all tied together.
- Grief can be anticipatory, meaning that we know it is coming so we are hurting every moment until the loss finally happens. And it doesn't hurt any less from all the anticipatory hurting.
- Grief can be disenfranchised, meaning that the grief is not recognized in its depth by others in our social network or larger culture. We have cultural rules for the amount of grief we are allowed to feel, don't we? A miscarriage is considered less of a loss than that of a child. A pet is considered less than a person. A neighbor less than a parent. A former partner versus a current one. Grief can also be disenfranchised when the relationship

wasn't a healthy one. Sometimes relief is mixed in with that grief which can in turn cause guilt. For example, the loss of a parent who was abusive is often a disenfranchised grief.

- Grief can be delayed, meaning that we push it aside and continue to function until the point when it comes back and knocks us sideways. We use busyness as a protective mechanism . . . until things explode.
- Grief can be displaced, meaning we duck and cover on the real source of our grief and have a strong reaction to something else that seems out of proportion. For example, someone may seem stoic at the loss of a parent, then weep uncontrollably after finding a dying bird in their yard some months later.

The Platitude Bullshit People Say That Doesn't Help

"Time heals everything, you know?"

Fuck yes, I know it will eventually get better. But that's not right now, is it? So stop talking.

"It's a blessing. He was in pain, he was hurting, he was ready to go."

Maybe so. But I wasn't ready. Or maybe I was ready, but now my anticipatory grief just jumped off the high dive. No matter how good a death it was, or how much it had been prepared for, it STILL FUCKING HAPPENED.

"God never gives us more than we can handle."

God (or any higher power) is not some kind of dickhead setting up pain and struggle litmus tests. If She wants to get my attention or encourage my personal development, there are far better ways to go about it. Things happen to people that they can't handle all the time. That doesn't make us failures in the eyes of our system of faith. Don't short-change anyone's spiritual journey by throwing this in their face, FFS. And don't set them up to feel like they shouldn't ask for help.

"We must be strong."

Why? Why must I? Why can't I be as small, and hurting, and knocked out as I feel? Why am I not allowed my experience? Why do I have to pretend to be better than I feel? Fuck inauthentic strongness. I'm not strong right now so I'm not going to pretend to be.

"You're holding up so well."

This bullshit goes with "being strong." Whether I am or not is beside the point. You have no idea of my private moments or my internal reality. And I don't want to be praised for making everyone around me more comfortable by not wailing and weeping. Because I may need to wail and weep at some point, and now I will be afraid to do so in front of you.

"I know how you feel."

Oh my fucking Buddha, you do NOT. Do not compare your loss to mine. Whether it was less, about the same, or worse. Just don't try to hijack my experience. Everyone's grief is unique. You may have a good idea of what I feel but I promise you do not have the same exact experience as me. Allow me the validity of being the only person who knows exactly what I'm going through at this particular moment.

We've all said this shit and we've all heard this shit. It may not have been offensive to whomever the receiver was, but it certainly wasn't helpful. So please, bite your tongue on the platitudes. If you don't know what to say, just shut the fuck up and be there.

If something stupid slips out, own it. Say "I didn't mean to say something so stupid. I feel awkward and unhelpful and I was trying to come up with something that would make you feel better when there isn't any magical thing to say. I'm so sorry."

What Actually Helps

Here are some things that you CAN say. None of these statements are magical emotional Neosporin. They may not help. But they won't diminish or demean the grief experience of someone else. They won't shape or control their behavior to your expectations or social goals.

- You must feel as if this pain will never end.
- I'm so sorry that all this happened to you.
- This must seem like more than you can handle.
- Don't feel that you need to be strong when you are hurting and need help.
- It's OK to cry. Or be mad. Or feel numb. Anything you are feeling is OK.
- Some things just don't make sense.
- I don't have anything to say to make things better for you right now, but I will be here with you.
- I am happy to help in any way I can, but I don't need to do something for you to make myself feel better. I will offer help, but will also not do anything if that's what you prefer.

Or you can just be quiet. You don't have to chatter away to be a healing presence in someone's life.

Here are some more ways to care for someone who is grieving.

- Listen differently. Give people space to tell their story if they want. Don't interpret or add your own filter. Show openness and receptivity to what they are saying to show you can be with them as they process. Reflect what they are saying and how they are feeling. Ask open-ended questions that encourage them to continue speaking if they so desire. Validate their experiences. Show that you care and are concerned for them. These are all the basic tricks that therapists use in building relationships with their clients because they are just good humans connecting to other humans skills to have.
- Offer specific support that will actually fill a need. Don't make empty, vague offers of support. Sometimes when we are grieving we don't know what would help, but if someone offers to bring the kids to the pool or do the dishes, we realize that would be wonderful.
- Ask what would help. It's also OK to say you don't know what to offer that would actually be helpful, but if there is something that WOULD help you would be happy to do it. If someone else in the grieving person's life is acting as their primary support/ point person, ask THEM.
- If they say no, back the FUCK off. Tell them that the offer remains open but don't nag or perseverate.
- Don't expect people to be able to answer questions or make decisions. Avoid asking as much as possible when they are in the first few days of their grief experience. When you feel completely fragmented, pulling the pieces together to be rational feels overwhelming.
- Sit with the person's pain and suffering with compassion. Do this instead of offering positive stories or trying to fix, giving advice or suggestions. Be willing to do nothing, just be with, acknowledge and honor the person, their pain and their suffering. Just having told one's story can often be powerfully therapeutic.
- Attend their story and experience rather than your idea of the truth or what you think they should experience or do.
- Be aware of the bias our culture has toward redemptive stories. Do not try to change, rewrite, reframe or invalidate the person's non-redemptive, non-happy ending stories.
- Give credit for small or large efforts, endurance or strength in facing challenges without being patronizing. If someone is spiraling toward depression, encouragement for the behaviors

that are showing movement to healing is important, rather than just rescuing them when they seem overwhelmed.

Keep one foot in acknowledgment and one in possibilities, but do not insist on always speaking the possibilities.

Speak to the complexity of the situation, including seeming contradictions. Like, You can't go on suffering like this AND you don't want to die. Or, You want to give up AND you don't want to give up. The AND statement is infinitely more powerful than a BUT statement. Anytime we preface with a "... but ..." what we are REALLY saying is "you're wrong" rather than sitting with the contradictions we all feel when grieving.

Don't forget the forgotten grievers. Oftentimes many people are impacted by a loss, but we focus on certain, primary people.

Take Action: Honoring Grief Through Ceremony

We've talked about how the human brain is wired for story. And music. And connection. Is it any wonder, then, that we crave ceremony? Cornell anthropologist Meredith Small calls ceremonies the punctuation marks of life.

This makes sense, right? If our operating memory can only hold seven (yes, plus or minus two) items of knowledge at a time, is it any wonder, then, that we think in symbols and navigate the world within that reality? That we make meaning through creative expression?

We have certain cultural ceremonies for grief. Funerals being the obvious example. But funerals are often more and more soulless. A box to be checked off, rather than an opportunity to grieve. And so many grief-filled events do not get a closure ceremony. Not because we don't need it, but because there is no language for that need.

And this is where we fill in the gap.

What are you grieving that you don't even have words for? What symbolizes your experience? How can you use these symbols to create meaning? What would your ceremony entail?

Conclusion: The New Normal

Shit gets better. For serious it does. Not perfect, not pre-trauma innocence. But better. And sometimes richer and deeper for the experience of taking back your power on your own terms.

Certain things will probably trigger you. Anniversaries, life circumstances.

But your relationship with your trauma will change. It won't be the beast that controls your every move, anymore.

Your trauma will be more like that pain in the ass neighbor with too much time on their hands.

You know the one.

Who reminds you that the trash pick-up is changed because they are on a holiday schedule. Or tells you that your dog cries a lot when you are at work. Or that the new guy on the floor below totally looks like the drawing of that man that was on the news for robbing a convenience store. You know, it just might be him.

They are a well-meaning pain in the ass.

And you make friends with this person the way you do with your trauma.

Sometimes they give you good, useful information. You say thank you. You take the important information and act on it. And you dismiss the rest.

If you don't need to act on it, you tell them thank you for sharing information that is thoughtfully intended to help keep you safe.

You listen, you smile, and you think "Fuck you, Amygdala" and go back to living your life.

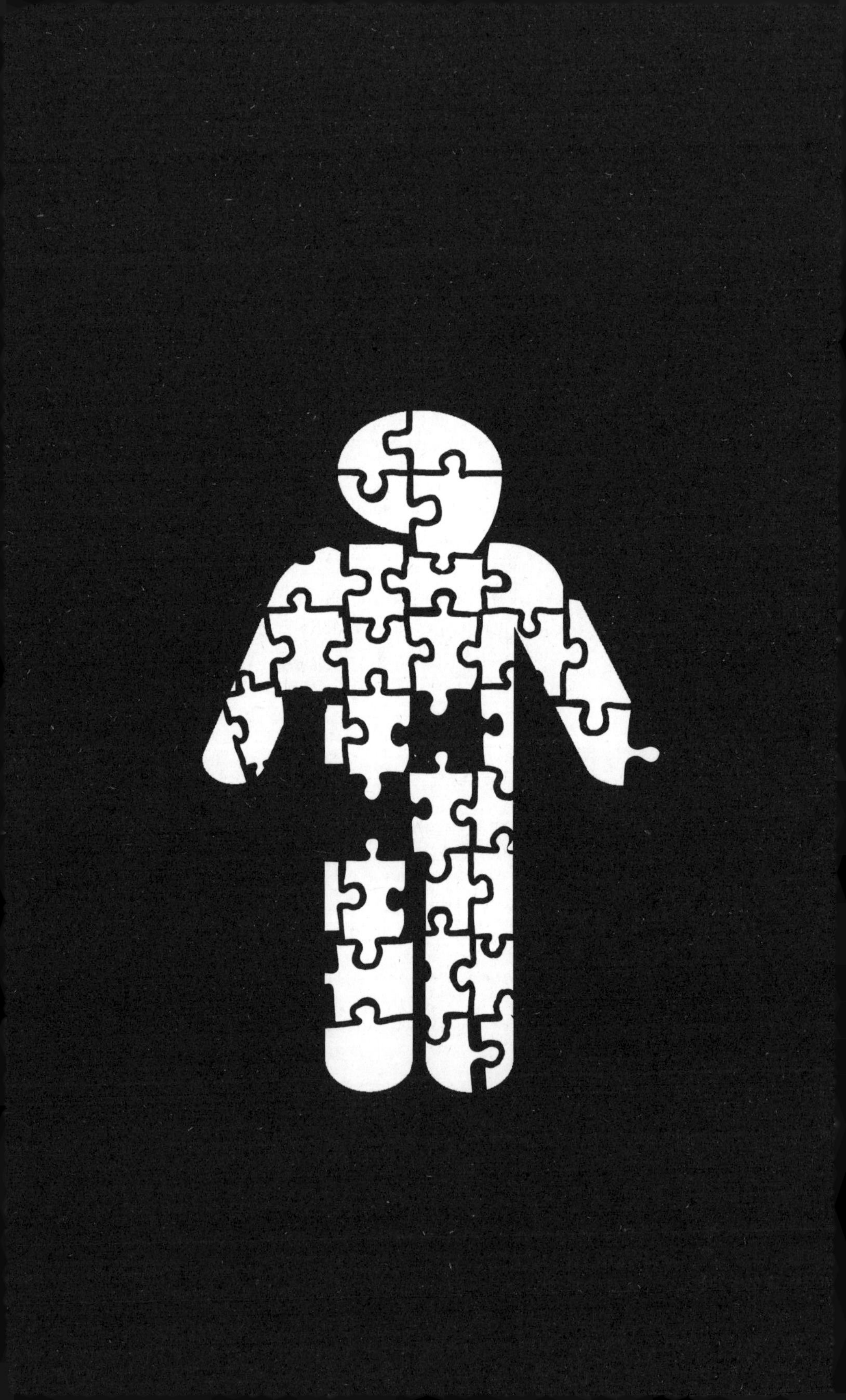

Unfuck Your Body: Using Science to Eat, Sleep, Breathe, Move, and Feel Better

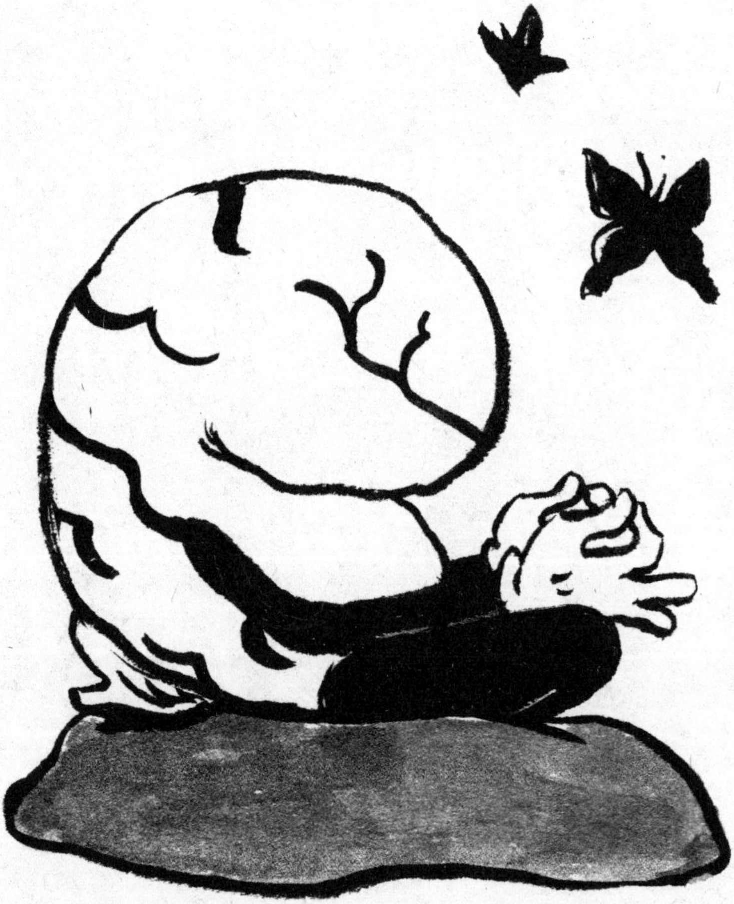

INTRODUCTION

Where do we even start with talking about how bodies get fucked up?

We get sick or injured. Trauma takes root, directly affecting our physical body as much as our brain. Stress seizes us up. Our toxic environments and food systems poison us. We experience pain. Our immune systems freak out and we don't know why. We have kids, or don't. We get busy and stop exercising. Years of insomnia catch up with us. We have surgery or take medication that changes our bodies. Or, most common of all, our personal meat puppet gets older and less tolerant of our bullshit.

We can't talk about bodies without talking about our brains, and vice versa—because our bodies and minds influence each other in every area of our physical and emotional lives.

This book is about how the body and mind communicate with each other using the vagus nerve, and the enormous role trauma, inflammation, toxicity, and stress play in that communication and our overall health. And most of all, it's about how we can feel better, by improving our body-brain awareness, developing habits that support the brain and body, and accessing treatments that serve our physical and mental health.

When my first book, Unfuck Your Brain, came out, there was so much I wanted to include about the mind body connection that there just physically wasn't room for. I swore that this book would follow up where that one left off.

Unfuck Your Brain is about trauma. So is this book. Trauma is a physical event, an injury to the nervous system. In that book, I did talk a little about the impact of trauma on the body (like with the physical symptoms of PTSD, anxiety, depression, and anger) and in some cases recommended physical treatments. I focused mainly on mental and emotional sources of trauma, as well as ways of working with those issues to promote healing.

But so much of trauma is a bodily experience that it merits a deeper dive and its own book. Stuff that we have known is incredibly helpful to mental health (like yoga, breathwork, somatics, and dietary changes without the BMI body shaming bullshit) as practice-based evidence is now collecting more and more data to back it up as evidence-based practice. And we are gaining ground at light speed at answering the "but why" questions of the body-mind connection. So much so, that I have to dial it down a bit and not write the 12 volume Encyclopedia of Body Unfuckening that will then be sold in late night commercials by Time

Life Books (and if you are old enough to get that joke, you are as middle aged as I am).

There was some concern that if I wrote this book it would get shelved as another "change your body, change your life" diet-and-exercise regime book with tips like gargle with lavender essential oil, sleep upside down like a bat, and live on a diet of bee pollen and kale. Or whatever idea is fresh at this moment. But one thing that has happened in the years since Unfuck Your Brain first came out, is a bigger cultural awareness of the mind-body connection and how we support whole health by recognizing both. This means it isn't weird and woo-woo for us to recognize our gut as being our second brain. Or that polyvagal theory explains so much about how our bodily reactions fuel our thoughts and feelings. Stuff that nutritionists and other complementary practitioners have been yammering on about for a century or more is now entering the mainstream with enough energy that I can tell this story with hella research and without the presumption that I am trying to sell you on a fad regime that includes wasp stings, protein powder, and astral projection.

So here is the goal. To dive into the science of the mind-body connection. To really look at how and why the body impacts (ok, actually is in charge of) our mental health. To separate fact from fiction on body-based treatments and holistic care (with the best research we have at the time of this writing) as ways of supporting/enhancing other traditional treatment options. To help us all consider what wellness looks like beyond fads and beyond bullshit cultural norms and standards. To create space to personalize a wellness plan that suits you.

We'll also talk about a lot of practical things you can do to unfuck your body, including coping skills, food, meds, movement, sleep, breathing, and mindfulness techniques. I'm all about the practical. I also busted my booty to approach each topic without all the shame and blame crap we're all used to getting served to us. I know these are loaded topics, but we're going to make them all as un-loaded as possible. And you can skip whatever chapters you aren't up for dealing with right now. There isn't an order you need to do things, it's all about finding what works for you.

A note about my expertise and its limits: Much of what you'll find in this book falls into the category of "complementary medicine." Complementary means just that: adding to, shoring up, augmenting, and helping us heal. As well as working many years as a therapist and now working in the field as a coach, I fall into the nutritionist/complementary practitioner category. I have a post doctoral certification in clinical nutrition. I've also trained in yoga (including trauma informed yoga), meditation, mindfulness, breathwork, and a lot of the other stuff I talk about in this book. So I recommend them with a solid understanding of what I am recommending and an understanding that they are not intended to diagnose, treat, cure, or prevent any disease. When I talk about supplements, this information is based on available research and my own training coursework, not statements that have been evaluated by the Food and Drug Administration. I expect that most of you have a doctor who is an MD. I am not an MD and am not looking to replace MDs or discourage you from going to one. Your MD is doing the diagnosing and treating, I'm providing ideas that can help support your body's capacity to heal. In my own practice, it's just as much a part of being a trauma-informed mental health coach as the talking part. Ultimately, anything in this book you try should be done in concert with a trusted medical provider and your own inner voice telling you what most nourishes you.

Context and Deeper Inquiry

Much of what I write about in this book has deep cultural and spiritual roots. Western medical and psychiatric practitioners (and philosophers) have argued for over a century about how minds and bodies are connected. Historically there was no separation, meaning treatment protocols were as much about the soul or our place in society as they were the mind and body. These are roots that modern scientists keep trying to appropriate and distance themselves from at the same time, rather than appreciate and embrace.

Take this example from a peer-reviewed journal:

> The psychophysiological coherence model draws on dynamical systems theory. We use the terms cardiac coherence and physiological coherence interchangeably to describe the measurement of the order, stability, and harmony in the oscillatory outputs of the regulatory systems during any period of time.

Any idea what they are talking about? They're talking breathwork. Specifically about nadi shodhana pranayama (which already had a perfectly usable English translation, alternate nostril breathing). Oscillatory means breathing in and out. Regulatory systems? Your heart and lungs. The fuck, right?

One of my clinical nutrition professors jokingly told us that the word "herbs" chokes scientists up so badly they had to change it to "polyphenols" in order to stomach studying them. And polyvagal theory may only have existed for a few decades, except that it also exists within 10,000 years of Traditional Chinese Medicine, in forms still used today.

Dr. Candace Pert once said that scientists would rather use each other's toothbrushes than each other's words. But in this case it goes even deeper than branding. As I mentioned above, there is a distancing from the cultural roots of these earlier modes of healing. The bestseller The Relaxation Response, first published by Herbert Benson in 1975, intentionally decoupled spirituality from transcendental meditation in order to encourage non-Buddhist individuals to use it for its health benefits, essentially cherry picking from a religious practice.

But here's the thing—you don't have to subscribe to a belief system to have a deeper experience (and appreciation) of a practice. I worked hard to acknowledge these roots throughout the book, but reviewing 10,000 years of Traditional Chinese Medicine isn't practical. I tried, my editor said "girl, no." And honestly, that work has already been written way better than I could have written it.

So here is my invitation and encouragement to explore deeper. If you already have practices that you engage in, or if you find some in this book that you connect with, you will gain more from the practice by recognizing how it developed in context. For example, I would encourage my yoga people to read books like Embracing Yoga's Roots and The Myths of the Asanas. At the very least, we will have a lot fewer people ending class with "namaste," which is actually a term used in greeting.

There isn't much new under the sun, and we can always benefit from learning about the practices that have provided so much healing across so many generations, right? Respecting what inspires us and heals us is never wasted time.

Section One: What's Happening with Our Bodies?

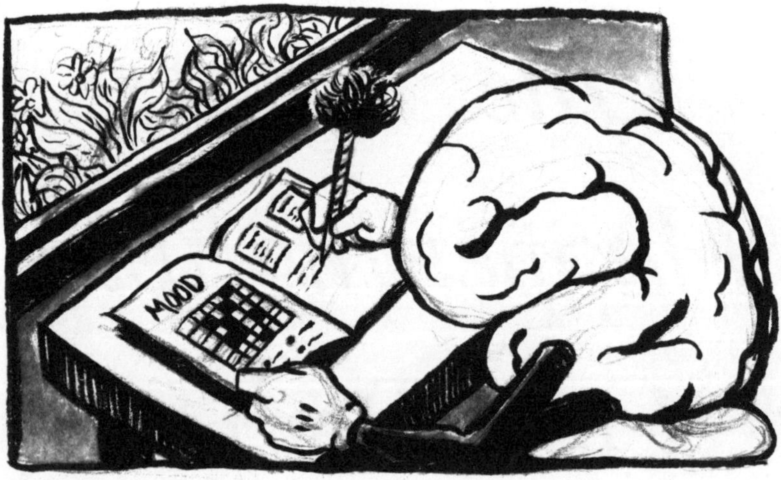
MOOD

HOW THE BODY AND BRAIN COMMUNICATE

Our bodies and brains really are not separate things, even though they are typically treated thusly. We tend to think of the body as the meat sack the brain is in charge of hauling around, when in fact they are as dynamic and interreliant a duo as Pancho and Lefty.

One of the major pathways of brain-body communication is the tenth cranial nerve, otherwise known as the vagus nerve, (historically referred to in Traditional Chinese Medicine as the du channel) which serves as the foundation of polyvagal theory. All methods of body-brain intercommunication appear to organize through this channel.

The vagus nerve is the part of us that most of this book rests on. It's the nerve that physically creates the mind-body connection, linking your brain and your gut and the rest of you. It's the body's communication system. It's how information, inflammation, and relaxation spread. And because our whole body is involved in our emotional health, understanding the vagus nerve helps us understand both our physical health and our emotions, and how they are connected. In the next part of the book, we'll look at trauma, inflammation, stress, and toxicity and how the vagus nerve mediates them all.

The vagus nerve's information flow is designed to help us stay alive and stay safe. But like every other safety process, it is designed to err on the side of caution by embedding memories of past threats and overcorrecting juuuuuuust in case something might be dangerous. Hence, the prevalence of trauma-informed responses and fuckery galore.

In this chapter, we're going to take some extremely fancy science and boil it down into something a normal-but-nerdy-enough-to-be-reading-this human can understand. If you can understand these ideas, then you'll have the key to understand so much about how our bodies and brains work, how they get fucked up, and how they can heal.

Is the Vagus Nerve a New Idea?

First, a little bit of history. Because vagus theory is seen as cutting edge in the scientific community right now, but it goes back thousands of years.

We've known forever that there is a governing mechanism that delivers information throughout the body to include the brain. The oldest records we have of a singular, governing bodily system are from the Mawangdui (206 BC to 9 AD) and Zhangjiashan (196 to 186 BC) tombs of the Han-era Changsha Kingdom. These texts describe 11 pathways that carry the same names as the acupuncture meridians described in later works. The idea is that these meridians are pathways through the body in which our vital energy (Qi) circulates. They are still widely used today in Traditional Chinese Medicine to treat a wide array of ailments, physical and mental.

The idea of a singular, governing system within the body wasn't missing from Western culture, either. In 1543, Flemish anatomist and physician Andreas Vesalius, the "father of modern physiology," wrote and illustrated a seven-book series called On the Fabric of the Human Body that included amazingly detailed drawings of the nervous system showing a mind-body connection similar to what Chinese physicians had long been aware of.

Back in 1872, Darwin wrote specifically about the expression of emotions, noting the bi-directional neural relationship between the brain and the heart. But the founders of modern psychology and mental health treatment must not have read this, or they must've done the thing scientists have been doing since the beginning of sciencing—ignoring anything that didn't fit their paradigm.

What did fit this new, modern research paradigm? The work of British physiologist John Newport Langley, who wrote the "definitive" guide to human physiology in 1921 (still in the middle of the emerging field of psychology) which shifted the whole focus of physiology away from the idea that our brains and bodies are in constant communication back and forth with each other. Modern medicine was the future, therefore studying how X pill affects Y organ became the standard practice.

It wasn't until the 1990s that a research scientist named Stephen Porges started studying the autonomic regulation of preterm infants, which led to a serious reexamining of how our bodies affect our brains and vice versa throughout our lifespan through the central organizational structure of the brain-body connection.

How Does the Vagal System Work?

The vagus nerve is the information highway between the emotional-cognitive centers of the brain and the body, including our intestinal functions.

Right off the bat, one of the most important things to know about the vagus nerve is that it swings both ways (heh): It carries information and activates response both from the brain to the body and from the body to the brain. We like to think of the brain as being in charge, but we have four times more messages going up to the brain rather than down from the brain—80% are body-to-brain (afferent messaging), and only 20% are brain to body (efferent messaging).

Junior high science flashback: Nerves are cells that have special communication functions. Like telephone lines that run all over your body, they communicate throughout the body as bioelectrical signals. Like, what happens if you touch a hot thing? The nerves in your hand send a message of "FUCKING OW!" to your brain, which then sends a message back saying: "WELL PUT IT THE FUCK DOWN THEN! THAT'S THE LITERAL MEANING OF DROP IT LIKE ITS HOT!!!"

Nerves exist throughout our body and serve to transmit electrical impulses for intra-body communication. Our sensory and motor functions in the body are specifically tasked to 12 cranial nerves. Some of these cranial nerves are super specific. Like the olfactory nerve, unsurprisingly transmits information about what we smell to our brain. But number 10 of 12, the vagus nerve, is the longest, weirdest, and most complex of the twelve pairs of cranial nerves. The name itself (vagus) comes from the Latin word for "wandering" because this nerve wanders all around the damn body, sending information to organs and tissues. It wouldn't be irrational to say that this particular nerve is an information superhighway.

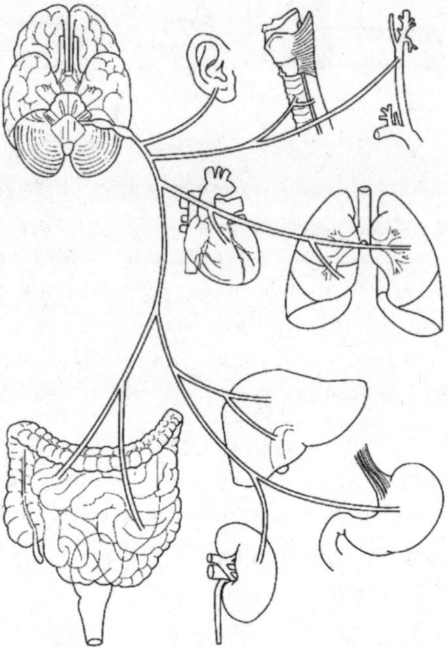

This? The Fancy Fucking Diagram of the Vagus Nerve. So You Can See How the Brain Communicates with Every Major Organ in Your Body. No Pressure to Remain Calm Then, Right?

Nerve cells don't just bop around aimlessly like your useless ex. They are organized into systems. Nervous systems are the networks of the nerve cells and fibers that transmit messages. These systems make the messages transmit more efficiently. So that you will, indeed, drop it like it's hot when need be.

Now while the vagus nerve is the messenger for an entire nervous system, it is only one of several nervous systems that create the entire human nervous system. So, the humazn nervous system can be broken up into the central nervous system (brain and spine) and the peripheral nervous system which connects the brain and spine to the rest of the body. The peripheral nervous system can be split again into two parts:

- The somatic nervous system, which we have voluntary control over
- The autonomic nervous system which is the part that we do not have voluntary control over, which regulates all of our organs and endeavors to maintain bodily homeostasis

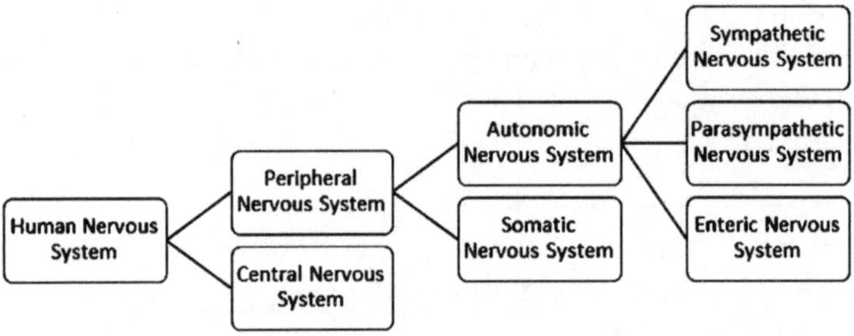

Bodies. So complex and so absurdly simple at the same time. Am I right?

The autonomic system is the one we are focusing on in this book. All autonomic means is self-governing. These nerves work involuntarily and are not under conscious control. So you are not allowed at any time to decide whether or not you are going to drop the hot thing. That's the kind of shit that will get you killed. Your body is not interested in negotiation, shit's just getting dropped. You're starting to feel me on why this is important info, yeah?

The autonomic nervous system has three components: the sympathetic, parasympathetic, and enteric nervous systems. And the vagus nerve is their communication pathway. It's important to understand how they work in relation to each other.

The sympathetic nervous system governs our fight-flight-freeze instinct, which is critical to our survival. It is activated in the face of a threat or perceived threat, whether it be to our actual, physical safety, the individuals we love and care for, our possessions, or our needs, wants, desires, well-being, and belief systems. Essentially, anything that challenges the core of who and what we are and who or what belongs to us invokes a protective response. It has nothing to do with how mentally or physically strong we are or how much we love the person or people that we are with. That ability to be engaged and connected goes offline.

If we perceive aggression as a means of escape, we will fight. If our instincts tell us we can't fight effectively but we can escape, we will flee. If neither of these responses are likely going to be effective, we will freeze.

All of these strategies, even fighting, are purely defensive ones. The intent is not to win against or overwhelm the threat, but to survive. The body's job is to size up the situation and figure out the best means of staying alive. It chooses a strategy based on the information it is receiving and past understanding of the threat. We may move back and forth between strategies as we take in information and gauge our effectiveness at managing the perceived imminent threat. All three responses are part of our defensive, survival instincts.

I'm focusing so much on the freeze response (official science-y term: dorsal-vagal response) because it's talked about the least. And it's the one that most human beings are embarrassed about, although it makes just as much sense as a protective strategy as fight and flight do. It's also the most physically dangerous: the freeze response can actually kill you if it goes on too intensely, too long.

So why does the body do something so dangerous? Peter Levine (until Porges, he was one of the few theorists to talk about the body's survival mechanism and trauma) states that there are four potential evolutionary survival benefits to the freeze response:

- Most predatory animals won't eat an animal they believe is already dead unless they are really hungry. Most animals have encoded information that meat that is already dead may be spoiled and therefore is a risk to eat.
- It is more difficult for predators to detect prey that is not moving. Immobilization shuts down all movement responses. Even if we are trying to be still and quiet it is difficult to do so unless we have become biochemically immobilized.
- When one animal collapses in a group, this distracts the predator from the rest of the group, allowing their escape.
- The freeze response releases a numbing agent in the body that makes the pain of attack more bearable.

Now obviously, it makes sense that the sympathetic nervous system should not be in charge all the time. It would make us fall apart at the seams pretty quickly (and this is why people who don't have conscious ways to cope with chronic stress do fall apart at the seams pretty quickly).

Our second nervous system, the parasympathetic nervous system, is the one associated with social relationships and bonding. We're pack animals. We need to connect to other human beings for long-term survival, not just for mating season, and be able to navigate the world without feeling batshit crazy and threatened by our surroundings all the time. Being relaxed and alert is how we best engage with the world around us. This means that when the parasympathetic system is in charge, we are able to connect and communicate and form social relationships because we feel safe to do so.

The foundation of Porges' research on the vagal system is the finding that our nervous systems work in ranked order (a hierarchy). Safety and connection and relationships—the functions governed by the autonomic nervous systems—rank highest on the hierarchy. But because these processes are managed outside of conscious thought, our ability to remain calm and engaged and relational is the first thing we lose when our bodies perceive threat. In order to be our best selves, to live and work in cooperation and build relationships, our bodies have to perceive us as being safe.

But when something challenges our sense of safety at a bodily level, the parasympathetic system goes offline. This works because the sympathetic nervous system is myelinated, while the parasympathetic nervous system is not. I know, I know with the science textbook words, but this is actually an important point. Myelination provides insulation, which speeds up the sending of the messages. So the nervous system that is in charge of our stress response works faster than the one that is in charge of our chill response.

Both systems operate involuntarily. And the sympathetic nervous system has to be turned off for the parasympathetic nervous system to work, meaning it has to determine that there is no stress or threat and that you are allowed to go about your day. But even when it's not running the show, the sympathetic nervous system is still humming in the background, watching for danger. And it works faster than the chill system, so it will shut shit down on a moment's notice.

Any of us with unresolved trauma histories are far more likely to have our parasympathetic systems go offline, putting us into survival mode. We'll get more into this in the trauma chapter coming up soon.

The stomach is called the second brain for a reason. The third part of the autonomic nervous system is the enteric nervous system, which resides in the gastrointestinal tract and is the largest of the three autonomic nervous systems and has its own unique microcircuits. It receives feedback from the other two systems but is also able to operate independently of them. There are people out there with severed vagus nerves and their enteric nervous systems work just fine. This is some zombie science shit.

Because many neurotransmitters, signaling pathways, and anatomical properties are common to the enteric nervous system and the central nervous system, it's safe to say that the vagus nerve is actually messaging our "gut feelings" to the brain.

And those gut feelings are loud. Our internal bodily state is communicating continuously with the brain far more than the brain is communicating back with the body (4 to 1, remember?). The brain is dependent on the physiology of the body to manage our breathing, our heart rate, whether or not we are hungry or full, and the nervous system activity related to our emotional states. This isn't something we think about (pun intended), which is why Dr. Candace Pert, the neuroscientist who first became known as the person who discovered the opiate receptor in the brain as a freakin' undergrad, stated that the entirety of the human body operates as the unconscious mind.

If the vagal system is the body's information superhighway, how exactly does that relate to stuff like being scared, activated, or experiencing a trauma trigger? We know that memories of past events are stored in the amygdala, but how exactly is that memory file being pulled up? Is it just within the brain or is it also in the body?

Dr. Pert's research described and explained how human moods, feelings and emotions are mediated and experienced through peptides. Peptides are made up of amino-acids (the organic compounds that combine to form proteins in the body) but can be best thought of as information substances because their common function in any form is to distribute information throughout the body.

Yes, there is a high concentration of peptide receptors in the amygdala. But there are also high concentrations of them at the back of the spinal cord (vagus!) and any place in the body where information about the five senses enter the body (vagus vagus vagus!). Peptides are what activate the vagal system in order to send and receive messaging. Our body-mind is using peptide cues to choose or discard both emotions and behaviors. And the vagal system is the mechanism for how the information travels.

This is how, as Dr. Pert put it, traumatic emotional events put down deep roots in the body, not just as episodic-autobiographical memories. She noted that "while we may not remember something consciously, the psychosomatic network in the body does."

And that, smart cookie, is exactly why we're talking about this in so much scientific depth. Your feelings are real. It's not a made-up discomfort, it's biochemical and bioelectrical messaging happening between your body and mind on a constant basis. And the system is wired to err on the side of caution to keep you safe. So if you have been through some deep shit, your whole body becomes wired with a hair-trigger invader detection system. That doesn't mean healing is impossible. It's completely fucking possible and I see people do it every day, which is why I love my job so much. But we have to understand what healing entails for the entirety of the body, how to change our relationship with past events in our lives, and how to move forward as healing survivors.

Recognizing Your Personal Vagal Responses

Ok, so there was a lot of blahblahblah about scienceblahscience. We're about to get into a whole lot of the ways your vagal system can get fucked up, but before we do that let's start putting this knowledge into practice so you can recognize what's going on in your own body.

You're going to see the lolwut-inducing term vagal tone quite often throughout this book. So just to let you know now, that really just refers to the activity of the vagus nerve. Its ability to communicate quickly and effectively. The better its ability to communicate, the healthier we are both physically and mentally. The word tone comes from how the effectiveness of vagal communication is measured in terms of heart rate variability, which is interesting (to me) and super-techy and not important to this discussion (for everyone else).

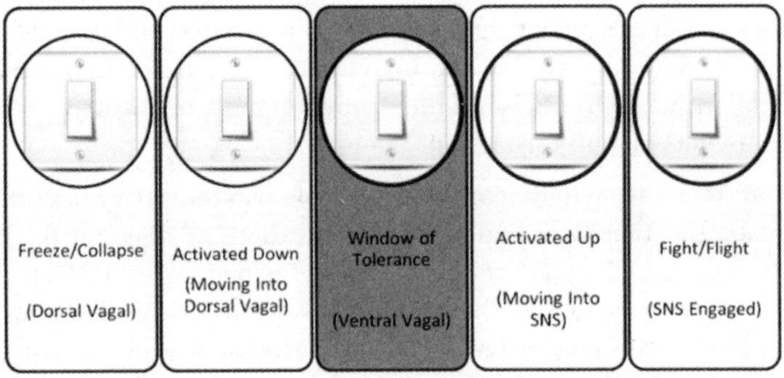

Our body's vagal response has an array of "options." Visualize a series of light switches, with "safe" in the middle and "too low" on one end and "too high" on the other, and a couple of switches in between for when you're moving down or up.

Remember how I said fight, flight, and freeze are all survival instincts, and your body is going to read the room and choose the physiological response that makes the most sense? Porges's work visualizes the response options as existing on a ladder, which presumes that we enter and exit certain states in a certain order. I've found this personally confusing and instead visualize a series of flip-switch options rather than a spectrum.

Depending on the level of threat detected and previous experiences, the body will flip one switch rather than another which is why you can go from fight/flight to complete collapse so quickly. The body has to make snap decisions. I have worked with people who only freeze up, others who only fight, and people who run the gamut. Remember how I mentioned earlier it's about what the body recognizes is its best bet for survival or pain management?

On the "too low" end of the spectrum, you have the freeze/collapse response switch, scientifically known as the Dorsal Vagal response. On either end is the sympathetic nervous system switch. On the "too high" end, you've got your fight and flight responses, or as we call it "SNS Engaged". In the safe center, you have your window of tolerance switch, where your vagus nerve sees no threat and your parasympathetic nervous system is engaged. That's your baby bear just right switch. Like any spectrum, there are shades in between—you can be activated down into dorsal vagal or moving up into SNS and notice that and bring yourself back into your window of tolerance if you need to. That's what we'll be working on here.

Our goal is to stay within our window of tolerance, and learn to expand our window of tolerance as much as possible. In a perfect world, we would become activated enough to deal with potentially threatening situations, but we wouldn't become SNS Engaged or Dorsal Vagal unless we were under a real attack, right? But a trauma response trains our bodies to presume attack based on the traumas we experienced. So it may not be real in an external world sense, but is very real to our internal world.

Window of Tolerance

In our our window of tolerance state (ventral vagal), our muscles are relaxed, our breathing is easy, our heart rate is resting, our blood pressure is normal, our skin is our "normal" rosy hue (which is obvs different for everyone, but there is blood flow to the skin enough to give us some color), our pupils are normal sized, our eyelids are relaxed, and our digestion is functioning. Our eyes and mouth are moist and our skin is dry. We can differentiate individual sounds from background noise (the muscles of our middle ear have tone). Emotionally we are calm. We can feel love and pleasure. More complex emotions are bearable (e.g, we can be sad or frustrated but process through the experience with a sense of it being manageable). Our prefrontal cortex (thinking brain) is engaged. We are able to connect with self and others, and feel integrated within our own bodies. Our parasympathetic nervous system is in charge and it's doing a great job.

Think about:

- What signs tell you that you are in your window of tolerance?

- What activities, coping skills, and behaviors help you remain in your window of tolerance? Which can you do for yourself? Which do you need support from others to do? Who are your go-to support people?

Fight / Flight

As we start getting into the the danger zone heading toward fight or flight (with our sympathetic nervous system activated), our muscles become more tense, our breathing gets faster and comes more from our upper chest (hyperventilation), our heart rate and blood pressure go up, our skin gets paler (under whatever level of melenation we have) because blood is rushing to our muscles away from the skin, our pupils become dilated, our eyelids get tense, and our digestion halts (this is why the dorsal vagal is called fight/flight and ventral vagal is referred to as rest/digest). Our eyes and mouth start to become dry while our skin starts to get sweaty (though it may be a cold sweat). Sounds become overwhelming, and it becomes harder to pick out individual voices (we lose tone in the muscles in our middle ear to make it easier to pick out low frequency predator sounds). Emotionally, we start to feel angry or fearful and our ability to connect with others becomes increasingly limited and eventually almost nonexistent. Concomitantly, our thinking brain goes increasingly offline and we find it more and more difficult to connect to our own bodies.

Think about:

- What signs tell you that you are in fight or flight mode?
- What helps you move out of this response and back into your window of tolerance? Which can you do for yourself? Which do you need support from others to do? Who are your go-to support people?

Freeze / Collapse

As we move into the shutdown state of freeze mode (dorsal vagal activated), our muscles become rigid instead of tense, and we will move from hyperventilation (getting too much oxygen) into hypoventilation. Our breathing and heart rate can bottom out to very slow (bradycardiac). Our blood pressure will also get very high and then bottom out. Our skin will often become even paler, our pupils get very small, our eyelids will start to move from very tense to either completely closed or stuck open. Our eyes and mouth will get very dry and our skin may go from extremes of hot to cold, though will eventually become very cold if we continue in this state. All auditory stimuli can become loud and overwhelming and we may shut all sound out completely because of it. Emotionally, we may feel terror or complete dissociation. Our thinking brain moves into being inaccessible, and connection with others and our own bodies moves to being impossible.

> NOTE: Once you are in hypofreeze (bradycardia) this is now a medical emergency, and emergency medical care is required. You've probably heard about seeking medical attention if someone is "in shock" and that's exactly what's going on here.

Think about:

- What signs tell you that you are in freeze mode?
- What helps you move out of this response and back into your window of tolerance? Which can you do for yourself? Which do you need support from others to do? Who are your go-to support people?

In Section Three of this book, we'll have a ton of exercises aimed at recognizing that your body is reaching for a particular switch, when it's been flipped and how to work with that state, and how to expand our personal windows of tolerance. But first, let's go into some of the reasons our vagal system regularly goes wonky to begin with.

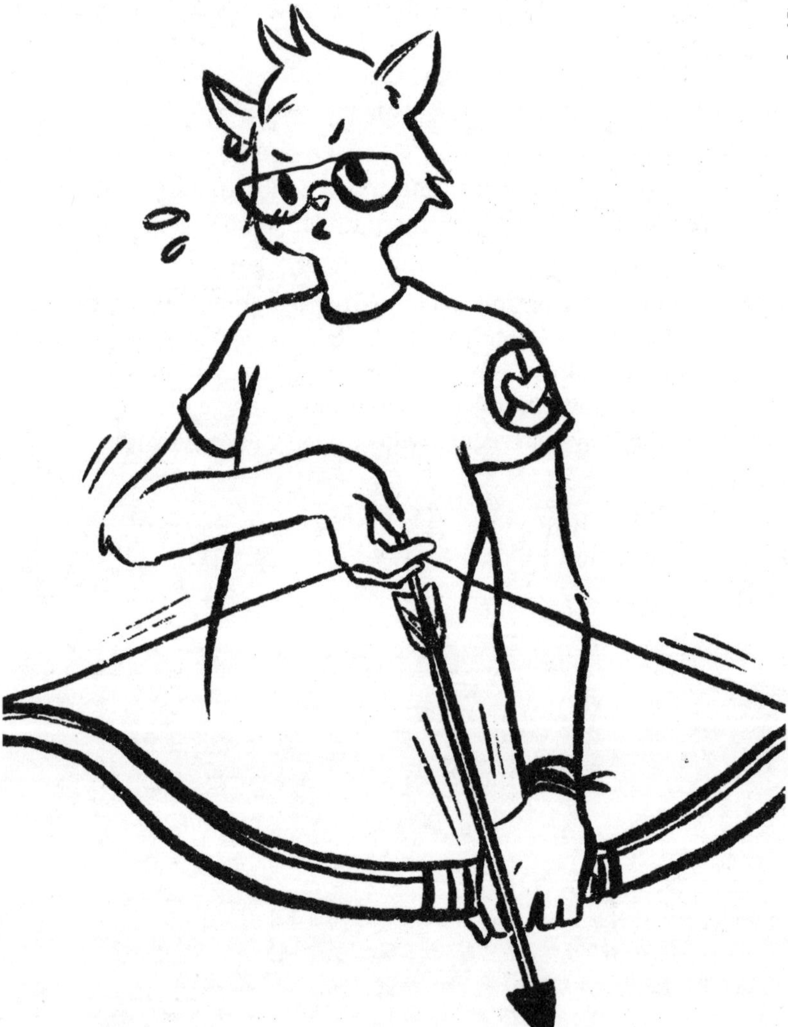

HOW DO BODIES GET FUCKED UP AND WHAT DOES MENTAL HEALTH HAVE TO DO WITH IT?

I think everyone feels that their body is enemy territory. We feel a sense of frustration and even failure at our inability to "be healthy," by whatever health standard has been established in that regard. And while there is a lot of information out there on how to "be healthy" so much of it is contradictory and extreme and unhelpful. And it rarely takes into account how much our bodies are taking in that is really out of our control.

The reason I carry such a big purse all the time is that I have a multitude of soapboxes I insist on dragging along with me. One of the biggest of the boxes involves all the systemic ways humans struggle with physical and mental health issues that have little or nothing to do with their personal choices.

Yes, I know. Mainstream media will insist otherwise. As will a lot of medical and health practitioners. Or programs trying to sell you a new smoothie as a quick fix. When reality is so fucking complicated that everything I am about to cover is only the tip of the iceberg.

But first things first. I want you to take a couple of pieces of scrap paper and write "because fat" on one and "because lazy" on another. Now crumple them up and throw them away. Or stomp them. Or set them on fire (but safely, of course).

Because bullshit.

While dietary changes and movement can help us combat the systemic problems I'm about to throw down about, oversimplification and victim blaming have no place here. I am so over that bullshit and I hope you're with me.

Now, we all know our food system is crap. And the crappier it is, the more it is subsidized. The Standard American Diet is SAD for a reason. And if you are poor? You are so truly, deeply fucked within the current system, I don't have a purse or a soapbox big enough to even begin to get started. But this is stuff we all know, and I want to go even deeper than "genetically modified soybeans, amiright?" because it's bigger than all that and the solution-generating depends on understanding it.

But before we start getting granular with doable solutions, let's get into the physical mechanisms that are causing body fuckery to begin with. The biggest culprits? Trauma (surprise!), inflammation, environmental toxicity, and our relationship with stress.

Trauma

Short answer: It's trauma. It's always the fucking trauma. Trauma is something I write about a lot—it's the whole point of these books.

When we talk about our five senses, we talk about how we use them to organize information from the outside world, but rarely do we use them to register what is going on inside of us. In reality, we are receiving internal sensory information on a constant basis but are rarely connected to that experience simply because that's how bodies are supposed to act. All of it. Walking, talking, breathing, avoiding a crack in the concrete that we could trip over, recognizing that the milk is spoiled as soon as we open the container and not drinking it. It would take too much of our physical and mental effort to do all of these things consciously and continuously. These behaviors have to be automatic for our survival.

Any living animal will respond to changes in light and shadow. From amoebas to Homo sapiens, we perceive a threat and duck. The difference between us and amoebas is that we can (at least on a good day), become aware of our instincts and challenge the efficacy of our ducking patterns. This means being more aware of the interplay between our external and internal sense messages. And learning to tolerate our duck response without needing to always duck.

We need this duck response to survive. But sometimes the wiring goes wonky. You know. Our body and mind are over-eager and over-protective and start sending haywire messages that are overanalyzing current experiences and anticipating dangerous and damaging future experiences based on our past experiences.

That's the very definition of a trauma response.

And sometimes the duck response gets stuck on. And when it sticks around for the long term, we call it PTSD, which is a fear response that gets switched on but never gets switched off.

You can read all about trauma and PTSD in Unfuck Your Brain. In this book, we're going to focus more in depth on how they affect the body.

Of course, trauma affects our health at all stages of life, but childhood trauma is more likely to change our epigenetic structure, according to a 2014 Yale University study. The world is unsafe from the get-go, and when things happen to us as kids—either one big event or a lot of bad things—our stress response gets set to high alert, which can persist through our adult life if left untreated.

One term being thrown around on the regular now to account for the impact of childhood trauma on our bodies is "ACEs." An ACE is an "adverse childhood event" which is a fancy way of saying childhood trauma. The Center for Disease Control and Kaiser Permanente conducted one of the largest research studies on the impact of ACEs on health and well-being over the lifespan, and developed a questionnaire which is widely used for determining how much childhood trauma might be a part of your life now.

The ACE questions are looking for information about your life prior to your 18th birthday, specifically regarding abuse, neglect, and what are termed household challenges. Abuse questions ask about physical, emotional, and sexual abuse. Neglect questions focus on physical and emotional neglect. And the household challenges include having family members with a mental illness and/or substance dependence, having family members incarcerated, witnessing interpersonal violence, or witnessing separation and/or divorce.[2]

Researchers have linked ACEs to the onset of chronic conditions and early death in adulthood. The more ACEs that occur, the more an individual is at risk for negative health outcomes. If you experienced an ACE (just one!), you are twice as likely to suffer depression. And also twice as likely to suffer cancer, heart disease, and diabetes.

Studies have also shown that ACEs mean you are far more likely to suffer with migraines and irritable bowel disease, as well. Women who'd faced three types of childhood adversity had a sixty percent greater risk of being hospitalized with an autoimmune disease as an adult. Suffering six categories of early life stress shortened one's lifespan by twenty years. ACEs are also tied to the adoption of health-risk behaviors (smoking, not exercising, eating gummy worms instead of broccoli, etc.).

So the CDC looked at the data and came up with a fancy explanation for the data. They created a graphic[3] that endeavored to explain the relationship of ACEs to the physical and mental health issues that we see co-occurring with them. It shows a pyramid with ACEs at the base, and then several levels building on each other, starting with social,

---

2 The ACEs assessment is easily found online, and free to use (just not free to republish in a book so I didn't). The original assessment uses more gendered language (did you witness your dad beat up your mom), so I prefer the state of California ACEs Aware version, which uses more general terminology about parents, guardians, and partners. Additionally, their website has free training you can enroll in, which actually does go into epigenetic changes, how emotional trauma impacts the physical body and the like. It's the only ACE materials that I have seen discussing that information (besides my own), team science!

3 Since it's a government graph it's public domain so I can reproduce it just to yell about it. Woohoo!

emotional, and cognitive impairment, leading to the adoption of health-risk behaviors, which produce disease, disability, and social problems, all culminating in early death.

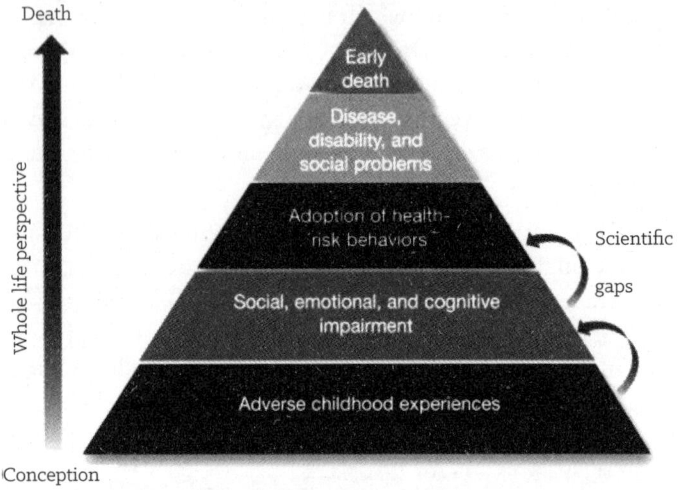

I call bullshit.

This model leans heavily on the trope that trauma fucks us up so we don't take care of ourselves. The implication is that we are fat and lazy (and whatever else), which is making us sick. Because of trauma, sure, but it is still very victim-blaming.

This graphic refers to research gaps that seem to show that science doesn't know how ACEs lead to impairment or how that leads to risky behaviors. This is bullshit too. By the time the CDC published this graphic in 2014, there were already plenty of studies to explain what was going on and there are even more studies backing up the understanding that trauma alters the immune system and metabolic system and these changes persist over time, increasing our chances of developing disease. Everything that we will discuss in this book in terms of upregulated inflammation and vagus system messaging can also be ACE-activated.

The body does not differentiate how it responds to physical and emotional trauma. We already recognize that if we are in a car accident, and our chest hits the steering wheel, that causes pain and inflammation, and that injury can lead to more health problems down the road. And now it is time to recognize that growing up in a household where you didn't feel safe and loved and secure causes the same pain and inflammation.

That's a little heavy, I know. When I teach this class, people generally need a minute to breathe.

What we also need to know, though, is that just like we can treat physical injuries and recover from them, emotional injuries aren't our destiny either.

Inflammation

Inflammation is another one of those buzzwords that you hear all the time and to be fair, nutritionists looooove to blame inflammation for everything, sorry about that. We have this idea that inflammation is inherently bad and is to be avoided. In reality, inflammation is just as important and life saving as our fight/flight/freeze responses. Inflammation is the result of our bodies fighting off infection and external invaders like viruses and bacteria. This fighting-off battle is mediated substantially by chemicals in our body called cytokines that signal our white blood cell count to rise and the like. And? That inflammatory reflex response in the body? Is mediated by the vagus nerve.

As with the vagal system, the body remembers past threats and can stay upregulated long past when you need to fend off attackers. Cytokine production can get stuck on, resulting in chronic inflammation. Chronic inflammation leads to tissue damage, disease susceptibility, and autoimmune issues. The World Health Organization recognizes that chronic inflammatory diseases are the most significant cause of death in the world.

Inflammation can result not just from physical injury, but psychological injury—like trauma. And chronic inflammation leads to this higher risk of diseases. High rates of inflammation are found not just in individuals with heart disease and cancer and autoimmune disorders, they are found in individuals with diagnoses of PTSD, OCD, depression, and anxiety disorders. According to a 2012 study in Biology, biomarkers for inflammation are higher in individuals who have experienced adverse events.

So, I'm gonna say this again because this is one of those "thesis statement" ideas that I want to stick with you even if you don't remember fuck-all about the rest of this book. The body responds to physical trauma with inflammation, right? If you smash your thumb with a hammer (by accident, not a suggested experiment or anything) it hurts like a motherfucker and it becomes inflamed to protect the area while it is healing. The body also responds to emotional trauma with inflammation. The body doesn't differentiate where the injury is coming from or the type of injury it is. Inflammation is part of the body's healing mechanism and it responds to physical and emotional injuries in the same way. We need this response in order to be able to rest and recover after an injury.

Another important thing to know is that this response majorly slows us down. If the body recognizes itself as injured—physically or psychologically—its first line of defense to ensure healing is to conserve energy for the healing process. In order to make sure that that energy is available, it reduces our natural drive to perform other tasks, even simple stuff like taking a shower and brushing our teeth, because task performance takes energy.

In fact a study from Emory University found that inflammation doesn't just make us tired and sore, it directly reduces the dopaminergic signaling system in the brain, which assists us with a multitude of tasks including spatial working memory, cognition in general, motor function and other shit humans need . . . and is a necessary part of having the energy and motivation to do shit. Fancy terminology? The body engages in an immune-mediated disruption of the dopamine pathways using inflammation as a mechanism to decrease dopamine production.

How would the world be different if we recognized that inflammation is stripping away our ability to "function normally?"

Our microbiome (that's our bodies' internal soup of bacteria, fungi, and viruses, both helpful and harmful) changes constantly throughout life based on our exposures. These exposures include toxins (that's the next chapter), foods (which can operate like toxins), and our stress hormone cascade (which is a whole complicated process in and of itself and therefore has its own upcoming chapter, exciting right?).

Inflammation problems often start in the gut and/or are reinforced in the gut, allowing them to run rampant through the body. It's like having a wound on the inside and every time we eat or drink (and we kinda have to in order to do the staying alive thing) we are poking at the wound.

Our gut is full of organisms. Most of them are not trying to kill us, but live with us happily, keeping us healthy. The mechanism in play here is that the chronic activation of our stress response (traumatic events, adverse childhood events, fucked up shit happening on the regular, call it what you will) is fucking up the balance of these bacteria (as are toxins, don't forget the toxins!). More and more research is focusing on the gut microbiome of individuals with childhood trauma (the ACEs again) or PTSD and finding that they have significantly lower levels of Actinobacteria, Lentisphaerae and Verrucomicrobia. Coprococcus and Dialister (all good bugs for the tummy) have been found to be consistently depleted in individuals struggling with depression, whether or not they were undergoing treatment.

Imbalances in our gut bacteria can lead to damage of the lining of the gut. The fancy term for this process is leaky gut (Finally! An easy one to remember!) because gut lining damage means that toxins, bacteria, food particles, etc, can leak through the intestinal walls into the bloodstream. Then the body says "Wait, what? Invader!" and launches an attack (immune system response) which perpetuates the cycle of inflammation.

Inflammation spreads like wildfire once the on switch becomes stuck (the molecular switch for chronic inflammation is a cluster of immune proteins called the NLRP3 inflammasome that was just isolated in a laboratory in 2020 by scientists), and it lights up through multiple pathways in the body, using the vagus nerve as its superhighway.

More and more research is demonstrating that inflammation is a trigger for many mental health and physical health diagnoses. When we recognize that, we can perceive healing in a different light. Integrative medicine expert Dr. Mark Hyman views disease as having processes, not causes. When I wrote Unfuck Your Brain, the whole point was to explain "if this is how our brain is wired to process, we need to change how we approach healing in order to be effective." And we need to approach the body-mind in the same way.

How Inflammation Affects our Mental Health

So how does inflammation affect our emotions? We already talked about how our enteric nervous system comes into play, and how our gut bacteria can give us feelings. But a lot of mental health problems start in the body before they end up tearing up shit in our brains.

The brain and spinal column have their own, unique immune system (the neuroimmune system). Until recently, researchers assumed that inflammation of the brain (neuroinflammation) was pretty rare, because there's a wall of cells, called the blood-brain barrier, between the neuroimmune system and the rest of the body's immune system.

But we are now finding increasing evidence that neuroinflammation may be as common as cornbread (that's not a real expression, I just made it up, pass it on). When inflammation stays upregulated (turned on for long periods of time) and crosses the blood-brain barrier, we can get a ton of mental health problems, including depression, by the looks of it.

Let's back up and look at how the neuroimmune system works. It's managed by these tiny brain cells called microglia. Microglia make up about 10% of the brain and serve various protective functions depending on the part of the nervous system they are in. One of the things they do to protect our brain is secrete cytokines (inflammatory chemicals) when they detect a threat. The swelling caused by the cytokines serves as a buffer while the microglia attack and destroy whatever crosses the blood-brain barrier.

Scientists are now finding increasing evidence that microglia can remain upregulated even when the original invader is no longer present (just like the inflammation process in the rest of the body) . . . and, at that point, are no longer serving their reparative function. For example, researchers have found that individuals who engaged in binge drinking as teenagers, had upregulated microglia far into adulthood even when they were no longer binge drinking. In another recent study, researchers found that many individuals who suffered an ACL tear (a pretty horrific tear of a ligament in the knee that is caused by a torquing motion, which is why you see it in athletes a lot) also suffered neuroinflammation afterward. And those with that higher level of upregulated microglia after the tear had slower bodily recovery and were more likely to reinjure their ACL.

Does this mean every injury can cause a neuroimmune response? And if you are klutzy as I am, are you entirely fucked for time eternal? Scientists don't know enough to answer that question with precision. But it happens often enough that we need to be aware that it is a possibility that could be impacting our continued physical health as well as our mental health.

One of the most studied impacts of inflammation on our mental health (and an example of how complicated it can be) is depression.

The brain is the least understood organ in the body, which means that we have a lot of theories about depression and a good number of the puzzle pieces, but we haven't fit everything together yet. For a half a century, the idea was (and depending on who you ask, sometimes still is) that low serotonin causes depression. This is what antidepressants were created to address, and why their effectiveness varies wildly. Research that endeavors to monitor the influence of serotonin typically leaves us with more questions. When the metabolization of serotonin was studied in human spinal fluid back in the 70s, there was no difference in the levels between depressed and non-depressed individuals. And just in 2019, scientists removed the stuff in the brains of mice that produces serotonin, thinking they would exhibit signs of depression when they did so, but they continued micing along as normal.

Does serotonin play some role in depression? Of course it does. In my book This Is Your Brain On Depression, I wrote about how serotonin transmits messages between nerve cells, and therefore has a role in the coordinated function of the nervous system. When you're depressed, something gets janky in that process, but we don't really know what. Low serotonin may create depression, or depression may be creating low serotonin. Either way, inflammation seems to be a likely stakeholder in the process.

While lower levels of serotonin are correlated with depression, researchers are realizing that the causality is not cut and dry. Serotonin is a chemical that is found throughout the body. In fact most of it is found in the gastrointestinal tract, ninety percent of it, in fact, produced by the enterochromaffin (EC) cells that line the digestive tract. Some research shows that taking an antidepressant creates more serotonin in the stomach, not in the brain directly. Which isn't necessarily bad. A study done on mice found that when the gut-brain connection is severed (this is the vagus nerve), the antidepressants also stopped working, leading to the theory that serotonin is gut-produced and the vagus nerve is the mechanism of travel up to the brain.

To get a different perspective on how depression digs its claws into us, let's start with where inflammation itself starts, in the body. Those same EC cells that make serotonin in the lining of the gut also relay information to the rest of the body and brain about our diet, our microbes, and possible inflammatory factors. Like, "dumbass is eating hot cheetos again even though we've warned her a thousand times, release the kraken!" These EC cells serve to activate responses within the gut-brain axis and they influence a batrillion important parts of our physiology: cognition, metabolism, you name it.

There was a great scientific journal article published a couple of years ago called "The Bowel and Beyond" (I knoooooooow, this is what I read for y'all!) in which the authors stated something that many of us have intuited for a very long time: that if we recognize that the gut-brain connection has a significant impact on keeping us healthy, it also must have a significant impact on how and why we become ill. This begs the question: the "social, emotional, and cognitive impairment" that the CDC likes to remind us is a result of childhood trauma—that sounds a lot like depression, doesn't it? And that loss of energy to complete tasks? Is depression a product of inflammation? Is depression actually a body illness rather than a mind illness? And is the body trying to protect us from further pain by slowing us down?

This is deep mind-body connection shit that we are just beginning to wrap our science brains around. But we know that inflammation causes "sickness behavior" in that it slows us down to create opportunities for healing. And we know that neuroinflammation increases the chances of nerve cells dying and not regenerating. And we can see a decrease in the effectiveness of the brain's ability to communicate (which happens in part through serotonin, which is a neurotransmitter).

There is far too much data out there to stick with the classic model of "take an SSRI and the magic happens," especially when research shows that antidepressant medications are not effective for many, many people. This isn't me dissing antidepressants. I know they have been life-saving for many people, and if you are one of them then that's awesome. But because they aren't helpful for everyone, we need to step up our treatment strategy game, right? We want to keep everyone on Team Alive and Happy. And adding immuno-psychiatry (to borrow

Oxford psychiatrist Edward Bullmore's term) to our range of treatment options increases our chances of finding effective treatment strategies for people, especially the people who haven't benefited from traditional antidepressants.

Inflammation and Chronic Pain

According to an NIH study in 2012, 11% of U.S. Americans (over 25 million people) reported having some form of pain every day for at least three months in a row. That's a lot of people suffering all the fucking time because we are struggling to find treatment options that bring relief. These numbers are also super relevant to everything I wrote about the mind-body connection. We know that pain and depression share the same neurophysiology, meaning the parts of the brain that are involved in perceiving pain also affect mood. So while being in constant pain is reason enough to experience depression, it's more insidious than that; they actually end up together more often than not, like peanut butter and jelly.

There are two types of pain that we're going to be talking about here, nociceptive and neuropathic.

Nociceptive pain requires a physical interaction or a physical stressor, like a sports injury, a papercut, or chronic muscle tension due to how we sit at work. This is the sort of pain that shows your body is working correctly, giving you information about an injury. But if you've been following along, you'll notice that a lot of the body's signals can get stuck on.

Neuropathic pain doesn't always have a physical component. This could be when the nervous system keeps sending pain signals to the brain after the physical injury has healed, or as a result of conditions that don't have an external physical injury component (like diabetes, cancer, multiple sclerosis). Lots of things can set off a neuropathic pain response, like being reminded of your injury, being inactive, your immune system being activated, or even changes in temperature.

While there are numerous neuropathic chronic pain conditions, the one that is finally being taken more seriously and studied more intensively is myalgic encephalomyelitis (ME), also known as chronic fatigue syndrome (CFS), which is characterized by extreme fatigue, joint pain, dizziness, and difficulty with memory and focus, among other symptoms that go on for months and months. I'm going to talk specifically about ME here, because research in this area has led to huge breakthroughs on where it comes from and new ideas on how to treat all types of chronic pain.

So where do ME and other neuropathic diseases come from? The Mayo Clinic defines ME as "a complicated disorder that can't be explained by any underlying medical condition." First of all, um, thanks? This lack of definitional clarity (and the presumption that it's all psychosomatic) is a big contributor to the reason that while there are an estimated two million U.S. Americans with ME, 90% of them have not been diagnosed.

ME affects twice as many women as men.[4] It's most common among people over the age of 40 and doesn't seem to favor individuals of certain races or socioeconomic status. Because of the physical and psychological distress associated with ME, there are much higher rates of unemployment among people with the diagnosis, meaning that this disease alone is causing an economic loss of 9 billion dollars per year in productivity. Not that our human worth has anything to do with our productivity but damn you'd think this would make treatment a higher priority for the overlords of capitalism.

ME was originally termed chronic fatigue syndrome, but the disease isn't just being "really tired." According to the CDC, other conditions should be ruled out first, and a diagnosis requires a significant drop in regular activity levels due to severe fatigue that has lasted more than 6 months, a spike in symptoms when you engage in physical or mental activity, and trouble falling or staying asleep. There also needs to be either impairment of short term memory or dizziness, faintness, or weakness when standing or sitting upright.

There are also physical, measurable pathologies associated with ME (meaning we can diagnose it with more accuracy). They include:

- Altered gut microbiome with less colony diversity
- Hypermetabolic response to stress (presumed to be the result of mitochondrial dysfunction)
- High level of immune cells (especially NK cells)
- Chronic or reactivated infection with a virus such as Epstein-Barr
- Elevated levels of oxidative stress, especially after physical activity
- Bacterial infections such as a Mycoplasma species or Borrelia burgdorferi

4 Women account for 80% of the autoimmune diseases in the US overall. It turns out that there is an inflammation reason for that as well. Individuals with wombs, predominantly cis women, have bodies anticipating the existence of a placenta, leading to the pregnancy-compensation hypothesis. Pregnancy requires downregulation so the body doesn't consider the placenta and embryo an invader to be attacked. Therefore when the body is not pregnant, the immune system gets spikey to protect from germs. Since we don't have near the number of pregnancies we did in the past (thanks birth control!) the spikey levels stay higher for longer causing more inflammation and autoimmune disruptions.

- Lyme disease, FM, or postural orthostatic tachycardia syndrome (POTS)

Why are we talking about chronic pain syndromes in the middle of all this shit about inflammation and the vagus nerve? Once again, it's the vagus nerve. The vagus nerve is the nervous system's conduit of information throughout the body as it connects all of our major organs. And all of our organs have likely at one time or another harbored the herpesviruses (not just the STD, but also HHV6, HHV-5 (cytomegalovirus), and HHV-4 (Epstein-Barr virus))[5] which has been thought to be associated with ME/CFS for decades.

If any of these viruses lying dormant in the body wake up, then they start replicating in different organs in the body and using the vagal system to reach the brain. The brain's first line of defense is to combat them with glial cells. The glial cells are the scaffolding for the vagus nerve, and they also assist in regulating nervous system messaging. So the presence of infection causes them to release cytokines, free radicals, and glutamate, causing system wide inflammation. Constant production of these chemicals is what tells the body we are injured, making chronic pain likely. This can add up to the otherwise unexplainable joint aches of ME, and if it remains untreated can become something termed allodynia, meaning any touch, no matter how slight, will cause the nervous system to react with pain signaling.

When dealing with treatment-resistant depression and pain, we are moving more and more in the direction of treating chronic inflammation in the brain and body. Strategies for this include antiinflammatories, glial cell inhibitors, and vagus nerve stimulation. A series of journal articles by medical doctor and researcher Sota Omoigui posits a unifying theory of pain which states that all pain (whether acute, chronic, peripheral, central, nociceptive or neuropathic) originates with inflammation and our bodies' response to inflammation. Inflammation is mediated by all the stuff we've been talking about thus far (cytokines, neuropeptides, and neurotransmitters) creating our own unique inflammatory profile, which varies person to person and even varies within the same person over time. If we can understand our inflammatory profile, Dr. Omoigui states, we can treat our pain effectively.

Tl;dr: Our inflammatory response is not designed for modern society. It's very likely that many of our "modern" ailments, including mental illness and chronic pain, are the result of inflammation running rampant and we should be focusing on treatments that mitigate these issues at their source.

Some Signs of Chronic Inflammation

---

5 Most humans carry several of these herpesviruses in latent form unless some stressor or biological event allows them to become reactivated.

Acute inflammation is pretty obvious, right? Pain, swelling, redness, heat, and complete loss of function. Chronic inflammation is more subtle.

Stuff you might notice

- Fatigue
- Sore joints
- Chest pain
- Lower back pain
- Mouth sores
- Rashes (Livedo Reticularis, a purple marble-y rash is especially common)
- Insulin resistance (which you will notice either through checking your blood sugar or recognizing it in your body when it's unstable)
- Muscle weakness (myositis)
- Bowel inflammation (abdominal pain, diarrhea, cramping, constipation)
- Dry eye
- Mental fog
- Memory issues

Stuff your doctor might notice

- Hardening of the arteries (arteriosclerosis)
- Excessive blood clotting (hypercoagulation)
- Insulin resistance noted in bloodwork (high fasting glucose, high fasting triglycerides, high A1Cs (amount of red blood cells that have sugar coated hemoglobin)
- Increase in erythrocyte sedimentation rate (ESR), C-reactive protein (CRP) and plasma viscosity (PV) in your blood work (they demonstrate elevated protein, which is related to higher levels of inflammation)[6]

If you think chronic inflammation might be something that is up with you, find treatment providers who specialize in this area. If your regular doctor has blown you off, look for people who specialize in

6 This is easier to find than artery plaque build up and the like. I always suggest to clients to find out how much blood work is covered under their well care if they have a large deductible and get as much as possible. Generally only a basic panel is requested unless your doc is doing diagnostic labs, but get a full panel and differentials if they will prescribe it (and if it doesn't cost you thousands out of pocket). As a nutritionist, I look for patterns of elevation in lab work, not just numbers being completely out of range, as a clue to inflammatory fuckery taking hold.

pain management who aren't just medication pushers. Ask online and join groups of individuals with similar diagnoses to hear about new treatment options. You aren't doomed to live a life in bed, we are getting better and better at treating chronic pain.

Toxic Environment

Toxins are antigenic substances. Antigenic means anything that produces antibodies in the body as part of our immune response. That is, toxins are poison. They fuck up the internal workings of our bodies, even when present at low concentrations. Even when they are not producing a specific disease (though that happens quite regularly too) they are pinging our immune system and upregulating our inflammation levels on the regular.

Toxins can be a lot of things, but for our purposes, I am not referring to unique poisonous events like snake bites or the cinnamon challenge, but instead the various chemical compounds that have entered our everyday environment and our bodies in the last 200 years (but especially post World War II) as a byproduct of pesticides, industrial waste, burning fuel, and other crap modern technologies create. We are barraged by toxins every day in the air we breathe, the water we drink, the food we eat, and the products we use.

Avoiding toxins is something you might hear people talk about or read about in magazines—but it's not as simple as a personal choice to buy organic or use an expensive stainless steel water bottle. Some of our exposure is within our control—like broccoli being a better meal choice than gummi worms. But even the broccoli we are eating today is often sprayed with pesticides. And even the fancy organic kind doesn't have the same micronutrients that it used to have. The earth's atmosphere is a closed system, the soil is slowly being depleted, and the toxins are recycling into our food supply (among other places).

Even though chemical pollutants have been accumulating on the planet at accelerating rates in the last 75 years, we have only begun to start monitoring how it is affecting the environment, animals, and us. We may bump into an article in our daily scroll that demonstrates how air pollution is destroying the gut microbiome and cardiac cellular structure of individuals as young as three years old in Copenhagen (this is a real thing, not a made up example) and think that's pretty fucked up. We may read up on how many of these chemicals are not just toxic in general, but either mimic or block the work of certain hormones in our body (endocrine-disrupting chemicals, also a real thing, not a made up example). Just in 2020, scientists discovered that there are traces of microplastics in human organs and traces of nanoplastics in human tissue. But it's difficult to fully grasp the impact of how toxins are fully affecting our body-mind since most of the research has been done on animals. Additionally, there is tremendous variability between people and how they react to certain chemicals.

We know that we all have a bioburden of these chemicals and there is likely an additive effect of their existence in our systems that builds up over time and is impacting our physical and emotional health. We won't know the extent of it until we start monitoring this data on a significantly larger scale. It's important to recognize that our body burdens are not short term. For instance, if we paint our bathroom, the chemicals we inhale can be found in our system for a couple of weeks after. Many of us hold these chemicals for indeterminate amounts of time. The most in-your-face example of this issue is among the Inughuit peoples of the Arctic who still eat an Indigenous diet of foods they fish and hunt. Quebec epidemiologist Dr. Éric Dewailly was studying the effect of toxic exposure on breastmilk. He decided to use Inughuit women as his control sample, presuming them to be a "clean" standard to compare to other women because of their Indigenous diet. So he took their blood, expecting it to be free of toxins. He was shocked at what he discovered: that Inughuit women have an incredibly high level of toxic compounds in their bloodstream—in fact, they're significantly higher than those of women in industrialized settings.

The Inughuit are not the only Inuit peoples with these high levels of toxic compounds. Because the industrial emissions, pesticides, and chemicals from the rest of the world are unable to break down and weather patterns allow them to eventually travel into the polar ecosystem where they are absorbed into the animals that are eaten by the peoples who subsist off of them. As a result, nearly all Indigenous individuals living in Greenland and northern Canada have mercury and PCB levels that exceed international health guidelines. Their bodies contain the highest human concentrations of industrial waste found anywhere on earth—so much so that Inuit women have been told not to breastfeed their children. Their breastmilk and their tissue could be classified as toxic waste. The exposure of babies in the womb alone is affecting their immune systems and brain development. Dewailly's studies were done in 1987, and many of the babies he was studying decades ago are now mothers themselves.

But that doesn't mean people south of the Arctic Circle are living toxin-free lives. Bill Moyers submitted a sample of his blood as part of his investigative piece Trade Secrets: A Moyers Report, a 2001 investigation into the chemical revolution and the companies that drove it. His blood sample was returned from the Mount Sinai School of Medicine with the information that there were 84 distinct toxic chemicals found in his body. These 84 chemicals make up his personal "chemical body burden." Some of the chemicals found in his blood were ones that have been banned for several decades and some were so obscure that there was no information even on what they were.

And 84 really wasn't that bad. According to the Environmental Working Group (EWG), the average newborn baby has 287 known toxins in their umbilical cord blood. Eighty thousand toxic chemicals have been released into our environment since the dawn of the industrial revolution. We are each exposed to just over 2.5 billion pounds of toxic chemicals and 6 million pounds of mercury alone each year.

Now we add to that the common toxins humans experience in their lifetime. Not all of these toxins are human-made chemicals—there are certain naturally occuring substances like mold, fungus, or tick bite transmitted bacteria that operate as biotoxins for the human body. And some toxins we welcome into our bodies as treatment for something more insidious—like cancer treatments—but they are still toxic. And then there's your everyday stuff. Toilet cleaner in a spray bottle, pesticides on food, car exhaust, off gassing from new furniture, those plug-in air fresheners, the plastic in your face lotion . . . .

These toxins cause, you guessed it, inflammation. And all the issues that can come along with it, including mental and physical illnesses and chronic pain. They can even influence our trauma responses by decreasing treatment efficacy.

Take all of these together, add our own unique genetic make up to the mix and we get varying degrees of total load. Total load is the total amount of stressors (which includes toxins) to your system at any given time. There is only so much we can handle without overflow and illness. And some of us have gene patterns that make us more susceptible to overload. About 25% of people have the specific gene pattern that means their bodies don't have adequate mechanisms to deal with these toxins, which makes them more likely to be susceptible to chronic inflammation and increased likelihood of illness.

A lot of people with a high toxin load may have normal labs, or may show signs of candida, bacterial overgrowth, or a parasite infection. They get treated but then it keeps coming back. The aforementioned mercury numbers? People without the GSTM1 gene which is critical for mercury detoxification are far more susceptible to that total load tipping point. The people who are genetically more susceptible or have more exposure (such as individuals who work with harsh chemicals or live in especially toxic environments like the Inughuit women) are the same ones that are more susceptible to Chronic Inflammatory Response Syndrome (CIRS) because their bodies can't naturally shed all of the toxins they are taking in.

Physical Symptoms of Toxic Overload

Some signs that you might be dealing with a greater toxic load than your body can handle include:

- Fatigue
- Concentration difficulties
- Muscle aches
- Headaches
- Joint pain
- Sinus problems (congestion and/or postnasal drip)
- Gas, bloating, water retention, constipation, diarrhea, or extra Stinky Poops[7]
- Heartburn
- Sleep problems
- Food cravings (quick carbs usually because blood sugar is wonky)
- Trouble losing weight, toning up, or increasing energy (you're doing the right things but your body isn't feeling any better)
- Skin problems (rashes, eczema, psoriasis, acne, canker sores)
- Halitosis
- Puffy, dark circles under the eyes
- Premenstrual syndrome or other menstrual disorders

If you have a suspicion this might be a major issue for you (especially if you've had identifiable exposures, like living in a major agricultural area or growing up in a moldy house or a war zone), working with a clinician that specializes in shedding a toxic load can be hugely beneficial. There are treatments (medications, supplements, and specialty diets) that help you significantly lessen your toxin load. As does doing everything in your power to control your toxin exposure as much as possible by whatever means are available. When it comes to detox, everything within this book applies. Movement and eating strategies, treating inflammation, and the like can help you better mitigate the things you can't control so they don't affect you nearly as much.

Stress

Like inflammation, stress is an example of something that isn't inherently bad for the human body but becomes problematic because

7 I mean, all poop stinks. It's poop. But if it's that chronic "something crawled up my ass and died" smell then that may mean toxins your body is working to dispel.

of modern life. We talk about stress and being stressed probably more regularly than we discuss any other aspect of our health and wellness. However, it has become so big and so vague that we lose sight of the fact that stress isn't external events. And we have far more control over our stress response than we do over our toxin exposure.

Stress is how our body responds to life events with the appropriate output of resources. Stress is heavily influenced by our life events (stressors), the chronic nature of them, and even our perceptions of them. And understanding all of this isn't as complicated as most research papers would have you believe and is a very important part of anyone's personal wellness plan.

What Is Stress?

Stress affects us all differently. Some people thrive on it and use that energy to get shit done. Others feel overwhelmed and check out. Maybe you get energized and motivated. Maybe your shoulders get tight. Maybe your whole body gets tight. Maybe you yell at people or drive recklessly. Maybe you space out. We all respond differently based on our previous experiences.

Physiologist Walter Cannon first proposed the idea of the "acute stress response" in 1915. He also termed it the "fight or flight response"—which is going to sound familiar; remember, the fight or flight response (which is, yes, also called the SNS vagal response) is what becomes trauma if it gets stuck. His use of the term "stress" comes from the engineering field. Stress, in the context of engineering, refers to the pressure or tension imposed upon material objects. Because (no shit) we are also material objects and experience pressure or tension on our state of being.

In the 1930s, a physiologist named Hans Selye's inability to do basic lab draws led to our first understanding of the effects of stress on the body. He was trying to study the effects of ovarian extracts on rats but sucked horribly at the injections. He kept dropping the rats and ended up chasing them around the laboratory for hours on end. Fortunately, he was a far better physiologist than rat handler, and he noticed that his ineptness was causing enlarged adrenal glands, fucked up immune systems, and ulcers in all of the rats that were fried by his continuous bullshit.

Our bodies are quite able to manage occasional stressors and have a nice orderly way of doing so. But as Selye discovered through his dumbass behavior, our bodies are not designed to respond to stress all the fucking time. When that happens our bodies get overloaded and we get sick. Selye referred to this overload as general adaptation syndrome, which today is called "adrenal fatigue."

But in a clinical sense, stress is a more neutral term that refers to any event that requires an output of resources.

Stress can be good (output of resources to create art, run a race, or finish school) or it can be bad (coping with a car accident, an illness, or being terminated from a job). Kelly McGonigal, in her book The Upside of Stress defines stress in terms of meaning. Things are stressful to us because they fucking matter to us.

Whether the situation is good or bad, we can hit a point where we run out of the resources that we need to cope with the situation. And that is what distress is. The point of resource depletion. The point where we need support. It isn't something you can do on your own. It isn't a term that identifies someone as tragically fucked up. It's a clinical term that we understand to mean this person needs some help.

If you have tipped into distress, maybe it's because life has been throwing you too many curveballs and then you also just spilled your coffee and it was the last fucking straw. Or maybe it's a lot of great stuff happening, like you're on a fun trip and you hit exhaustion/sensory overload and the ziplining event reduces you to tears even though you were the one who planned it. They are both distress, not because they're equivalently upsetting but because they're overloading your system.

And it's distress that researchers are talking about when they say that our "stress" numbers are through the roof, worldwide. The numbers were bad when I first wrote about them a few years ago, citing Gallup's 2018 Global Emotions Report. Then things got so much worse. The American Psychological Association partnered with the Harris Poll in 2022 to see how numbers stood two years into the pandemic. What's up right now? The world is on fire. We have a global pandemic, enormous racial tensions, worries about mass shootings, money problems in general, inflation specifically, and the war in Ukraine. Issues around Covid were reported as stressors, including confusion about mandates and vaccines. But even more importantly, Covid and the ensuing shutdowns drew back the curtain on relationship problems for many people. More than half of the people surveyed reported relationships either ending or becoming incredibly strained during the pandemic.

How Does Stress Work?

Stress—or distress—is regulated by something called our "HPA axis", short for *Hypothalamic-Pituitary-Adrenal Axis*, which is basically our central nervous system as it is intertwined with our endocrine system—which produces our hormones.

The HPA axis is designed to keep our body balanced (or as scientists put it, in homeostasis). This means, weirdly enough, helping us react appropriately to stress. In order to stay on an even keel, we are meant to deal with problems quickly and efficiently so we can go back to point chill. Two of the main hormones that the HPA axis deploys to deal with stress, however, cause problems when they are activated regularly and run rampant. They are adrenaline and cortisol.

Adrenaline

When our body determines an event to be stressful, a cascade of events is set off. The amygdala—the emotional center of the brain—starts the process, sending a signal to the hypothalamus in the brain stem region, which has the task of releasing hormones to help us level up to respond to the stressor. The hypothalamus flips the switch for the sympathetic nervous system to get ready to engage and tells the vagus nerve to shoot a message down to the adrenal glands that they need to pop the tab on an energy drink.

The adrenal glands say "bet" and release adrenaline into the bloodstream. Adrenaline (also called epinephrine) ups our heart rate and our blood pressure, expands our ability to take more air into our lungs, makes our pupils expand so we can take in more visually, and redistributes blood to our muscles. It gets us ready for action. Adrenaline is our first line of defense. It's such an immediate response that it happens pre-awareness. Whatever we are looking at, hearing, or smelling, we haven't even processed the information in the prefrontal cortex—the thinking brain—but the body is already chugging Red Bull. Because it happens so quickly, it also wears off really quickly. It's that flush of energy you get when you have a really bad scare. Then when you feel kinda nauseous 20 minutes or so later, that's the adrenaline wearing off.

Cortisol

After the adrenaline kicks in, if the amygdala says "nah, not done yet, need more juice" we end up with cortisol production.[8] Cortisol is also a flip-switch for the sympathetic nervous system, causing rapid heart rate and breathing and all the same energy drink feelings, but even more sustained.

Cortisol is slower-acting in the system than adrenaline, since it's the second line of defense and is designed to keep our nervous system on the gas to deal with a longer-lasting situation. It takes more time to build up in the body, and takes longer to dissipate back out. When we are trying to test someone's chronic stress levels, we look at cortisol. Cortisol levels going up are also correlated with vagal tone going down

8 This is where we really see the complexity of the whole system. Cortisol doesn't release on its own. The continued threat signals the hypothalamus to release corticotropin-releasing hormone (CRH), which travels to the pituitary gland (*there*'s the P part of HPA!), triggering the release of adrenocorticotropic hormone (ACTH). Then the ACTH runs to the adrenal glands, prompting them to release cortisol. I refrained from putting this in the main text of the book because *ugh* it's a lot of science.

(as measured by heart rate variability), meaning we are far less likely to remain in our window of tolerance.

You've probably heard about how cortisol causes belly fat and heart attacks? That's because it changes the body's metabolism by altering our blood glucose when it is in our system all the damn time. Cortisol also increases amygdala activation and brakes hippocampal activity (which keeps the hippocampus from going in and telling the amygdala to calm its tits), which leads to more cortisol production (Thanks, brain!).

Continuous cortisol build up makes our thinking brain (the prefrontal cortex) far less effective. Just like trauma, chronic stress changes the blood flow in the brain because the blood flow is going to the muscles of the body to prepare us for an attack. Decreased blood flow means decreased brain activity which creates "holes" in our prefrontal cortex.9 It fucks with our ability to think clearly and remember things that aren't related to stressful situations. Which is why you feel like you can't think straight when you are really stressed out, because you can't think straight when you are really stressed out.

Cortisol is a total asshole, BTW, if it's something we have in our system on the regular. This whole response of the body makes evolutionary sense. It protected us from predators, right? But that's not modern life and we are not suited to having this chronic chemical cascade going all the time in the face of everyday stressors.

It's like driving a car and you get stuck in 5th gear. You may still technically be the one driving, but the actual amount of control you have over the car is pretty low. You're kinda just looking for a pile of hay to crash into to avoid as much damage as possible, right? (Hi, yes, I grew up on The Dukes of Hazzard, why do you ask?)

The Consequences of Chronic Stress

The question, then, is how exactly does a normal, protective stress response lead to chronic, unhealthy distress? There is no one, singular answer because we are talking about really complex fucking systems. But Western medicine has been catching up in the past decade to what Eastern medical professionals have been saying for about three thousand years and functional medicine practitioners have been saying for over a hundred years—that there is quite likely a huge role being played by inflammation.

So we know inflammation is how the body responds to perceived threats through the production of cytokines activated by the stress response. And we know that the cytokines can stay upregulated when

---

9 As determined by measuring blood flow and electric activity in the brain through SPECT imaging (Single Photon Emission Computed Tomography, if you're nasty).

stress is chronic, creating the perfect human body soup in which to cook up some physical and mental health issues.

Stress is hell on our guts. That chronic production of cortisol is telling the body to get ready to fight, right? And the opposite of the fight/flight response is the rest/digest response. We can see how the body not having time to do the resting/digesting part affects the gut's ability to protect us from other illnesses. The gut does this through an immunoglobulin called secretory IgA. Once that system starts going down, pathogens in the gut start running amuck.

Additionally, all that cortisol starts eating the glutamine, which is an essential amino acid, in our gut lining, which strips away another layer of protection. Then we get gut permeability (meaning pathogens get through the gut lining into the rest of the body). Yes, the leaky gut thing again. Because this is another cause of the breakdown to our gut lining (and other tissue in our body, such as our muscles) and we are now more likely to have food sensitivities, less able to handle toxin exposures, and have more trouble absorbing nutrients in general.

All of this (waves arms around wildly) is modulated by the vagus nerve—both the emotional component and the inflammation component.

Pretty much everything that can go wrong with us, in terms of physical or mental health, has a stress connection. Naming them all and detailing the connection would be a multiple volume book series. WebMD (everyone's favorite internet diagnostic tool) will tell you that chronic stress causes (to name just a couple) heart disease and asthma. And on the "mental" health side, depression and anxiety are strongly correlated with chronic stress.

Physical Symptoms of Chronic Stress

- Cardiovascular issues like abnormal heart rhythms, high blood pressure, heart disease, heart attacks, and strokes
- Disordered eating patterns and weird weight fluctuations due to jacked up hunger signals from cortisol
- Menstrual problems
- Loss of sexual desire, sexual dysfunction, impotence, and premature ejaculation
- Problems with hair and skin (hair falling out, skin problems like rashes, eczema, acne, etc.)
- Gut upset (IBS, gastritis, ulcers, nausea, GERD, etc.)
- Low energy
- Headaches, other aches and pains (chronic or acute), and tenseness throughout the body

- Upset stomach, including diarrhea, constipation, and nausea
- Racing heart and rapid breathing
- Other nervous behaviors (fidgeting, picking at cuticles, etc)
- Changes in sleep
- Changes in appetite
- Getting sick more easily than usual (colds, flus, infections)

Emotional/Mental Stuff

- Mental health problems, such as depression, anxiety, PTSD, and thought disorders
- Feelings of agitation and frustration
- Uncontrolled mood swings, racing thoughts
- Thinking you are losing control, being out of control
- Low level depression, hopelessness, helplessness, worthlessness
- Unable to relax or enjoy things you usually enjoy
- Avoiding people and situations you generally enjoyed in the past
- Inability to focus, feeling disorganized and forgetful
- Incessant worry
- Making bad choices and judgements
- Always framing things through a negative lens
- Struggling to stay organized and/or focus your attention
- Procrastinating and avoiding responsibilities
- Increased use of substances to manage mood (drugs, alcohol, nicotine, caffeine)

So for those of us with all kinds of continued stress-response upregulation of the HPA axis and its hormonal compadres, we start seeing the effects in our lives. It can also be complicated, because many of the symptoms of stress can be symptoms of other things. Is it stress or is it immediate death butt-cancer?

Saying it again for the people in the back who are worried about going all woo-woo and ignoring other serious medical issues: We always need to rule out other medical stuff that might be going on. And even if it isn't immediate death butt-cancer, it's still serious. Your body is trying to get your attention. Because early stress symptoms turn into chronic problems within the body which can lead to serious illness (and yes, more on that later).

Additionally, you may have already had some of these issues and then they got exacerbated by stress. Everyone with a chronic physical or mental illness is totally nodding their head right now. When you look back at all of the chemicals associated with the stress response and look at how they operate within the body, this list starts to make tons of sense.

Stress affects everyone differently, and clearly, the more chronic the stress, the more likely it is to cause a cascade of issues. Which brings us to . . .

When Chronic Stress Becomes Worse

When chronic stress starts to cause more severe issues, we have what's long been referred to as *adrenal fatigue* (which I touch on in *Unfuck Your Brain*). Except you won't find that diagnosis on your medical records anywhere. The problem is although it sounds clinical as fuck, adrenal fatigue still isn't an accepted medical diagnosis. Adrenal insufficiency is something that can be measured on lab work, while adrenal fatigue cannot.

Whether we call it adrenal fatigue, general adaptation syndrome, or hypoadrenia, there is no real diagnostic criteria to determine it exists; you won't find it in your medical records anywhere. It's a catchall term for a set of symptoms like body aches, fatigue, nervousness, sleep disturbances and digestive problems. It's hard to define what we can't measure. And the medical establishment understandably worries that there is another medical illness causing those symptoms that are being left untreated, like major depression, Addison's Disease, or even ME.

And that's entirely fucking fair. Other serious medical issues should always be ruled out first. But if we do rule out other stuff and are still feeling low-level shitty all the time, we are doing ourselves a disservice by not considering that we might be experiencing a physiological maladaptation to stress causing a chronic dysregulation of the HPA axis.

Our bodies are not designed for being in a constant state of stress. Modern living and anticipatory distress have made it far more likely that we remain in this state of disequilibrium on an ongoing basis. And with more and more research linking patterns of adrenal hormone output to other chronic illnesses, I think that we are doing ourselves a disservice by dismissing that the cascade of events caused by the stress response, if activated constantly, causes dysregulation of the HPA axis. One term I've seen more recently in response to this idea is HPA-D (HPA-Dysregulation) as a replacement term for adrenal fatigue.

So rather than looking just at adrenal output as a measure of disease, we are looking at the entire system becoming hypo-activated.

That is, slowing down from overuse.[10] It's the body's way of adapting, physiologically, to the constant influx of stress hormones—by decreasing production of those same stress hormones. Just like the whole HPA axis activation is a complicated process, so is the adaptation of the process to chronic stress which appears as HPA dysregulation. And when we slow down on producing stress hormones, our body is less able to effectively respond to stress (which remains a legitimate need), which causes more stress, and begins the cycle again. This can lead to more complex physical and mental health issues, like . . .

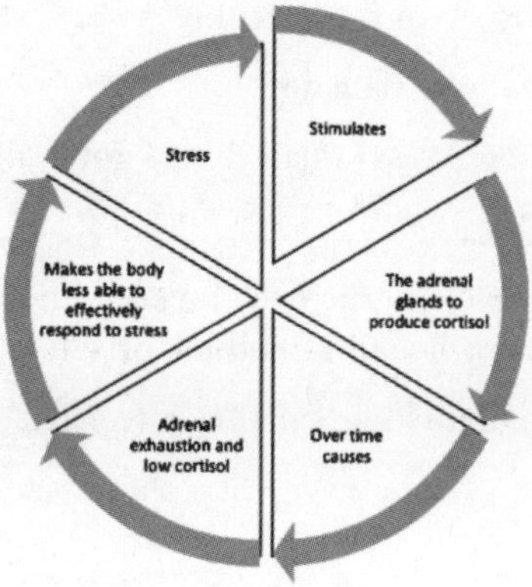

How We Think HPA-D Continues to Self-Reinforce

While we can't measure issues within the adrenal glands until they are shutting down (which then gives us a possible diagnosis of a disease like Addisons, Cushings, etc), we can measure for patterns of elevated cortisol with a fairly simple saliva test. We can also measure an individual's Cortisol Awakening Response and their Cortisol-to-DHEA ratio.

Even easier than that? Another common symptom of HPA dysregulation is orthostatic postural hypotension. Meaning, a drop in blood pressure when you stand up. If I suspect HPA-D, I will have someone lie down on the floor and take their blood pressure after resting there for a few minutes (the floor in my office is clean, though, it's cool). Then I will have them stand up and take it again. Normally, someone's blood pressure should go up when standing up, but if it drops (especially by 10 or more points) that's a sign of HPA-D. The bigger the drop, likely the bigger the problem. I know this sounds a little redonkulous, but a recent study of patients in Poland found orthostatic hypotension in all of the study participants who had both adrenal insufficiency and adrenal crisis.

Long story short, there are usable testing techniques that we can employ to recognize a body overloaded by stress before we develop

10 I have a middle aged body and I resemble this.

an even more complex and chronic mental health issue. I see it akin to treating chronic allergies before it becomes a bronchial infection or pneumonia. We can also look at good old clusters of symptoms in our lives.

The symptoms associated with HPA-D may feel super vague to you, but they are still a good starting point. And when we see certain patterns in symptoms we can get a better idea of what's going on. Symptoms of HPA-D due to chronic stress can look somewhat different from stress symptomatology. Here's what we look for:

- Difficulty getting up in the morning
- High levels of fatigue each day
- Inability to handle stress (small things get really big, really fast)
- Cravings for salty foods
- Higher energy levels in the evenings (and not just because you are finally away from your stupid job or school day)
- Overuse of stimulants like caffeine (I feel attacked)
- A weak immune system (every bug that makes the rounds, you get)

If this sounds super familiar to you, it's another case where it's good to find a doctor who takes this stuff seriously. Not one who says "Hahaha, just relax, it's not that bad!" Plus, everything we talk about later in this book about supporting a healthy body, was written with stress hormones in mind, not just vagal response (cuz it's a system that self-references constantly, right?). Making lifestyle changes is hard work, but you're already doing the hard work of living with an exhausted body, so this will be a cakewalk in comparison!

Section Two: Unfuck Your Body

The first part of this book was about how our bodies (or rather, our body-minds) can get fucked up. You made it through some hella science, gold star!

The second part is about the fixing. Yesssss, fixable! Or at least, pretty damn manageable! Yaaay for hope! If we change how we view the creation of those issues, we can change how we approach supporting the body's ability to heal, right?

We're going to start with working on the vagus nerve itself, and directly addressing the stress, inflammation, and toxicity that throws us for such a loop.

Then, we have chapters that cover various aspects of bodily unfucking, so we can go right to where we are feeling it the most: eating, movement, and sleep. And we're also going to talk about meditation and breathing.

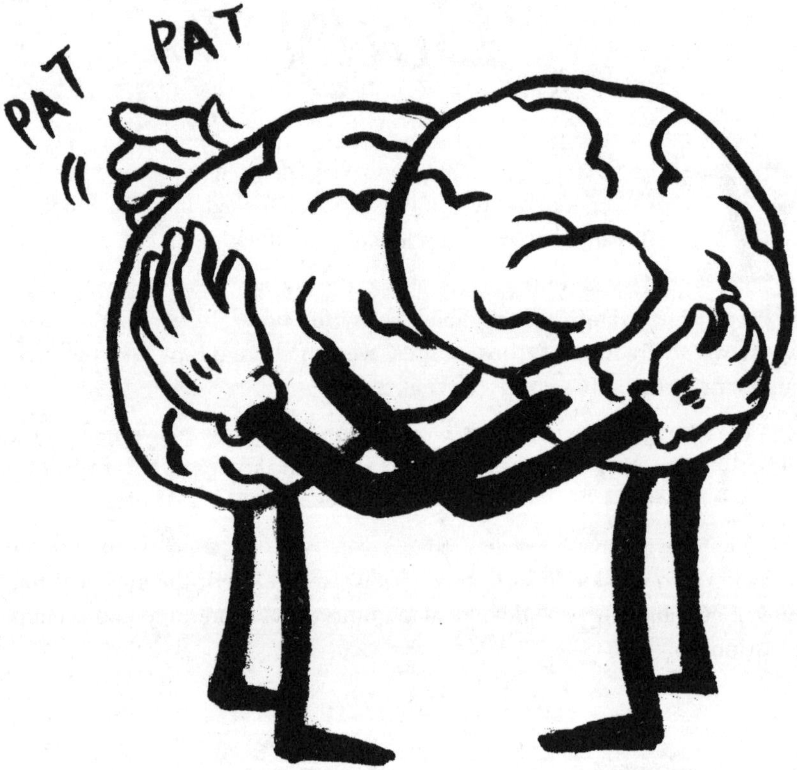
PAT PAT

UNFUCK YOUR VAGAL SYSTEM

Okay, so if the vagus nerve is the body fuckery superhighway, we should start our healing journey there, right?

It turns out that we can influence our vagal tone directly, which can go a long way toward getting us back into that window of tolerance we talked about in Section One—a state where our nervous system isn't primed to respond to immediate threats and we are able to be relaxed, social, creative, and curious instead of just preparing for attack. Learning to recognize your body's responses to various situations and work toward managing them is foundational to body-mind healing. And here you thought I was going to tell you to eat more kale and go breathe in a salt cave!

If you have spent a lot of time being dissociated from your body, even recognizing how your body is responding can be really difficult. So it definitely needs to be said—it's okay if you aren't aware of your body's responses right now and/or don't have good coping mechanisms to deal with them. Cuz the next couple of chapters are going to teach you some. This is designed to help you start recognizing your body's responses in a conscious way and figure out what may already be in your toolkit and what tools you need if yours is currently empty.

How to Stimulate the Vagus Nerve Directly

All of the other chapters in this book relate in one way or another to healing the body-brain connection, and much of that relates to the vagus nerve (even when we are focusing on physical inflammation in the body, that is still largely affected by vagal tone).

One of the best, most direct ways to regulate the vagus nerve is through breathwork. There is a whole chapter about this coming up. I've studied breathwork pretty intensively, so I kinda geeked out and there was no way it would all fit here, so feel free to skip ahead if you want to get right into working on that. But there are other mechanisms for vagus stimulation that don't require a dissertation that you can start experimenting with right away.

Directly calming the vagus nerve is becoming a more common (and drug free) treatment option. The FDA approved a vagus nerve stimulation (VNS) device in 2005 as a treatment for severe, treatment-resistant unipolar and bipolar depression. The device gets surgically implanted underneath the skin near the collar bone and stimulates the vagus nerve much in the way a pacemaker stimulates the heart muscle.

So impacting the vagus directly is obviously hugely beneficial. And we can make that happen without going half-Borg in the process.

Ear Stuff

The most direct way to improve your vagal tone is through stimulating the auricular branch of the vagus nerve (ABVN) which runs through the skin of the outer ear canal and parts of the ear. I know this seems like a weird place to be able to access the vagus nerve directly through the body, but that's because it's actually a remnant of our embryonic nerve, which supplied the first branchial arch.

It is also known as Alderman's nerve, a centuries-old historic reference to London politicians who would activate the ABVN with rosewater to encourage digestion. Besides helping with indigestion, stimulating the ABVN has shown to help with migraines, panic attacks, and our stress response. Stimulating the ABVN is being investigated as a medical intervention for chronic heart failure, so it's the real deal. This impacts the vagus nerve directly, telling the body to activate the parasympathetic response system again, which puts us back in our window of tolerance.

If you are looking at an ear, and consider the ear canal 12 o'clock, the ABVN runs 1 to 3 o'clock from it. You can feel the cartilage from the ABVN which leads down to the ear canal if you are poking your finger around in there, looking like a weirdo in the middle of the grocery store.

Pressing on that area or wearing an ear seed (an acupressure ball that you stick onto your skin) are both ways of stimulating the ABVN. I also know several people who have had that area pierced and found it hugely beneficial for their anxiety and migraine headaches. I'm not recommending ABVN piercing necessarily (an ear seed is way less invasive), but if you were kind of wanting to get one anyway it may have benefits beyond the aesthetic.

Tongue Stuff

The tongue is so weird, y'all. The deeper we get into this, the weirder the body seems to be. The tongue is part of the autonomic nervous system and part of the somatic nervous system. So the tongue is activated both consciously and unconsciously. And it is thought to be part of all three components of the autonomic nervous system. Not just the sympathetic and parasympathetic, but also the enteric—which makes sense, because our tongues are an essential part of our eating and digestive process. The tongue represents the gateway to the enteric system, due to the presence of specialized ganglia on the anterior and posterior area of the tongue; it would act as a chemical "spy," letting the stomach know what fuckery we have put in our mouths.

And remember when I talked about the difference between afferent and efferent information?

Meaning brain-to-body and body-to-brain communication? The tongue becomes a crossroads of efferent and afferent information.

Because the tongue operates involuntarily and voluntarily, this is another place we can activate vagal tone. One of the simplest ways is tongue positioning. When we push our tongue up against the roof of our mouth (even if we do it subconsciously) we are activating the sympathetic nervous system, moving us into fight/flight. Moving our tongue out of that position activates us going back into our ventral vagal window of tolerance. If your tongue tends to get stuck and clenchy when activated, take a sip of water and hold it in your mouth, letting your tongue "float" in the water. Or stick your tongue in a glass of water to help detach it from your hard palate.

The Felt Sense

Another important way of working with our body-brain connection is to deepen our recognition of how our bodies react to stimuli. We started with some physiology basics in the first part of the book, like about how our heart rate and skin color respond to different vagal states. Now we are going to get a little more nuanced.

The felt sense refers to the inner feelings of the body. It's also termed interoception. It includes things like noticing when your chest is tight or your stomach is rumbly.

The idea originates with Eugene Gendlin, who was a couples therapist in the 1950s who was trying to find the common thread in why some of his couples were able to achieve their goals and heal their relationships, and others ended up getting divorced. He couldn't find an obvious thread regarding the type of problem that brought them to counseling, so he started going through hundreds of hours of tapes of therapy sessions and had an aha moment after some time. The people who "got better" were the ones who were able to go quiet and still and listen to their bodies rather than just stay in their brains and listen to their thoughts. He termed this the felt sense, and thought, "Well what if we teach people to do this?"

So he created a technique called Focusing and published a book by the same name in 1978. He has a six-part system, but has always maintained that anything that helps you get to the felt sense is totally awesome, which means that many tricks and tips have been formulated over the past several decades. And as the connection between polyvagal theory and interoception has become clearer more recently, felt sense work has become more common.

Interoception Exercise

This exercise helps us feel into our bodies in a deliberate way, which can be helpful when we are either hypervigilant to external information or dissociating and shutting down. Learning to connect to our felt sense helps us develop a better working relationship with our vagus nerve, so we can recognize when we are out of our zone of tolerance and work to get back into it.

I use this exercise (adapted from Peter Levine's book In An Unspoken Voice) all the time with clients as a skill for managing trauma reactivity, internal overwhelm, and dissociation. Want to get an idea of where I'm going with this?

- Hold out one of your hands. It doesn't matter which one, but take note of your choice.
- Hold it in the air, without letting it rest against another surface (like a table top or your leg) for support. If you cannot comfortably do so, then absolutely use a surface for support.
- Open up the palm of that hand, facing back toward your body, and use your eyes to observe it.
- Slowly make a fist with that hand, watching the whole time. Take note when your hand feels completely closed into a fist.
- Without breaking eye contact, open your hand back up.

Now close your eyes if it feels safe for you to do so. If not, try softening your gaze so you aren't looking at anything in particular (instead of focusing on your hand) and repeat this exercise.

Feel what having your hand open feels like from the inside, then the act of closing your hand into a fist, then reopening. Pay attention to all that you notice in your body that wasn't present when you were focusing on your external sight messages.

How did your awareness of the experience change once you were entirely dependent on your internal sense messages? Was it disconcerting at any point? Comforting? Did anything shift or feel different in how you connect with yourself?

I have also had clients use their feet with the exercise, but making sure to keep them connected to the floor for grounding. Try flexing and wiggling your toes with and without visual stimulus and see if the experience changes for you any.

P.A.T.H.

This is another interoception exercise, with the goal of connecting to the felt sense and recognizing your body's messaging. It adds some parameters to the sensory data you are paying attention to, which is helpful if your senses feel overwhelmed. This exercise is less for calming yourself when things are crap, and more for gaining more clarity over how your body communicates in all kinds of situations.

Turn your attention inward instead of toward the environment around you. Part of you will continue to pay attention to the environment to keep you safe, while you relax your body and soften your gaze but leave your eyes open.

Now, ask yourself the following four things about your body right now.

P. Where can I feel pressure?
A. Where can I feel the air around me on my body?
T. Where is there tension?
H. Where can I feel heat?

Finding the Words

As you feel more comfortable in working with your felt sense you can expand your awareness of the sensations you are experiencing. Just like emotions, sensations are intended to give us information not to last forever.

Here is some sensory vocabulary:

Burning/Hot/Cold/Warm/Chilly/Icy/Cool/Clammy/Chilly/Sweaty/Gentle
Sharp/Dull/Rough/Smooth
Shaky/Trembly/Tingly/Twitchy/Butterflies/Jittery/Jumbled/Jangly/Itchy/Jumpy
Weird/Off-Kilter/Off-Center/Edgy/Tearful/Owie
Hard/Soft
Stuck/Weak
Strong/Tough
Small/Large
Sour/Sweet/Bitter/Salty/Pungent
Relaxed/Calm/Peaceful/Flowing/Spreading/Silky/Still/Tranquil/Comfortable
Undisturbed/Chill/Still/Quiet/Peaceful Empty/Full Fast/Slow/Still
Tight/Tense/Pressure/Vibrating/ Dizzy/Fuzzy/Blurry/Woozy/Faint/Light-Headed
Numb/Prickly/Tickly/Goose-Bumpy/Uncomfortable
Light/Heavy
Open/Closed/Loose/Tight

Some of the body sense words that may help you define your experience include:

Pressure, Air Current, Pain, Tingling, Itching, Temperature, Size, Weight, Shape, Motion, Speed, Texture, Earth Element, Color, Smell, Taste, Sound, Lack of Sensation

Because this is a pretty big list it may feel like writing a thesis on your body. Start by just noticing a couple of things. Maybe start with two or three opposite possibilities and decide which fits best. For example, does it feel tight or loose? Heavy or light?

Self-Holding

The goal of this exercise is to remember that our body is a container for our sensations and feelings. Dissociation sometimes leads to us not even realizing we have edges. A holding exercise helps us recognize our container, connect to it, and ground within it. It helps us "settle" even when experiencing uncomfortable emotions and sensations.

There are several ways to do this exercise, here is a basic version, but keep in mind it can be done laying down, sitting up, or some kind of in-between reclining.

Self-hug: Place one hand under the arm on the opposite side of your body, and the other hand over the upper part of the other arm. Give yourself a hug. The light squeezing can soothe the nervous system the same as getting under a heavy blanket. Now just pay attention to your body. Don't try to force any reactions but see what shifts within you.

Positive Thinking

Positive thinking sounds cheesy, but it works. This is different from being pollyanna-ish and pretending things are just fine when they are a shit-show. By contrast, positive thinking frames our experience around whatever control we do have in any given situation, which helps us activate our own ability to not just survive but thrive.

One proven method you can use to shift your thinking is journaling. There is so much research out there on journaling and how it affects mental health. Probably because it's a cheap thing to study. But also because it is an activity humans have engaged in since we developed the ability to read and write, which way predates the field of psychology.

Journaling has been found to be helpful with specific struggles with anxiety (trait anxiety) as well as with low-key continuous anxiety (state anxiety). It helps us manage stress and maintain a positive mood (read: window of tolerance).

One specific journal exercise designed to build a positive mindset has been shown to have a direct impact on vagal tone:

> Each day for three days in a row, reflect on a positive experience in your life, and imagine yourself back in that experience. Think about your emotions and how you felt in your body when it happened. Write about the experience in as much detail as possible, especially focusing on the thoughts, feelings, and sensations that went along with it.

Even better news? You only have to journal for three days to see results. Not thirty. Just three. We can all handle that. And if you are the student who is always going for extra credit, you can absolutely continue past day three.

Aromatherapy

Working with scents really is a whole other entire book, or at least zine, especially when we get into essential oils and all that weird misinformation out there co-mingled with valid scientific data. Suffice it to say that there *is* valid scientific data that shows that aromatherapy directly affects the body-brain connection. So much so, that certain therapeutic interventions use scents as part of trauma recovery work.

We now know that scents are recognized midbrain (in the amygdala), enhancing our sympathetic response—which is why we can respond so strongly to smells without our thinking brains even realizing what is happening. Researchers have also found that smells directly impact gastric vagal nerve activity. So we can use them to physically activate a feeling of safety and calm.

Certain scents have been studied for their impact on the vagal system more than others. Lavender likely has the most research behind its effectiveness at calming the nervous system, with citrus scents following right behind. The gastric vagal nerve activity study was conducted with grapefruit essential oil, FWIW. And we don't have to engage specifically with essential oils, obviously. Smelling plants in a garden, making a fragrant tea, and using a nice scented bubble bath are all aromatherapy. Essential oils are strong and portable, so that's what you will see used in studies, but the hot tea I make for people in my office is just as scent-soothing as the oils I keep for people to use if they so desire.

Even though there are certain oils that have been shown to be efficacious for calming the vagus nerve, we all have our own unique history with particular smells. It can be helpful to go to a store that has samplers, so you can test out different scents and see which ones are best for your window of tolerance.

The easiest way to use essential oils is to put a drop on the palm of one of your (clean) hands and cup your hands around your nose and mouth, breathing deeply to inhale.[11] If you feel calmer, that scent works for you.

Once you've identified a soothing scent, start using it when you feel calm to connect it to your window of tolerance. Then move on to using it when you are activated, to help you get back into your window of tolerance. A couple of drops on a cotton ball that you store in a ziplock bag and carry in your pocket makes it portable without bringing the whole bottle with you. A low-tech version of a diffuser is to drop a little on the lightbulb of whatever lamp you're using. You can get fancier and high tech from there, but aromatherapy can get expensive so I always suggest (like with everything) experimenting before investing!

Purchasing quality essential oils and avoiding pyramid schemes, scams, and crappy products is a book in and of itself. Start with companies that are well reviewed online, that are selling therapeutic grade oils, and that you can just . . . buy from. If they try to get you to sell the oils, buy a bunch of weird crap to go with them, drag ten of your friends over to your house for an oil party, or whatever, walk away. We're just looking at helping you find tools to manage your body-brain connection, not looking to start a home business that requires thousands of dollars of investment in some kit.

11 Look up contraindications for any essential oil you are thinking about using. Some of them shouldn't be used while pregnant or if you have certain medical conditions. Some shouldn't be applied directly to the skin. While the palm of the hand isn't particularly sensitive skin for most people, you can blend any oil with a carrier oil before applying it to your skin, particularly if you haven't done a patch test on that particular oil or blend yet.

PAIN AND THE MIND

First of all, it's important for me to say and resay x1000 that pain isn't all in your head. Pain is a very concrete, physical reality for many people. So when I talk about mental health approaches to pain management, I'm not saying, "Don't be crazy, the pain doesn't physically exist," I'm saying, "The human mind has great capacity for self-healing when we recognize the validity of our experience and focus on our own self-care." And research is backing this approach up.

One of the best known names in pain research is Dr. Sean Mackey, who runs the Division of Pain Medicine at Stanford. Some of his findings include the benefits of using cognitive behavior therapy—he found that 30% of people with fibromyalgia report a reduction in pain after using CBT. He has also studied the effects of mindfulness meditation—study participants reported a 40% reduction in pain intensity when using this technique (there's an entire chapter on this coming up). Another strategy he looked at was conscious distraction—study participants reported a 44% percent reduction in pain intensity when focusing on an external soothing cue.

Remember when we talked about nociceptive vs neuropathic pain? Mental and emotional techniques can help us with the management of nociceptive pain that comes from immediate injury, and they can help heal us long term from neuropathic pain, by helping us convince our brains that the threat has passed. So I'm including two pain-specific techniques here, and the techniques in the breathing and meditation chapters were written with pain management in mind, not just trauma.

ACT for Pain

The two big mental components that help with pain are 1) recognizing the influence of thinking patterns on our pain and 2) being mindful of our bodies in the present. Acceptance and Commitment Therapy (ACT) combines both these strategies in a way that has gained a lot of traction in the last decade.

ACT was been described by its founder, Russ Harris, as "a type of therapy that aims to help patients accept what is out of their control, and commit instead to actions that enrichen their lives." I have peppered my previous books with ACT exercises. And there are plenty of people out there incorporating ACT interventions in their lives without going to an ACT therapist by focusing on the six mechanisms for creating more psychological flexibility in your life and seeing how they are influenced by chronic pain.

Acceptance: This includes recognizing the thoughts and behaviors that are associated with trying to either control or avoid the pain that are not the healthiest long-term solutions for pain management. I spent years trying to control my pain by ignoring it. Instead of avoiding pain by doing nothing, I pretended it didn't exist at all, constantly overdoing it and making it worse. In my practice I would say this pain response is just as common (if not more common) than trying to control it into submission with medications.

Cognitive Defusion: Activities that help disconnect feelings and thoughts that surround our experience of pain from the pain itself, in order to decrease its influence on our lives. (There is an exercise for this in the Mindfulness chapter.)

Being Present: Mindfulness of your immediate environment rather than being hooked into the pain preoccupations.

Self as Context: A perspective about your life in general with pain as only part of it.

Values: Identifying what matters to you that you want to prioritize above the pain. This helps you recognize how your pain-adaptive behaviors have gotten in the way of your goals.

Committed Action: The determination to achieve certain things based on your values while experiencing pain.

Investigating Our Relationship with Pain

One of the first things we can do is pay attention to our relationship with pain. I know, as someone who has lived with chronic pain for decades, that it gets very easy to just live in it, rather than try to engage with it in new ways. When I've engaged differently, I've seen huge changes in my ability to manage it on a day to day basis, and been able to tolerate spikes with self-compassion and consideration. While having no pain would be lovely, I don't have that expectation. I just want to be able to continue to live a full and active life, and recognizing that pain is a part of my human experience helps me do that.

Ask yourself the following questions:

- How have you put your life on hold because of pain?
- Is it the pain or the fight with the pain that is getting in your way?
- What are some pain controlling thoughts or strategies you engage in?
- What are some pain avoiding thoughts or strategies you engage in?
- What are some alternatives that you are willing to try that allow you to honor your pain but still be engaged in your life?

UNFUCK YOUR STRESS

While we all know a few stress divas who seem to have a homing beacon for inviting stress in, most of us don't choose stress, we just have to deal with it. Whether it's everyday stress, life events stress, or disintegration of society stress, this is the shitshow we've been handed. And research shows the more we try to avoid stress, the worse it gets. So what does help?

There's good news, I swear there is good news. Research supports that we have far more control over our experience of stress and how it affects our bodies than you'd think. Not by chucking everything and living in a van down by the river, but by changing your perception of stress.

Remember how we talked earlier about how stress is just your body perceiving that something is important and upping its resource game? Some smart people compared National Health Interview Survey data to mortality data in the US. Guess what they found? Stress alone isn't so bad for you. But if you think that stress is bad for your health and you perceive yourself as having a lot of stress, you have way worse physical and mental health outcomes. The increased risk of premature death for those folks was 43%. So if you think about stress in a negative way you are far more likely to die of a stress related disease.

There are tons of studies of this nature, if you start digging. In 1998, 30,000 adults in the US were asked about the levels of stress in their life and whether or not they felt that stress was harmful to their health. Eight years later, researchers scoured public records to see which of the 30,000 had died. While high levels of stress increased their risk of dying by 41% it was only true if these same people believed that stress was harmful to their health. Stress plus the belief that stress is harmful is what makes stress the 15th leading cause of death in the US. Our belief system has more impact on our longevity than quitting smoking or taking up exercise: while exercising and smoking cessation are consistently shown to add 4 years to our lives, having a positive outlook on aging adds 8, according to a Yale study.

And several of the studies show that there is a cascade effect on our behaviors, not just our health. For example, one study of Crohn's patients found that a patient's perception of their illness had a direct effect on their stress levels and their stress levels had a direct impact on the types of coping skills they used. That is, the more stressed they were, the more likely they were to use coping skills that were more harmful and costly in the long run, such as disordered eating, dissociating via overuse of social media and the internet, and abuse of drugs and alcohol.

Consider your own history with stress:

- What kinds of avoidant coping skills have you used in the past?
- What other kinds of coping skills have you used that aren't avoidant of the stressor but are ultimately unhealthy for you?
- What opportunities have you missed in an attempt to avoid the stress that would come along with them?
- How might you be limiting your future?

Embracing challenges and facing the problems in our lives proactively increases our likelihood of remaining in our ventral vagal zone of tolerance. The opposite of fight/flight is known as rest/digest in its passive state, but is also known as tend/befriend in its active state. Meaning we are engaged in connection with others toward the betterment of all. People who have suffered the most in life are also the people who jump in to care for others. Stress can actually increase our courage and our capacity for caregiving and strengthen our social relationships. Changing our individual lives, as well as the world around us, requires us to have a mindful relationship with our stress response.

Embracing Stress Through Mindset Training

The author of the book The Upside of Stress, Kelly McGonigal, (whose research is the starting point for a lot of what I write about here) states: "Embracing stress is a radical act of self trust."

We've been told not to though, haven't we? We're told to avoid stress, to calm down, that it isn't good for us. Harvard Business School professor Alison Wood Brooks asked hundreds of people the same question: If you are anxious about a big presentation, what's a better way of handling it? Feeling excited or trying to calm down?

91% of people said "try to calm down."

But, as mentioned eleventy times above, the stress isn't in and of itself bad—it's not necessarily a problem you need to solve or get away from. This is borne out by multiple studies, including the one mentioned above, where the researchers found that just saying "I'm excited" out loud can reframe stress as excitement. Despite what most of us have been told, it's easier for the brain to jump from anxious feelings to excited ones rather than calm ones. Cortisol is going to be activated because something matters to you. But you can consciously label it as excited instead of stressed, which changes how you interpret and experience your own body.

The practice of reframing our thoughts from those of overwhelm to those of empowerment is known as mindset training. This doesn't mean bullshitting ourselves, but recognizing that we do have the capacity to handle tough situations, or at least the capacity to give it our all and try our best. The term mindset is one of those words we associate with those performance coach guru types. Tony Robbins isn't wrong, though. Mindsets are really nothing more than the beliefs we have about ourselves and the world that shape our realities. This isn't negating the fact that we may be dealing with really fucked up situations, but is about taking back whatever power we have in our own responses when dealing with shitshow scenerios.

Mindset training has a direct impact on our stress response. One study found that a stronger physical stress response was associated with higher test scores in school situations, but only for people who have had mindset training. Another study demonstrated that just by telling people "You're the kind of person whose performance improves under pressure" increases their task performance by 33%. One of the biggest predictors of stress overwhelming us is our perception of not being up to the task, so focusing on the fact that we are, indeed, up to it shifts our thinking.

And yes, individuals with anxiety can absolutely benefit from mindset training. Since stress is one of the biggest anxiety triggers, researchers have demonstrated that the stress response (at least the beginnings of it) is the same for people who have anxiety and those who do not. It's our perception of what it means that differs. So a disruption of that stress response can end up circumventing anxiety and panic attacks.

Psychology researcher Salvatore Maddi termed this mindset-building a form of hardiness, meaning the courage to grow from stress. This is how someone can be "good at stress." It doesn't mean that difficulties don't get to us and stress doesn't bother us, but rather that we value growth, accomplishment, and being an active participant in our own lives enough that we befriend our stress response when we can and learn from it when it overwhelms.

Any stressful situation can become an opportunity to practice a mindset shift. When you notice your stress response activating, you can remind yourself that your body is reacting to something because it's important to you. Then, use that energy to help carry you through the situation. Whether you are getting through a stressful interview or fighting fascism, being alert, engaged, and present is vital to success.

Mindset training seems awkward at first, but once you build that neural pathway it becomes more natural and more likely to be your automatic response. As you practice, you won't have to work so hard at it over time. Your stress mindset will also change how you react to others' stress. Mindset leads to resilience. And emotional resilience is one of the first lines of defense against mental illnesses like depression and learning what behaviors build that up could clue physicians in on how to treat those illnesses.

Having a GOOD Mindset

You can practice mindset training as part of your daily self-care routine. I like the GOOD acronym of mindset training since it doesn't involve any kind of fake hype about shitty situations, it really just is about being grounded in your own self-efficacy. And clearly you are a fucking survivor—you're reading this right now, which means your survival rate thus far is 100%, right? This is one of those internal work exercises that might be easier to make external by journaling through it, especially at first while you get used to the process. But I am, for once, not insisting you write everything down if you really hate that shit!

Gratitude: Focusing on gratitude is a really good part of our mental health in general and can create a perspective shift in our day. This doesn't mean discounting what's problematic, but focusing more on what's good in your life.

Openness to Possibilities: If we are gratitude focused, we are far more likely to be aware of solutions, support, and opportunities around us. In a negative mindset, we are more likely to dismiss things that are available to us (or not notice them at all) because we are overwhelmed and frustrated with life in general.

Opportunities in this Experience: No matter what experience we are having, we can focus on the opportunities that exist to help us grow. We can learn more about different situations and ourselves even if we don't achieve the success we were hoping for. As someone who does a lot of political advocacy work, I can tell you that every lost battle taught me a new strategy of approach for next time.

Determine: Visualize yourself successfully embracing the challenges ahead. This is hardiness in action. If you mentally set yourself up for success, you are in the right frame of mind to tackle the project. And no, you aren't more frustrated if things don't go perfectly. I've found that even when I don't succeed, I'm still proud of myself for going in prepared and positive because I feel like I really gave it my all.

But the Key Thing About Stress . . .

It's super important that you don't beat yourself up for not doing stress well. The entire engine of modern society operates on the psychic energy of people not doing stress well. The whole game is designed to work that way. If you are exhausted, burned out, depleted, experiencing adrenal fatigue, and the like, just changing your mindset isn't going to resolve all that.

It took years if not decades to get you to the point of exhaustion you are sitting at right now, right? You can't unfuck this level of attack on a human body by chanting "I'm not stressed, I'm excited!" Caring for yourself is going to be a constant (D) all of the above situation.

Befriending your stress response is way easier with a non-exhausted body, right? You need to treat yourself as you would with any other illness, giving your body the time and ingredients for recovery. Everything else in this book is designed to help treat the chronic inflammation, chronic toxic stress, and the mindbody experience of trauma.

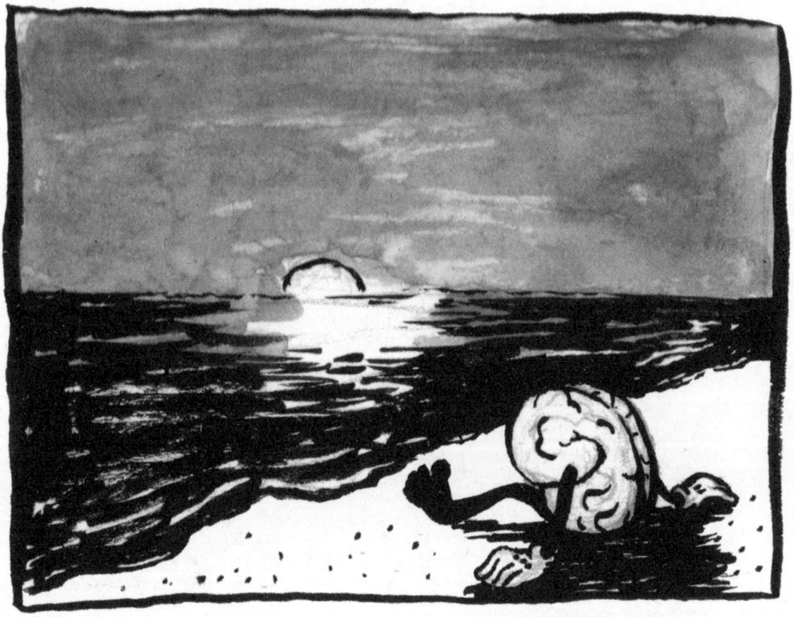

BREATHWORK

We're diving straight into what might be the most powerful tool we have to regulate our vagal system, expel toxins, heal from trauma, manage inflammation, and control stress: our breath. I know, that's some gross-ass hippie shit. I'm sorry. But it's true. Breath (pranayama), along with the topics of the next two chapters which are meditation (dhyana) and movement (the asanas), just happen to be three of the eight limbs of yoga. Now, I super pinky-swear I am not trying to trick you into doing yoga if that's not your jam, but when I was framing out this book it became pretty obvious pretty quickly that Patanjali figured out in the 2nd Century BCE, way before "modern" science did, that these are good ways to keep your body and mind healthy and connected to each other.

Some of these exercises come with contraindications. Just like something being a whole food supplement or herb doesn't make it a good choice for your body and circumstances, some breathing techniques may also be a bad idea. But hey, other than that? Breathing is free and you are already doing it anyway, so might as well get a little fancy.

This Is Your Brain on Breathing

Breathing is one of those things that we control with both our conscious and unconscious brain.

The unconscious part is managed by the brainstem, which I talk about more in Unfuck Your Brain. It's the keeping-the-body-alive part of the brain. It's often called the reptilian brain, though it's more complicated than that in reality.

An example is how the neural circuit in the brainstem affects the connection between breathing and brain control. That neural circuit is actually our "breathing pacemaker" because it adjusts itself based on alterations of our breathing rhythms.

If something activates our fight or flight response (like a big dog chasing us) our breathing will become faster and more erratic. Our heart rate goes up, our neural activity goes all kinds of wonky, and we have a strong emotional response, like anxiety, panic, fear, or anger. We all know that part, right? We've all lived that and some of us live it every day because of anxiety disorders that create imaginary big dogs on the regular. But here is the cool part: there is a bidirectional flow happening in this process.

Our experiences change our breathing, which changes our entire physiology. If we consciously change our breathing, we can also directly influence our physiology. Mindfully slowing our breathing increases our baroreflex sensitivity, which measures the amount of control over our own heart rate.

A recent study directly showed that changing our breathing can also change our emotions. If we control our breathing by counting breaths, we are influencing neuronal oscillations (super fancy way of saying brain waves if you are at a MENSA convention or looking to bore your Tinder date to death) throughout the brain, especially in the mid-brain regions that are related to the regulation of emotion. And according to a study in the journal of Cognition and Emotion, our breathing accounts for up to 40% of our emotional responses.

Controlling our breathing changes our vagal tone, triggering the parasympathetic nervous system which is the counterbalance of the "fight, flight, freeze" sympathetic nervous system response to stress (either real or perceived) which goes on to influence the entirety of our body and our long-term physical health (including activating the lymph nodes to better expel toxins), not just our short-term stress response.

Breathwork and Trauma Responses

Like any other intervention, those of us with trauma histories may need to take an extra special approach to breathwork.

I have over a decade of formal meditation practice and a pretty intense amount of clinical training in both breathwork and mindfulness. It can still be (it is still) really difficult. I know. I know. Conscious alteration of your breathing when you are triggered or activated may feel completely undoable. Someone telling you how to do it feels even worse. So if you have had an awful experience in a meditation class or a yoga class, with a therapist, or listening to an app, you aren't the least bit crazy, that's really common. So I want to talk a little about why that is and how to plan for it.

Trauma changes our breathing. When we are out of our zone of tolerance, our breathing becomes shallow (to change oxygen movement throughout the body to prepare for the perceived attack). And trauma survivors often hold their breath regularly without realizing it. And that creates tension and more body dysregulation than we are often even aware of.

We can learn from yoga practitioners who have been developing trauma-informed practices that can help you use mindful movement and breathing for trauma recovery, without being retraumatized or triggered by it. David Emerson's trauma-informed yoga is an evidence-based practice for trauma recovery, and there are several unique aspects to how he cues yoga that I use as a teacher and clinician.

One of the biggest differences in his approach is that he doesn't tell practitioners when to breathe in and out. He only suggests noticing it. If you have taken a more traditional yoga class, you'll remember being told when to breathe in and breathe out constantly. That's why the first breathwork exercise in this chapter is designed to help you just notice your breath, with no plan of altering it. Trauma survivors regularly struggle to notice their breathing at all, so beginning to do so is a really big deal. And it helps us notice when we are holding our breath as well. While an anxiety or panic response can include very rapid, shallow breathing, a trauma response may invoke a locked jaw, breath suppression, and abdominal inhibition.

Another really amazing resource is David Treleaven's book Trauma-Sensitive Mindfulness. If you are a trauma survivor or an individual who works with trauma survivors, this book is invaluable. He offers suggestions for managing trauma triggers and activation during mindful meditation practice, which can also be applied to breathwork to help maintain that polyvagal window of tolerance.

- Recognize your internal go and stop signals (thoughts, feelings, body sensations) as markers of how you respond to different breathing techniques. Which are most helpful? Which are activating?
- Take breaks when you need to or alter how you are holding your body. Move into a more comfortable position or wiggle in place a little.
- Open your eyes, if they have been closed.
- Change to slow, mindful breathing if you were trying one of the more complicated pranayama techniques.
- Focus on an external object that is in your line of vision.
- Shorten your breathwork practice period or otherwise adjust the practice itself (for example, the 4-7-8 breathing pattern can be altered to shorter breaths).

Learn and practice breathwork when you are in a relaxed state, rather than trying to do it when you are already activated. The more you practice when your body isn't under siege, the more likely you are to be successful with it when your body is under siege.

Breathing Exercises

We're gonna start with the classic breathwork techniques, then move into some more specific pranayama techniques, focusing on the ones that my clients have reported to be the most helpful over the years. I'm not just including pranayama because I'm a yoga dork. The impact of different pranayama techniques on physical and emotional health has been studied extensively in recent years.

Pranayama is the combination of three Sanskrit words: prana is our life force energy, ayama refers to lengthening and extending, and yama refers to containing or restricting.

This kind of breathwork is part of yoga, even though it doesn't fit what most of us see when we hear that word. When we think of yoga, we think of the bendy shit. But the poses and forms, which are known in Sanskrit as the asanas are in fact only one of the eight limbs of yoga and pranayama is another one of the eight. Many yoga practitioners will attest to the fact that pranayama is foundational to the asanas and the dhyana (meditation).

Pranayama is how we clear and cleanse our bodies, and the asanas and dhyana are how we test the efficacy of our breathing practice. And this is why the mindfulness and the bendy shit can be so difficult if you haven't gotten a handle on the breathing part.

A precaution about all of these techniques: If you have nose or throat irritation or congestion, it may not be a great breathwork day for you. If you have a strong negative response to any of the techniques, stop doing them immediately. Any specific contraindications for any technique will be listed with the technique itself.

Noticing the Breath

Settle your body into a comfortable position. You can close your eyes if you feel comfortable doing so, or settle into a soft gaze instead.

Bring your awareness to your breathing. Notice as you breathe in, and follow through as you breathe out. When your thoughts wander, just notice them, maybe label them as thinking, and bring your attention back to the breath. You can use Thich Nhat Hanh's breathing mindfulness technique to help center your focus on being mindful in the moment:

Breathing in, I know I am breathing in . . .

Breathing out, I know I am breathing out.

Breathing in . . . I know I am breathing in . . .

Breathing out . . . I know I am breathing out . . .

Notice the rhythm of your breathing, notice how it changes. Notice the sensations in the rest of your body and how they change. Don't do anything to alter your breathing or to "breathe better," just pay attention to where you are now.

No specific contraindications.

Three-part Breathing

We've all done a big inhale before starting a new task, right? The inhale is our sympathetic nervous system becoming activated, which gives us an energy boost to act. Someone in distress is breathing so rapidly they are constantly inhaling, building up an energy flow that tells the brain to become anxious or panic.

The exhale is the parasympathetic response, which lowers our heart rate and calms our energy.

The retention (the space between inhale and exhale) is the space where we connect with our body and what's going on inside it (interoception). So the 4-7-8 breathing pattern is designed to manage a stress response by lengthening out our periods of interoception and parasympathetic engagement.

- Breathe in for a count of 4
- Hold for a count of 7
- And out for a count of 8

You may feel a little light headed at first, and it's totally okay to sit or lie down. Another option is to use the same ratio, but shorten it:

- Breathe in for a count of 2
- Hold for a count of 3.5
- And out for a count of 4

No specific contraindications.

The Complete Breath (Dirgha Pranayama)

Dirgha is a good daily practice to help manage breathing errors that we have collected over time. While you don't (and really can't) breathe like this 24/7, practicing with it daily will help you naturally lengthen and deepen and relax your "regular" breathing naturally.

- Get in a comfortable position—seated is best for this practice. Hold your spine as straight as you are comfortably able to, and let your abdomen soften.
- Place your hands on your abdomen or bring awareness to that area. Gradually start to lengthen and deepen your breathing. Work to expand your belly like a balloon with each inhale, and deflate it back out upon exhale. This is abdominal (or belly breathing).
- Now shift your attention to your ribcage. If you are able to place your hands on the side of your ribcage, do so and focus your breathing into that space. Feel the flexibility of your ribs as you expand them on inhale and relax them on exhale.

- Now shift your attention to your upper chest. If you are able to, place the tips of your fingers on the front of your chest right below the collar bone. Focus breathing into this area, bringing awareness to your chest lifting slightly upon inhale, and softening back into your body on exhale.
- Try combining all three parts. Exhale fully, then focus on inhaling into the belly, up through ribcage, and then through the upper lungs. Gradually release the breath, noticing how the upper lungs, rib cage, and belly deflate as you do so.

Don't do Dirgha if you've had recent abdominal surgery, or if you have throat or sinus irritation or a respiratory infection.

Alternate Nostril Exercise (Nadi Shodhana Pranayama)

This technique is great for balancing the left and right hemispheres of the brain and balancing the vagal system. Studies of pranayama have demonstrated that alternate nostril breathing was the only type of breath work that was found to have a positive effect on the cardiovascular system (heart rate, respiratory rate, and blood pressure).

This breathing exercise involves breathing from alternate nostrils. It cleans nostrils and sinuses and is also helpful in the activation of the left and right side of the brain simultaneously.

- Get your body comfortable, sitting if possible.
- Place your left hand on your left knee, and lift your right hand up to your nose.
- Tuck your middle three fingers into the palm of your hand, leaving your pinky and thumb extended (the universal sign for "call me!")
- Complete an exhale, then use your right thumb to close your right nostril. Inhale through your left nostril.
- Use your pinky to close your left nostril while opening your right nostril and exhaling through the right nostril.
- That is one complete breath cycle. Continue for up to five minutes, making sure that you always finish your practice by finishing with an exhale on the left side.

Don't do alternate breathing if you have hypertension, an active migraine, or an active sinus or chest infection. Also generally be aware of discomfort if you have a full stomach.

Bee Breath (Bhramari Pranayama)

This technique has been shown to reduce stress and anger, help with sleep induction, and help strengthen the muscles of the throat.

- Get comfortable, sitting upright if possible.
- Take a full inhalation
- Hold for three seconds,
- Close your ears using your index fingers
- Make a soft humming sound on exhale (like the sound of a buzzing honeybee).
- Repeat 5-6 times if possible.

As an alternative to closing your ears, you can place your thumb on the cartilage between your cheeks and your ears, so you feel the vibration but aren't blocking off your hearing.

Don't do bee breath if you are actively suffering from a migraine. Also generally be aware of discomfort if you have a full stomach.

Ocean Sounding Breath (Ujjayi Breathing)

This technique is fantastic for centering and focusing concentration without the nervous system activation that usually comes along with increasing our attention.

- Sit comfortably, upright if possible.
- Relax your jaw and keep your lips closed.
- Start with some deep breathing to bring your body's focus back to breathwork.
- Now softly contract the back of your throat so you are making a "hhhhhhhh" sound upon inhale and exhale. Think of how you would use your throat to fog up a mirror. It can also be helpful to hold your cupped hands in front of your mouth and breathe into them so it sounds like holding a seashell up to your ear.

If it's hard to hear yourself, some people do well using headphones to block out other noise so they can hear the sound from inside their head. It's much easier to create the ocean sounding breath on exhale than inhale, so focus on the exhale first if you are practicing this technique and it's taking you a while to get it down.

No specific contraindications.

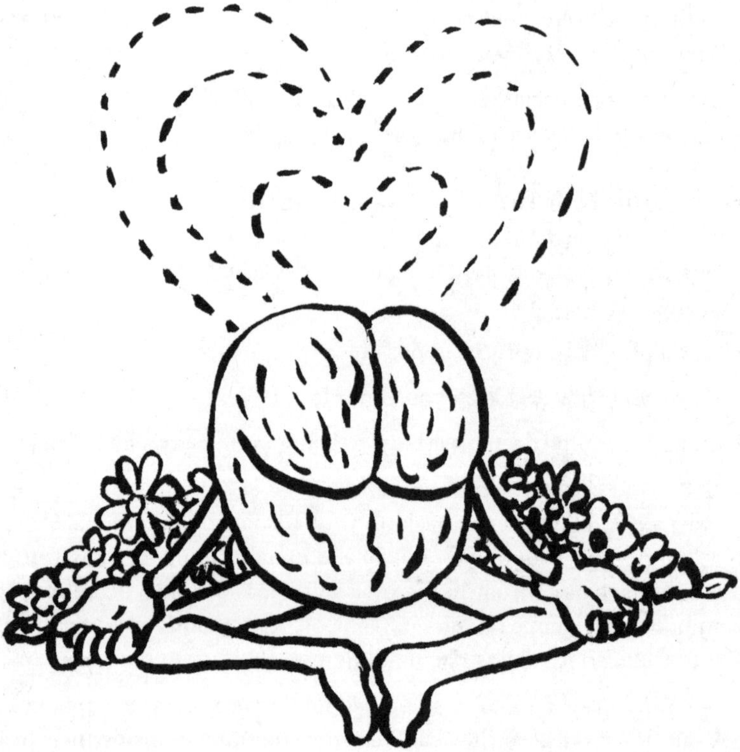

MINDFULNESS AND MEDITATION

In Unfuck Your Brain, I included a little intro to mindfulness and meditation. Let's get deeper into it here.

Mindfulness is the basic human ability to be aware and fully present in our own lives, to bear witness to the workings of our body and mind as well as what is going on around us. John Kabat-Zinn, likely the best known mindfulness instructor in the Western world, states that mindfulness is just awareness. It is the natural state of the human body, especially when we are young, but it is something we become trained out of when we developmentally get to the place where we realize we can escape our present reality and be somewhere else. In fact, we do that so often researchers have found that at least half of our waking hours are spent with wandering minds.

Mindfulness does not require meditation. Mindfulness is essentially the best path we have figured out for accepting the is-ness of our lives. This isn't to say that we should take shit lying down, it's about recognizing the reality of the current moment rather than getting so wrapped up in how we want it to be/how it should be that we get stuck. When we get stuck in how things should be we get stuck in unceasing judgment, which is not a place systemic change comes from.

Meditation, by contrast, is a formal process of focused attention and does not have to include mindfulness. Transcendental Meditation (TM) is probably the best known form of meditation that is not mindfulness-based. TM uses a monosyllabic sound as a mantra to help the mind get out of the loop of spinning thoughts (more on this in a bit). This seems like a nit-picky difference, but a mantra meditation is creating a new present moment with a specific repeated sound while mindfulness meditation is just about being in the present moment.

Mindfulness meditation is where the two meet. This is where that process of awareness is brought into the formal practice of focused attention. This doesn't mean perfect attention, but it is a process of recognizing when the mind wanders and refocusing awareness back to the present when it does, usually with some kind of anchor (the breath is the most common).

There is not a "correct" form of mindfulness, meditation, or mindfulness meditation. They all have the same goal of helping achieve a peaceful mind and manage stress so I am including a wide variety of practices for you to experiment with in this chapter.

You might have some beef with the idea of mindfulness and meditation. Which makes sense, because a lot of the breathless writing you've probably run across about it is about some kind of escape from reality into an ethereal higher consciousness. You might get the idea that you are supposed to go into meditating (or come out of it) empty-mind and completely calm. That it has to be done in a certain exact way every time which involves some weird pretzel contortion position. And probably shaving your head and wearing saffron robes. Or whatever. And none of that is true. None of this is about changing yourself. It's the opposite: meditation and mindfulness are about meeting yourself, finding yourself, and connecting to yourself exactly as you are in the present.

Will mindfulness and/or meditation change your life? Yes. But maybe not in the ways you expect it to or hope it will. Over a decade into practice, I still don't have a calm brain. But I do have space between my brain's chatter and my reactivity. I have a different level of awareness of how I'm reacting to myself and the world. I see different choices and different paths. You may think "that's it?" but as a person with a loud-ass brain, I can tell you it's still life-changing.

You know why mindfulness-based therapy is so brave? Because even when we are told that we will reach down and discover our innate goodness, we are still so fearful that isn't the case. What if we are the exception? What if we are the one person too broken inside to be worthy? What if the real truth is that I am that one person who is not ok?

Bravery is telling that voice to fuck off. Bravery is digging deeper still, past that voice, to listen through all the chatter. And to trust the goodness is there. And you (yep, even you with your broken, hurting, scarred, and fragile insides) are still innately, beautifully, and so deeply good.

You will find that space. Keep looking.

This Is Your Brain on Mindfulness and Meditation

Mindfulness has been so well researched at this point that the info on the research backed benefits would be an encyclopedia in and of itself. But here are a few of the big ones that are most relevant to what we're focusing on in this book.

Mindfulness has been found to:

- Positively impact overall human functioning (cognitions, emotions, physiology, and behavior)
- Improve attention and focus

- Provide greater empathy and compassion, positively impacting interpersonal behavior
- Reduce proactive interference (when old stuff we know gets in the way of new stuff we are trying to learn)
- Help manage caregiver burnout
- Help manage chronic pain (showing just as much benefit as CBT)
- Help overcome insomnia
- Help with the management of mental health issues, including depression, anxiety, and PTSD
- Increase the body's immune response

A lot of studies have been done specifically about meditation, and the results are fascinating. We have literally thousands of years of mindfulness and meditation practice documented in human history that include reported benefits of the practices. With the advent of fMRI (functional magnetic resonance imaging), we can actually see how mindfulness and meditation affects the functioning and even the neuroplasticity of the brain, which is the brain's ability to grow, learn, and heal damage.

When scientists have looked at people's brains while they meditate, they find that within a few minutes of beginning meditation, the ventromedial prefrontal cortex lights up, meaning that this part of the brain is electrically firing. This is the thinking brain, the "monkey mind"—the part of the brain that tries to connect every thought to our "me-ness" and plans for the worst all the time. This is why the first few minutes of meditation feel so grunge and funky.

If you stick with it past those first uncomfortable minutes, the lateral prefrontal cortex lights up instead. This is the part of the brain that has more equilibrium. Our thoughts become less chatty and me-focused, less obsessed with potential catastrophes and more accepting of what is actually happening.

If we meditate daily (or at least really regularly) for two to three months, then our dorsomedial prefrontal cortex starts to get activated during meditation. This is the part of the brain that is related to empathy. We become more compassionate in our daily lives toward ourselves and others.

Over time, meditation increases gray matter in the prefrontal cortex, which is brilliant for emotional regulation, focus, and ability to problem solve. It also thickens the hippocampus and decreases the amygdala response, which helps us stay anchored in the present (read: less likely to have our fight-flight-freeze response activated). The brains of meditators also show an increase in alpha wave activity (something people pay good money to induce with neurofeedback, hypnotherapy, and alpha stims). Meditation keeps neural connections strong and prevents atrophy. Essentially, the brain of a meditating middle-aged person is comparable to the brain of a 20 year old.

Meditation also changes the chemical structure of our body. It increases the chemicals that help us maintain calm homeostasis. GABA (gamma-aminobutyric acid), serotonin, and BDNF (brain-derived neurotrophic factor) are all chemicals that are of benefit to mood stabilization and all are increased with meditation. Additionally, the hormones associated with stress (cortisol and adrenaline) seem to be mitigated by meditation.

This gets us back to the idea of a vagal window of tolerance. More and more research is demonstrating that meditation not only helps while we're meditating, but also helps us remain in our window of tolerance in general by creating positive alterations in the neural activity and connectivity of the default mode networks of the brain (the storytelling brain). This means meditation is teaching the brain to learn process-specific states of calm (all the time regulation) instead of state-specific calm (we're calm when we meditate).

If you're looking for the benefits of mindfulness and meditation, but are uncomfortable with it being tied to a particular religious or spiritual practice, you can find therapeutic programs that utilize these techniques without being tied to "something bigger." Mindfulness and meditation practices have long been used in clinical settings like therapy, and there is a huge and growing amount of research backing this up.

The two that have been around the longest and studied the most are Mindfulness-Based Stress Reduction (MBSR) which was developed by John Kabat-Zinn and his colleagues at the University of Massachusetts Medical Center and Mindfulness-Based Cognitive Therapy (MBCT), developed by CBT specialists at the UCLA School of Medicine, using Kabat-Zinn's work as a starting point. MBSR has a more generic application and is applied to stress arising from a variety of life events including physical or mental illness. MBCT is a spin-off of MBSR, and tends to target specific conditions and vulnerabilities. It adds cognitive behavior therapy (generally considered the therapy gold standard) to MBSR in order to add focus to shifting patterns of thoughts, emotions, and behaviors that do not serve your emotional health. Other common modalities, most notably Dialectical Behavioral Therapy (DBT) and Acceptance and Commitment Therapy (ACT), are not mindfulness-based, but rely on mindfulness as a core skill.

Trauma Sensitive Practice

While mindfulness and meditation can be of huge benefit to a large number of people, it isn't magic for everyone, and may require trauma-sensitive modifications, just like any body-oriented practice. If you have a trauma history and try to sit down to meditate following any standard instructions, it's possible that it will fuck you up.

Things you may notice that are signs of dorsal and ventral vagal responses (either fight and flight activation, or freezing up) can include:

- Prolonged, uncontrollable crying
- Shortness of breath
- Trembling
- Clenched fists
- Getting very pale or very flushed
- Excessive sweating
- Depersonalization
- Derealization
- Fear
- Panic

Having a trauma history, or having a trauma response while meditating, doesn't mean you can't meditate or practice mindfulness. But those of us with intense trauma histories need to have space for choice. This means choosing to work through a trauma history in our own time and in our own way, instead of having memories flood our present moment and disrupt our lives. Traditional meditation practices encourage us to go back to the breath and to treat any triggers or activation as thinking that detracts from the present moment. Instead, a trauma informed practice helps us lean into uncomfortable feelings without losing our zone of tolerance.

If trauma is an issue for you, here are some tips, many of them inspired by David Treleaven's book Trauma-Sensitive Mindfulness. This may be familiar from the breathwork chapter.

1) Recognize your internal go and stop signals (thoughts, feelings, body sensations). You don't have to sit and stew in emotional pain. Some discomfort can help us grow, but retraumatizing ourselves fixes fucking nothing. Notice what practices are helpful and which are activating. Get up and take a break when you need to, but next time stay seated just a little longer.

2) You don't have to sit in physical pain either. Take breaks when you need to or alter how you are holding your body. Move into

a more comfortable position or wiggle in place a little. While meditation (specifically mindfulness meditation) has been shown in research to be incredibly helpful to pain management, it's not supposed to be torture. Support your body in whatever ways you need to to be as comfortable as possible.

3) Meditation exercises often suggest closing your eyes. This is totally optional. If you don't feel comfortable with your eyes closed in the environment you're in, leave them open. Or start with a soft gaze as a step towards closing your eyes.

4) If your practice involves attending a class, talk to the teacher. If there is any hands-on component (like if your practice involves yoga or tai chi), you can tell them not to provide physical adjustments (meaning, not to touch you).

Just like with everything else in this book, listen to your body more than you listen to me. Don't do things that are awful and upsetting for you. Meditation is a chance to work through crap without being overactivated. So if you are overactivated by something, it may not be for you, at least not right now.

How to do Mindfulness and Meditation

The rest of this chapter is devoted to giving you a taste of some of the variety of practices to see which resonate best with you. There is meditation without mindfulness, mindfulness without meditation, and practices that incorporate both.

The fact that there are such a wide variety of practices out there that have demonstrated effectiveness is really good news. If you have had a bad experience with any practice in the past, it means there are a variety of other methods you can experiment with.

Let's try some new stuff, yeah?

In chapter 4 of *Unfuck Your Brain*, I include instructions for a basic mindfulness meditation. If you're new to meditation, it would be a great idea to start there and then move on to the different variations of meditation I go over in this chapter.

Most research demonstrates that 15 minutes of practice is the amount of time it takes to gain the benefits of mindfulness meditation. If you can't tolerate it for that long, that's also okay. Practice working up to it. If you find that it's helpful and want to extend time out further that's also great, but not required.

Mindfully Eating a Raisin

This mindful eating practice is a classic MBSR (mindfulness-based stress reduction) technique. It gives you a different element to focus on, other than your breath.

- Place a few raisins in your hand. And no you don't have to use raisins, any food will do. I've found that even people who don't like raisins are not bothered by them in this exercise. But if they really gross you out, grab something else.
- Pretend this is your first day on the planet. This is a new food that you have never seen before, and you are an alien explorer that is going to make scientific study of raisins and raisin-ness. Use all five of your senses to explore it. Turn it around with your fingers, notice the color, the tactical sensations. How does it fold or reflect light? What does it smell like when you hold it up to your nose? Does it make any sound if you apply pressure?
- You will start having thoughts of the "Why am I doing this? This is fucking weird" variety. Totally normal. Just recognize them as a thought you are having and bring yourself back to the activity.
- Bring the object slowly to your mouth. Notice how automatic it is for your hand to bring nourishment up to your mouth. Notice whatever anticipation you are experiencing. Is your mouth watering? Gently place the raisin on your tongue without biting down. Explore the sensation of the raisin in your mouth.
- When you are ready, bite down. Notice the taste that is released when doing so. Notice how you habitually move it to one side of your mouth over another. Slowly chew the raisin. Notice how it changes in texture, and flavor as you chew. When you feel ready to swallow, notice your conscious intention to do so. Pay attention to the sensation of it moving down your throat, to your esophagus.

How did the experience of eating differ when you did so mindfully? What did you notice? What did you enjoy? What was uncomfortable?

Metta Meditation

Metta loosely translates to loving-kindness. In essence, it's a focus of general goodwill, friendliness, and open-heartedness. It's a way of engaging in the world without all shields up, without feeling defensive and ill at ease.

A metta meditation involves focusing not just on the breath, but on a series of healing statements about yourself, another person or group of people, or the world.

The original text from the Buddha on metta (as translated from The Discourse on Loving-Kindness) is:

> Wishing: In gladness and in safety, may all beings be at ease.
> Whatever living beings there may be, omitting none
> Let none deceive another, or despise any being in any state
> Let none through anger or ill will wish harm upon another.

These statements have an archaic language (and don't worry, we're gonna use a more modern format), but speak to universal human struggles across time. Specifically, the harm we experience just by being a human living in an imperfect world, and the continued harm (suffering) that we impose on ourselves in the process. Metta meditation allows us to work with the feelings we avoid the most, like aversion and despair. The Buddha stated that by working with uncomfortable emotions, we can transform them into something that serves us better.

When we don't like someone, doing a metta meditation on their behalf feels gross. My meditation instructor encourages focusing on the easiest people first, the people or living things we love and adore (yes, it can absolutely be your pup or your favorite tree in the park if you aren't feeling particularly people-y). After that, we can move to the people who are a little more sketch, and finally to the people we consider the most difficult as we build tools to release whatever it is about them that creates toxic emotions within us.

Also, we should offer metta to ourselves. Self-hatred is far more common than hatred of others. Buddhist meditation instructor Sharon Salzberg discusses how this is super common in Western culture as an offset of systemic oppression (defined by bell hooks as "imperialist white supremacist capitalist patriarchy"). Because no matter what set of circumstances or privileges we have accessed, no one measures up to these standards. We all struggle with not-enoughness and feel a continuous need to earn our space in the world, rather than recognizing that we deserve by the sheer fact that we are human.

Here are some more modernized metta meditation statements that you can use in your own practice, that are used more often now than the Buddha's originals. You can say these out loud or think them in your head, timed with your breath. Where there is a blank you insert "I" or "my" for doing metta for yourself, "you" or "your" or the name of the person you are focusing on, or "all" meaning the entirety of sentient beings.

- May _____ be protected and safe from harm from others
- May_______be protected and safe from self-inflicted harm
- May _____ be happy
- May _____ body support the practice of loving awareness

- May _____ be free from anxiety
- May _____ be free from anger
- May_____be free from fear
- May_____love themself/themselves/myself exact as they are/I am
- May _____ be free from suffering
- May _____ find peace in the world
- May _____ find balance between attachment and apathy

Mantra Meditation

Using a mantra to meditate is the best known form of meditation that isn't mindfulness based. In Sanskrit, man translates to "mind," and tra means "to free from." Mantras are used as a tool to free the mind (or to be freed from the mind). They help break the cycle of spinning thoughts that lead to anxiety, self-doubt and the like. Transcendental Meditation, which relies on mantras, got really big when Maharishi Mahesh Yogi brought the ancient technique to the US.

As with other practices that have spiritual roots, researchers in the US were interested in how the techniques themselves, outside a cultural context, can alter physical and mental states. Since the 1970s, Herbert Benson, professor of medicine at Harvard Medical School and founder of the Benson-Henry Institute for Mind Body Medicine at Massachusetts General Hospital, has studied what creates that meditative state, which he termed "the relaxation response" (with a bestselling book by the same name).

Benson has experimented with subjects repeating Sanskrit mantras as well as nonreligious words, such as "one." He's found that regardless of what the practitioner repeats, the word or phrase has nearly the same effects: relaxation and the ability to better cope with life's unexpected stressors. Mantras actually soothe the default mode of the brain, keeping it from going into storytelling mode creating anxious thoughts.

Sanskrit chanting is often part of many practices, including different branches of yoga. Sanskrit often has complex meanings beyond the literal translations. I've found that learning the relevance and meaning behind mantras like om mani padme hum lends depth to my practice. But, mantras in any language have the same effect. You can chant any contemplative expression from your faith system (like "Hail Mary, full of grace") or something more generally spiritual (like "I am Divine Love"), or any secular humanist phrase, and gain the same default mode benefit. Or maybe there is a certain mantra about your path of healing that you want to use.

Once you've decided on a mantra, find your comfy place and set a timer for yourself. Start with a few deep breaths and then start chanting your mantra (in your head is fine, outloud voice is also fine). If you catch your thoughts wandering, bring them back to the mantra.

Meditation in Motion

What we often refer to as "walking meditation" is really just "meditation in motion." Whatever device you may use for mobility will become part of the process.

- Find an unobstructed space in which you can move back and forth in a reasonably straight line for about ten feet (yes, you can also do a greater distance). If you are walking and are able to do so barefoot (and it's an area that is safe for you to be barefoot), you may find it helpful to gain more awareness of how your body creates balance for movement.
- If you are walking, bring your attention to your feet, shifting your weight from side to side and front to back, as far as you are able to do so comfortably. Lift your head and chest so you are facing forward, let your shoulders drop away from your ears. You can clasp your hands behind your back, hold them in front of you, or let them hang loosely at your side.
- Lift up one of your legs. It doesn't matter which, but take notice. Pay attention to how your weight shifts in your body when you do so. What does the other side of your body need to do to hold your full weight. Move your lifted foot forward, then place your heel on the ground and roll the rest of your foot down, ending with your toes. Pay attention to how your other foot begins to lift and move forward as well. Bring that foot forward and repeat.
- If you use a device for mobility, focus your attention on the sensations of movement. Connect the sensation of using your hands to connect to the mobility support and guide you forward. Feel the sensation of moving forward and your connection of being embodied and supported in that experience. If you are using a chair that relies on voice, facial expression identification, or the like, focus on how you engage your body and connect to the chair to create movement. What shifts do you feel physically and energetically?
- No matter how you create movement, your mind will wander as minds like to do. As your attention wanders off, you can bring yourself back to present practice with the thought of "attention engagement forward" or an anchoring reminder of your choice.

- When you come to the end of your path (unless it was a circle to begin with), turn fully around, face the direction from which you came, and start over. If you are moving in a circular shape, simply notice that you have completed one full round.

Meditation on the Soles of the Feet

This particular practice has been shown to be really beneficial for the management of aggression and anger.

- If you are standing, stand in whatever relaxed posture is most natural for you.
- If you are sitting, sit comfortably with the soles of your feet flat on the floor or another surface.
- Breathe normally. You don't have to do deep belly breaths or anything outside of how you regularly breathe.
- Now, think back on an incident that made you very angry. Stay with that anger. Let the angry thoughts flow through your mind without trying to stop them. You may notice your heart rate or breathing go up as you remember that anger.
- Now, shift all your attention to the soles of your feet.
- Slowly, move your toes, feel your shoes covering your feet, feel the texture of your socks or hose, the curve of your arch, and the heels of your feet against the back of your shoes. If you do not have shoes on, feel the floor or carpet with the soles of your feet.
- Keep breathing naturally and focus on the soles of your feet until you feel calm and the physical signs of anger dissipate, this will take probably 10 to 15 minutes.
- Slowly come out of your meditation, sit quietly for a few moments, and then resume your daily activities.

Cognitive Defusion

Remember earlier when I talked about how we can practice mindfulness without doing so in the form of meditation? And how some forms of therapy aren't mindfulness-based but still center mindfulness as a core skill? Cognitive defusion is a technique from Acceptance and Commitment Therapy (ACT) that focuses on mindfulness in managing being overwhelmed without having to sit on a cushion with it. As with the other practices listed here, this is one I use with clients regularly.

This skill is designed to help manage thoughts that are painful, overwhelming, unkind, or unhelpful. We tend to over identify (fuse) with our thoughts, so thinking something like "I'm terrible" or "I don't deserve love" can become the truths we operate within unless we approach them with mindfulness.

- Start by identifying a hurtful self-criticism that you want to work with. If you can shorten it into a phrase or single sentence, it's easier to work with than a rambling paragraph of self-recrimination (which is my personal speciality).
- Let yourself engage with the thought rather than try to push it away. You can repeat it to yourself mentally or verbalize it out loud.
- Now add this modifier in front of it: "I'm having the thought that . . . " so "I don't deserve love" becomes "I'm having the thought that I don't deserve love."
- Now take another step away from it by adding "I notice . . . " so we are now at "I notice I'm having the thought that I don't deserve love."
- It may be wordy and complex at first, but with some practice you may be able to shorten it into a sentence that really gets at the heart of the issue.
- Now reflect on whatever mental shifts you noticed as you defused the thought by recognizing it as an experience your brain was having instead of your life operating instructions. What did you notice?

Mindfulness and Pain Management

Mindfulness for pain, whether acute or chronic, doesn't mean learning to ignore the pain so we can go about our day (let's be real, we are already way too good at that). Trying to escape pain just gets us more ensnared in the long run. When we feel what's real in the present rather than trying to hide from it, we are more awake and alive to reality. It's how we bear witness to reality, to be curious and compassionate rather than shaming and blaming or prickly and protective.

Earlier, I wrote about how pain works in the brain. You can use mindfulness to specifically train your brain to cope with pain by recognizing its existence rather than trying to avoid it completely or get swallowed whole by it.

When we hurt, our breathing tends to get shallow, in an attempt to avoid the pain. We can breathe into and through the pain as a form of mindful recognition, allowing the pain to speak to us and pass through.

Mindfulness can also include "conscious distraction" which seems like a contradictory statement, but if we start with attention, we can then make a decision to feel into our pain or to let ourselves carve out a break from it which is far different from "ignore ignore ignore."

We can also breathe into the places that are not in pain, focusing on whatever areas of our body are not experiencing pain at this moment, even if it's just the middle toe of your left foot.

If the pain is wildfire, you can even choose a focal point outside the body and declare it your no-pain zone to focus on while breathing deeply. This gives the nervous system some relief from its constant messaging. I had a college professor that started each class with a candle and a vase of flowers as our focal point in the middle of the room. Nowadays, I have a tattoo on my right wrist that serves as my focal point/anchor/reminder to be present.

Humming for Migraines

Tony Bateson, a chronic migraine sufferer, recognized that his migraines dissipated when he ranted and raved out loud. So he started studying, first of all, how that could possibly be, and second of all, if he could gain the same effect without the yelly part. He found a good deal of literature on sound healing and came up with the hypothesis that humming at a particular frequency was the part that disrupted the headaches. He began to play with the technique, particularly with mantra meditation, and came up with something that has helped others.

Others have since studied what he came up with and stated that it makes sense. Pain takes control of our brain oscillations (brain waves) and if we use an acoustic that creates an oscillation of the opposite frequency as the pain oscillation, it would neutralize. Acoustic frequencies, like mantras, have been shown to change the brain. So electrophysiologists think it may help with other pain as well.

The frequency Bateson found most effective to hum is 140 hz, which is essentially a low C sharp. My Buddhist-y and yoga-y readers will recognize this as the same tone as the chanted OM (which is also known as the sound of creation). If you are trying to find that frequency, look for a YouTube video so you don't have to invest in a pitch pipe to get it right. You are going to hum with your upper and lower jaw held together, teeth touching, but not a clenched jaw. Try to keep the hum as regular a rhythm as possible.

- Hum for 10 seconds
- Take a deep breath in through the nose
- On the exhale, hum again for 10 seconds
- Repeat for 9 more cycles (ten cycles total of hums)
- Rest for two minutes
- Repeat the sequence (ten cycles and two minutes of rest)
- Then rest for 10 minutes before going about your day

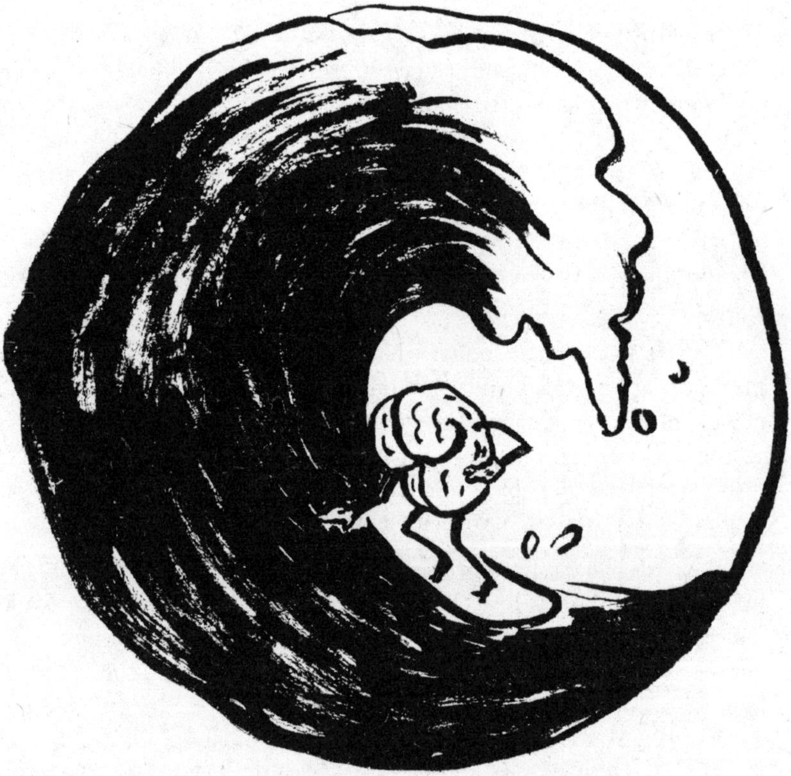

UNFUCK YOUR MOVEMENT

This chapter is about exercise. Wait, tho! Don't skip it! I swear there is not going to be any exercise shaming or body shaming! Quite the opposite, give me a chance?? I touch on exercise in Unfuck Your Brain, but here we're going to get deeper into it.

The idea of exercise often has a punitive connotation. Even the most benign definition of exercise I could find ("a subset of physical activity used for the specific purpose of promoting fitness and overall health") still reads as a chore to be completed, like: get your teeth cleaned, bring the dog to the groomer, and jump on the treadmill. Even if you like the results, the task itself being a chore is exactly the problem.

I'd like to change that. I'd like to reclaim moving our bodies because our bodies like to move. I want the process to be as joyful as the end result.

I grew up in probably the last unruly-gang-of-kids generation. As a Gen Xer, we ran in packs of bikes and Big Wheels and didn't come home until the street lights came on. If you got thirsty, you drank from the hose. In short? We played.

And I want to bring that sense of play back, in whatever way that makes sense to you. I happen to adore hiking, swimming, and yoga. And when I say yoga, I don't mean the sweaty kind that smells like feet and butts, but gentle practices. You may not like any of those things but maybe you adore basketball. Or gardening. Or maybe you are one of those people who digs running even when no one is chasing them with an ax. Or you used to. I want to encourage you to find that joy again. Or if you never had it, I hope that you can in some way find it.

This chapter is all about the positive effects of movement on our bodies. I'm including it all because it's extra motivation and I'm a research nerd. And if it motivates you to try something new or pick up something you used to adore then I did my job. But my hope is that you continue playing just because you love it.

How Does Movement Help?

Physical exercise is good for us, and not because of burning calories, or how it might make our bodies look.

We know this not just from people who took surveys and said they felt better after a boxing class. There is evidence of a biochemical effect of exercise on our mental health. Any kind of physical exercise is positively correlated with an increase in serotonin, the brain chemical that makes us feel good. You will read tons of stuff that says "exercise increases serotonin" and while that may be true, if you are a "show me the research" and "trust but verify" crank like I am, the mechanisms behind this assertion are super important to you. So let's look at that.

Some research shows that body movement increases the plasma level of certain branched chain amino acids (BCAAs) in the brain, which increases tryptophan absorption (which then bio-converts to serotonin). Another benefit: physical activity increases the protective cells and hormones (like endorphins) that mitigate our immune response, meaning the body releases fewer pro-inflammatory signals, which also ties in to better mental health.

Exercise has shown, time and again, to be of greater benefit than medications in managing dysthymia and milder forms of depression. Medications have a risk-benefit ratio that moving our bodies does not have. So much so that in the United Kingdom, the National Institute for Health and Clinical Excellence supports exercise as the first treatment option for these (again, milder cases). A study published in the Journal of Clinical Psychiatry in 2011 found that individuals who were being treated for depression and had sedentary lifestyles found symptom relief after a few months of a regular walking routine. Again, we're not talking about athletics, just whatever amount of movement feels good to your body.

Bonus points if exercise happens outdoors, where light exposure is also shown to be beneficial to mitigating symptoms of depression because you get the added effect of the vitamin D. I live in South Texas where it's winter right now but still sunny, bright, and will get into the low 70s. Not everyone has that option. People who live in places where there is less access to natural light are starting to invest in sun lamps to mimic the effect.

Other research demonstrates that exercise helps us build resilience to both physical and psychological stressors. Because only a complicated term will do, we call it the cross-stressor adaptation hypothesis. The idea is that physical exertion (not extreme but engaged in regularly) creates positive adaptations to both the HPA Axis and the sympathetic nervous system, making both of them less likely to become over-activated. This increased zone of tolerance may be a function of self-regulation. That is, exercise builds mindfulness of our autonomic state, helping us stay in that window of tolerance.

For individuals with chronic pain, movement can be very healing with some careful caveats. You have probably heard that exercise is incredibly helpful for managing chronic pain. This is absolutely true. But you have probably also experienced a significant worsening of your pain when you tried to exercise, which is absolutely real. Science backs you up. For normies, working out actually decreases the experience of pain. Things hurt less because endorphins are kicking in.

But the same wonkiness that causes chronic pain to begin with gets turned up even more when you first work out, which is why most of us end up avoiding exercise. It fucking hurts because the same mechanisms in your body that upregulated your pain response to begin with, get activated when you work out, especially if it's aerobic exercise and you haven't done anything in a while. The release of endorphins that actually help pain exists for normies, but not us.

So if it's true that exercise is making things worse, then why is all this data saying that it helps? There's a couple of things that we really have to consider when looking at movement for pain management. The first is the healing effect that builds over time. And that we need to focus on exercise that isn't aerobic in nature, and work with the duration and intensity that is manageable for our pain levels. This may mean swimming, where joints are supported by water. Or restorative yoga which is slower in movement and the forms are supported with pillows and props. There is a balance to be found between movement causing more pain and movement helping pain that is more razor-edge for individuals with chronic pain disorders.[12] But please don't give up. And don't think that gentle movement is a cop out. There are still huge benefits to be gained in making exercise part of your treatment plan, even if your legs up the wall in yoga just feels like a nice nap in the moment!

It teaches us, body to brain, that our body is not our enemy. And we all need more of that. Whether we struggle with chronic pain or not.

When clients ask me what forms of exercise I think they should engage in, my first answer is: anything you like or are interested in trying. If there isn't anything, try things that amplify that self-regulation process, such as yoga and qi-gong. That's not just because I like yoga—let me talk about why in a little more depth.

The Science of Movement

The human body is biochemical at one level, but at a deeper level it is electromagnetic. Everything contained in the human body is vacuum

12 Sciency stuff? Essentially, working out once, especially when it's something that is super bouncy-aroundy makes pain spiky if you have a chronic pain disorder because it increases phosphorylation of NMDA (N-methyl-d-aspartate) receptors in the RVM (rostral ventromedial medulla). But gentler and more regular movement reduces NMDA receptor phosphorylation, meaning it helps teach the body to be less pain activated over time. Then, over further time, it increases serotonin levels and our naturally occurring opioids in the body (including in the RVM which is what was initially causing the increase in pain). Your body eventually learns to use exercise to feel better the way it does for normies.

packed in between layers of connective tissue called fascia. Fascia connects organs to muscle, to spine, to nerves. The primary ingredient of fascia is collagen. Collagen is more than just strong – it's full of crystals, specifically, hydroxyapatite crystals, which are composed of calcium and phosphates therefore conduct electricity. Fascia creates impermeable compartments throughout the body. If you look at the main fascia structures throughout the body (you perv you), you see that they match up not only with the vagus nerve but the smaller pathways mapped by doctors of Traditional Chinese Medicine—the multitude of points used in acupressure and acupuncture.

This means that when we move our body, it causes an electrical charge in the crystalline material throughout our body. The connective fabric of our bodies creates a living electrical web.

So not only does our chemical body demonstrate a direct impact on our mental health, so does our electromagnetic body, communicating through an electromagnetic field. The intentional use of our body's electromagnetics (any kind of movement, and probably especially mindful movement) encourages interoception (our connection to the internal working of our bodies—our felt sense) and energetic discharge (a release of emotional tension from the body).

This is why movement is so effective as trauma therapy. When we exercise, we aren't just building serotonin, decreasing inflammation, and making our hearts healthier. We are reaching into where our emotions start and influencing their movement in the body. That is, we are teaching our body safety. And that is the foundation of trauma therapy: calibrating ourselves back to that physiological zone of safety.

Some Movement to Try

If you're new to exercise, coming back to it after a long time, recovering from an injury or illness, or have a history with exercise that's stressful or traumatic, I recommend starting with gentle movements. While there are very few times where I wouldn't suggest any kind of movement (being in traction in a hospital being the big one), I am big on the idea of "just move, whatever floats your boat." But there are a couple things I will specifically recommend to people in certain cases that I want to review real quick before we all take a taco break.

It needs to be said that in any cases where exercise is being used as part of a mental health treatment, jumping into it without any kind of clinical support can be dangerous. Activating sensations, thoughts, and emotions will come to the surface and you will need a space to process them out. Trauma informed exercise trainers and instructors are incredibly helpful, but also talk to your therapist, your sponsor, or whomever you are working with on your mental health as well.

Movement, just like working on sleeping, eating, medications, and supplements, is a process. Tracking what you do and what results you see is how you will develop a "best self" plan. So give it a whirl and track it like you're tracking any other changes you're making.

Gentle Movement

Some of the gentler forms of movement include yoga, tai chi, qi gong, or just plain walking at a pace and a distance that isn't painful for you. These are good ways of moving your body without causing strain or pain, plus they are the types of exercise that have been shown to have benefit to trauma recovery. When I started doing yoga in the 90s, it was not yet a ubiquitous practice (at least in Texas). Nowadays it's far easier to find gentle movement type classes, either online (live feed or videos) or in person. If you are looking to incorporate this work for trauma recovery, ask your therapist (if you are seeing someone) about specific teachers they recommend. Otherwise, start looking around. Some teachers are trained in trauma-informed yoga and other practices. Private studios may be out of your price range, but community centers may have free or donation based classes. The local "alternative" papers will usually have listings, as may your local library.

Functional Training and Corrective Exercise

If you have a history of physical injury or immobility that doesn't require physical therapy, but has still slowed you down, I recommend a personal trainer who specializes in functional training or corrective exercise.

Functional training is a workout with the purpose of improving certain activities in your life with more ease, less pain, and less chance of injury: like lifting heavy boxes at work or picking up heavy kiddos at home. Functional training is sort of between personal training and physical therapy, with the idea that resistance coupled with flexibility produces mobility. Instead of focusing on isolation training (targeting specific muscles in ways that don't necessarily support natural actions of the human body), functional training combines weight-bearing activities that build core muscle strength as well as compound movement exercises that focus on joint strength.

Corrective exercise works similarly, but focuses on fixing issues caused by imbalances and movement compensations as well as improving your functional mobility. For instance, if you have a condition that causes you to favor one side of your body, or weakness in an area due to a past injury or surgery.

These types of exercise aren't as fun and playful on the surface as something you inherently enjoy, but a good trainer can help you work in a way that helps you stay engaged while watching yourself progress.

Even exercise that is fairly prescriptive shouldn't feel bad, painful, or shameful. If it does, talk to your trainer or find a new one.

Strength and Muscle Building Exercises

Some people really enjoy a level of exercise that builds on getting strong, working up a sweat, and wearing themselves out enough that they feel a sense of having released negativity from their system. For them, gentle exercise isn't always the most therapeutic, and this isn't a one size fits all book, right? Weightlifting or another physical activity that requires a concomitant strength and muscle building program, like boxing, swimming, parkour, or circuit training programs like Crossfit or BodyPump may be more your speed.

While none of this is my personal cup of tea, there are a couple of situations where I highly recommend strength and muscle building. The first, is for individuals whose trauma history has left them feeling physically weak and overpowered. Feeling strong and capable in one's body can be an incredibly healing experience. The second, is for individuals recovering from certain eating and dieting disorders. When someone is engaged in an eating disorder, exercise is generally used as a means of influencing weight or shape. But in the case of anorexia or bulimia, that is exercise designed to burn calories (like running or aerobics). To be successful, strength and muscle building requires healthy energy consumption in the form of nutrient dense foods. The focus becomes on gainz instead of losses.[13]

---

13 However, it's worth noting that while this may be helpful for someone recovering from anorexia or bulimia, many facets of strength training may be at odds with someone recovering from muscle dysphoria (bigorexia), where the focus of the disorder is on building muscle. This is just one example of how the recommendations are going to vary based on each individual and their situation. Aaron Sapp and I have written more about muscle dysphoria in *Unfuck Your Masculinity,* information included also in *Unfuck Your Eating.*

UNFUCK YOUR SLEEP

I have people ask me how I get so much done in a day. I don't think I'm Superwoman by any means, in fact I think I'm pretty spoiled in that I really enjoy all the different things that I do. But it is a fair point, that I am juggling a lot of stuff that requires mental exertion and relational presence. And my answer to that question is a pretty simple one.

I get sleep.

Seriously, I prioritize and protect my sleep like it is absolutely necessary for my survival because honestly? It is.

When clients are presenting a big bundle of symptoms related to depression, anxiety, stress, stomach issues, chronic pain, chronic fatigue, and all those other things that mental health practitioners hear about, the first thing I ask is, "How's your sleep?"

And I usually get a double-take "WTF?" reaction. As in: "I just told you that running away from everything and living in a cave with the sasquatches in the Pacific Northwest seems like a good idea and you told me to have a juicebox and a nap?" And it's a fair question on the surface. What does sleep have to do with anxiety, depression, heart health, and inflammation? Probably a hell of a lot more than you realize.

What Sleep Is and How It Works

If you have read anything else I have written ever, you have accepted the fact that I like functional definitions that set the tone for what we're talking about. So here's one for sleep.

> Sleep is the brain's own meditative state that happens about 8 hours out of every 24 (if we are doing it right) in accord with our circadian rhythm. During sleep, some parts of the brain become way less active and other parts of the brain become way more active.

When I say circadian rhythm, I'm referring to the natural cycle that defines a day for us. Circadian just means "around day," after all. Every species on the planet (barring those that only live a very few days) has a circadian rhythm. It's generated by our internal time clock but informed by the earth's rotation. For my fellow science nerds, our internal time clock is an actual existing thing in the middle of the brain, called the suprachiasmatic nucleus.

Sleep occurs in four different stages that we cycle through during our time asleep. There are three stages of Non Rapid Eye Movement (NREM) sleep, moving from lighter to heavier and then there is Rapid

Eye Movement (REM) sleep which is the time period where most of our dreaming occurs.

The cycling through REM and NREM stages is weird AF. There is no symmetry to how it happens, except we do know that the NREM sleep is more dominant early and the REM sleep is more dominant later (and closer to the time we wake up). So if we stay up too late we lose more NREM sleep, and if we have to get up too early we lose more REM sleep. Both are important. Equally so. Let's get on with why that's the case, eh?

Why We Sleep

Understanding why we sleep has actually been one of the final frontiers of how-the-body-works science. And only in recent years do we have a better idea of what's actually going on.

When we are awake we are taking in all kinds of new information, right? NREM and REM sleep have different functions in terms of what our brains do with that information.

The brain is busy during the day, attending to all of our ongoing shenanigans. Sorting through those shenanigans takes time and energy we don't have when we are active. NREM sleep is our time to store this new info, strengthen some connections, and prune away the unnecessary bullshit. It reinforces remembering what we need to remember and forgetting what we need to forget.

REM sleep is the time where we integrate all the info we brought in with the stuff we already knew to be true about the world. REM sleep is essentially our emotional processing time. It helps us recognize patterns and fuels our creativity. This is the likely purpose of the dreaming we do in this stage. It helps us make more intelligent and thoughtful decisions in future days. The brain is figuring out what things are important to remember and what things can be let go of. For those of us working through our old crap and creating new, healthier associations and coping skills, sleep is an important part of all of that happening.

The latest research shows that essentially, sleep time is housekeeping time. Research published by Dr. Maiken Nedergaard in 2013 found that the brain's toxin flushing system (the glymphatic system) is ten times more active when we are asleep than when we are awake. If the brain is a city, the glymphatic system DR334 is our sewer system (pleasant image, right?). During sleep, our neuroglial cells (the cells that support our neuron functioning; the word "glia" means "glue" in Greek) shrink up, allowing our sewer system to flush out. The toxins are pulled out of the brain and into the bloodstream so the liver and kidneys can process the waste out.

It takes a fuck ton of energy to propel this process, and the brain doesn't have the energy to spare when it's busy processing information during our waking hours. Toxins build up continuously in our brains and bodies as the side effect of being alive on the planet. That's not a cause for concern, as long as the body is equipped to do the cleaning out part. For the brain, this process happens continuously as we move through different cycles of sleep.

You might be wondering what this has to do with the stuff we talked about in Section One. Many of the toxins being flushed are neurodegenerative molecules so there is clean space between brain cells, allowing better intra-brain communication.

Additionally, there's adenosine, a chemical that exists throughout every cell in the body and is one of the neurotransmitters (chemical messengers) in the brain. Adenosine has an important proactive role in the body—it's a nervous system depressant, meaning it suppresses arousal so we don't have panic attacks 24/7. It builds up during our waking hours and plays a big role in our feeling sleepy at the end of the day. One of the things caffeine does is block the adenosine effect, which is why it makes us so jittery. Adenosine also builds up in areas of inflammation, trying to keep our inflammation responses from killing us. And we are now aware that inflammation occurs from emotional trauma, not just physical trauma and that neuroinflammation is wayyyy more common than scientists previously realized. So sleep is imperative in managing our body's response to inflammation.

Every single one of these processes relates to trauma recovery. Dumping old ways of relating to the world and interacting in new and healthy ways? Reducing chronic inflammation and body toxicity? Flushing the built up crud that blocks the brain messaging correctly, and tamping down neuroinflammation so you can start the next day with a clean slate? Enhancing decision-making ability and creativity? Get some sleep!

Are You Getting Enough Sleep?

Don't fucking lie to me, now. You aren't, are you? And you aren't alone. Authors of a National Sleep Foundation report noted that two-thirds of all adults in the US do not get the minimum recommended amount of sleep (7 hours) at least on weeknights, and generally not at all. And it's not like everyone is coming close but getting 6.5 hours or something. Most people are clocking way, way less on a regular basis. This isn't just a US problem, however. The two-thirds number is exactly the same in Japan and nearly that in the UK. Other countries vary in their number count but it's still way, way too high. Even in Germany, where it's "only" 30% of the population who is sleep deprived.

Seven to nine hours: that's what adults are supposed to get. I happen to be a nine-hour person, but seven is the minimum to ward off all the ills I'm going to discuss below. This isn't a Dr. Faith number, this is a World Health Organization number.

"Bah!" a lot of people say. "I'm one of those people who don't need much sleep."

"Bah!" I say in return. Bullshit, alas. The number of people who actually are able to gain all the benefits discussed above on less sleep is minute. Like a fraction of 1%. And it seems to be related to a variant of a specific gene known as BHLHE41.

So why do so many people think they are just fucking fine? Several reasons, I'm guessing. The first is the cultural norm of sleep deprivation. We think we are supposed to push through things and be all tough and shit. Sleeping a full 7 hours is a cultural sign of weakness. Another reason is that it's the norm for us personally. We don't realize that this isn't our optimal self. It's just how it's been for so long. Finally, research demonstrates that we greatly underestimate our level of impairment from sleep deprivation. The rate of mistakes we make when sleep deprived has been tested and quantified in studies, but ask us to estimate our level of impairment? We think we've got it under control.

Because sleep is inextricably tied to pretty much every function of the human body, it is not a shock that not enough sleep (or disruption of quality sleep) is associated with a multitude of problems.

Here's a fun list of things we are far more likely to develop if we are sleep deprived:

- Reduced immune system function and immune deficiency
- Reduced motor function
- Cancer and the spread of cancer
- Diabetes
- Infertility
- Alzheimer's
- Depletion of our gut microbiome
- Cardiovascular disease
- High blood pressure
- Higher susceptibility to infections
- Stroke
- Congestive heart failure
- Depression
- Anxiety

- Bipolar disorder
- Schizophrenia
- PTSD
- Suicidality
- Shorter life span
- Vehicle crashes and traffic deaths. Drowsy driving accounts for more of these than drugs and alcohol combined.

Now some of these things are causal. Accident rates due to drowsy driving? We make mistakes when impaired. Period. But it isn't always a cause and effect situation. No one is saying (that I'm aware of) that sleep deprivation causes PTSD or any other emotional or physical illness. Correlation is not causality. But treating sleep can greatly reduce the symptoms of these other issues and help promote healing and recovery.

How to Sleep Better

Okay, first of all, if you have the ability to get enough sleep (as in you can fall asleep just fucking fine) but you don't let yourself get enough sleep (as in, you are binging on Netflix or some dumb shit instead of putting yourself to bed): stop that shit right now and get enough sleep.

There, easy fix.

Now, for the rest of you who are trying to get enough sleep but have trouble doing so and have for some time? Like you don't sleep well for several nights a week for months on end? Or maybe you're getting crappy sleep quality?

It's possible you have a sleep disorder you'll need to get medical intervention for. Talk to your medical doctor if you think this might be the case. But insomnia generally stems from worry, rumination, anxiety, and other types of emotional distress. It's common. 1 out of 9 people meet the criteria for insomnia at any given moment. The rest of this section is for you. Let's unfuck your sleep.

Set Yourself Up to Succeed

First, make sure you have appropriate sleep opportunity time. You need to give yourself a good 30 minutes to fall asleep. So if you need 7 hours, put yourself to bed 7.5 hours before wakey-uppy time. Have a regular going to bed and getting up time, even on your days off.

I know. The advice "have a bedtime routine" makes you want to throw up in your mouth every time you read it. But have a bedtime routine. If you didn't fall asleep during your 30-minute opportunity window, don't perseverate over it. Don't look at the clock. Don't toss and turn. Get up and go do something. Don't turn on the Xbox or anything super stimulating, and nothing with blue lights in general (read: anything with a screen). Read something dry and boring like a Dr. Faith book. Do a load of laundry, empty the dishwasher, something like that. When you feel sleepy again, go back to bed.

Don't take late naps. Naps in the early afternoon tend to be beneficial to us. Naps later in the afternoon or evening (I know a lot of after-work nappers) can disrupt your nighttime sleep.

Weighted blankets are superb for supporting individuals who live with anxiety, ADHD, ASD, and other issues. They have also been shown to support sleep. Weighted blankets provide deep touch pressure, which raises serotonin levels in the body, which as we know from above, promotes the generation and release of melatonin in the body. Weighted blankets used to be prohibitively expensive, but now can be found for under 100 dollars with some research. For adults, you generally want to get a weight that is 5-10% of your healthy body weight[14]. For kiddos, the general number is 10% of their body weight plus a pound of two.

Other weighting options can include "Korean mink" blankets (which I've seen available for up to 10 pounds for about 30 dollars, and no they are not actually real mink) or just piling on whatever blankets you have in the house. If you do the pile on trick, you will probably have to drop the temperature in the house some more because it will be significantly warmer. Weighted blankets use plastic pellets for the weight, therefore aren't as hot to have over the body.

Create a Good Environment for Sleep

Bedrooms are for two things and watching TV isn't one of them. It's bad for your partnership if you have one and it's really fucking bad for your sleep. A poll taken by a TV manufacturer (LG to be precise) found that 61% of people fall asleep with the TV on. Besides the blue light disruption, the cacophonous noise in the background is going to disrupt your sleep quality.

If you do better with noise at night, try a noise machine. Many of them offer different settings from white noise, like rain or heartbeats. A lot of people also use a fan or air purifier. Both make white noise while helping with air circulation and cleaning toxins out of your space.

Try to get natural sun exposure during the day and limit your blue light exposure in the evenings. Charles Czeisler of Harvard Medical School found that individuals who used electronic reading devices (like Kindles) before bedtime had a harder time falling asleep, had reduced

14 This isn't by BMI standards because, as we are going to establish in the next chapter, that's garbage. But the weight your body is healthiest at. If you are under or over that right now, adjusting the weight of your blanket accordingly probably won't be helpful, and will likely not feel right.

levels of melatonin in the body, and were groggier the next morning. We're talking like a 50% reduction in melatonin levels. That's a big deal.

It's the blue light coming from our screens, y'all. Whether it's an e-reader, our phones, or the TV, our constant exposure to the blue light confuses our brain into thinking it's daytime for longer than it actually is.

And if you're thinking "Fuck off, Dr. Faith, watching Netflix in bed is my low key reason for living, I'm not giving that up"? Studies have demonstrated that people who used blue light devices and wore blue blocker glasses for three hours before bedtime produced just as much melatonin as people who were not exposed to blue lights. And the glasses are super inexpensive, like under ten bucks a pair. You can also get them in different reading glass strengths, which is what I switched to a few years ago. I think they're actually kinda cute.

Another option is to download a program like f.lux on your computers. It will change your computer display's light settings to match what the sun is doing outside. I'm currently typing on my laptop at 8PM and the light is a dimmer pink so I don't need to wear my blue blockers of sassiness.

Temperature can help or hinder sleep. Your body temp needs to drop 2-3 degrees Fahrenheit (1 degree Celsius for anyone on the planet not in the US) in order to be able to sleep. Sleeping with a colder room can really help. Optimally, the room should be about 65 degrees. Most people keep their rooms warmer than that so 65 may be a big change. Try dropping the thermometer a couple of degrees from where you usually keep it and see if that helps. You can also take a hot bath since you will have a temperature drop when you get out of the warm water into the cooler air. And while exercise is helpful to sleep in general, exercising close to bedtime will raise your core body temperature and may disrupt your sleep.

Track Your Sleep

For about five minutes, everyone and their dog was wearing a FitBit, smartwatch, or other tracking device. If you still do so, use it to track your sleep! If you don't have one (or, like me, don't want the continuous shaming about your level of inactivity) you can use a sleep tracking app instead. I've been using the SleepCycle app for about two years now and it's been really helpful. It uses the mic on my phone to track my stages of sleep and quality of sleep. It also listens for distressed breathing and will record a small clip if you are snoring or if you've always wondered what you say when you talk in your sleep. It's caught me having an asthma attack in the middle of the night, which was very helpful information. If you notice chronic breathing problems, you could have sleep apnea and you need to get a sleep study to find out. Even if you pay for the premium version, an app like this is waaaay cheaper than another tracking device.

You can also keep a notebook by your bed and jot down notes about sleep time and quality.

Maintain Your General Health

A lot of sleep disruption is due to stomach upset, needing to use the bathroom more, and breathing issues. Using other sleep hacks without treating the root causes may help a bit, but in the long term is more like changing deck chairs on the Titanic than anything else. For example, if you have blood sugar stress, you will likely be up peeing in the middle of the night a lot more than you would otherwise.

Remember the hierarchy of interventions? First, try looking at dietary changes, lifestyle changes, and supplements that can help manage underlying issues. For example, food sensitivities might be impacting your health and your sleep, so try an elimination diet to figure out what those are. Or maybe you sleep better when you've gotten a certain amount of exercise. Or meditating right before bed could clear out the anxiety that keeps you up. Anytime we can give our body what it needs to heal itself instead of treating symptoms, the better everything works.

Prescription Medicine

If sleeping pills induced a natural sleep—meaning, appropriate cycling through NREM and REM sleep—that would be awesome. But they don't. According to studies, sleeping pills (Ambien, Lunesta, and the like) only demonstrate a small improvement in the time it takes to fall asleep and they don't create the brainwaves that we see in real sleep. And they have a fuck ton of side effects. You've probably heard about people doing crazy zombie shit on sleeping pills. There's also the grogginess and forgetfulness that happens the next day. And they're associated with higher rates of infection and higher rates of cancer too. Also? Higher rates of death. All the things that are more likely to happen because of lack of sleep also happen on sleep induced by prescription sleep meds.

But that's not to say that allopathic medicine can't help with sleep. Some drugs can treat the underlying conditions that disrupt our sleep, like blood sugar and anxiety. Night terrors are something people with PTSD are often (understandably) seeking to medicate away, but even though sleep medications can lessen the night terrors, they also end up disrupting REM sleep and you also lose all the things REM sleep gives the body, so it's not a good trade-off in the long run. There is a prescription option that may work better. Many individuals with PTSD have higher levels of norepinephrine (noradrenaline) released by the nervous systems. Meaning that the hormone/neurotransmitter that the body uses to engage the fight or flight response is swimming around in their heads, promoting alertness, even when they are supposed to be sleeping. Essentially, people with night terrors are trying to sleep through an activated sympathetic nervous system, and they aren't able to maintain a zone of tolerance even when they are conked out. So some docs are using a high blood pressure drug called Prazosin, which has the side benefit of suppressing the noradrenaline without suppressing REM sleep. Chat with your prescriber about it if this is something you struggle with.

Supplements

Supplements can be an effective alternative, but we should always take into consideration possible side effects and interactions with other meds. As we will see in the last chapter when discussing aspirin and acetaminophen and the like, over the counter doesn't equate to totally safe. Please read the Supplements chapter of this book and talk with your doctor before experimenting with supplements.

Melatonin is one supplement a lot of people find useful, especially those who have trouble falling asleep to begin with. Our body produces the hormone melatonin in the pineal gland. We generally have enough of it unless something causes a deficiency (as caused by the blue light usage, for example, which is everyone and their dog at this point). Melatonin works best if you take it 2-3 hours before you go to bed since it helps amp up the body's own natural melatonin kicking in as part of your circadian cycle. If you take it like you would a sleeping pill (swallow pill and lie down) you'll not get near the same effect.

For every person I've met who has tried melatonin and thought it was brilliant, I've talked to someone else who said it did nothing for them. There's a good reason for that. Even if you are taking it exactly when you are supposed to, you may notice that you fall asleep pretty well but the staying asleep portion of the program is still problematic. You're not the only one. Most melatonin supplements are fast-acting instead of continued release, so you get your little burst but then it wears off.

Melatonin is contraindicated for individuals with seizure disorders or high blood pressure. It also shouldn't be taken with a prescription sleep medicine. Like everything else, check with your doc and be safe.[15]

One of the other supplements I often suggest (and I talk about it more in the Supplements chapter) is L-Tryptophan (yes, the stuff in

15 I know, I am saying this a batrillion times, but I have had a doctor who did not give a *fuck* about my supplement schedule and wouldn't even document it. Fortunately, I knew because of my training to watch for certain interactions but his lack of interest was dangerous. I changed doctors. My current doctor doesn't just document what I take, she is super fascinated with it all and takes notes for herself because she wants to learn more about other avenues of treatment. This is totally the kind of doc to look for, if you have any decision making power in the process.

turkey). It is one of the essential amino acids that the body doesn't produce on its own (unlike melatonin). We have to get it from our foods or in supplementation. L-Tryptophan is used by the body to make niacin. Niacin makes, among other things, serotonin. And serotonin is instrumental in our melatonin production.

Now I know you're thinking, wait, what? Serotonin? Does that make L-Tryptophan an antidepressant? Some research shows that L-Tryptophan does demonstrate some relief of depression-related symptoms. If you are able to add it in, you may be able to talk to your prescriber about reducing or discontinuing other medications you have been taking for depression. But let them in on what you're doing before you start futzing with your dosages, mmmkay?

If you add L-Tryptophan, you may still use a little melatonin to help the falling asleep part but you won't need nearly the dose because the L-Tryptophan will keep it producing throughout the night like a champ. And, yes, there are multiple studies that demonstrate that L-Tryptophan supplementation works like a boss for promoting sleep. But L-Tryptophan is contraindicated for people with eosinophilia-myalgia syndrome and may have some level of interaction with other antidepressants since it is also involved in serotonin production. So all together now: Check with your physician!

Valerian root and the kava plant have both been used for their sedative effect for thousands of years and can therefore be beneficial for sleep. While I'm a fan of both, I am more cautious about the brands being used than I am with melatonin and L-Tryptophan. Both of these supplements are more expensive to produce, making it more likely that you end up buying something with a non-efficacious dose because the manufacturer is trying to amp their bottom line. I prefer the Mediherb brand because the quality is above and beyond and the manufacturing is so transparent. Annnnnnd because they water-extract their kava in order to eliminate many of the side effects associated with other extraction processes. If you've heard about kava being unsafe, you were reading about kava lactone toxicity. Essentially, some extraction methods used on the kava plant also extract glutathione, which can damage the liver. Clearly no bueno. Mediherb products are only available through professional treatment providers (as is another brand on my short list, Galen's Way). For over the counter brands that are good quality, I lean toward Gaia Herbs and Mountain Rose Herbs. You may also find an herbalist in your area that makes their own extractions so you can see their process up close and personal.

Finally, here are a couple of teas to try sipping before bed. Grandma was right to give you chamomile. It's generally really safe, per the FDA. Though if you have a ragweed allergy, you may react to chamomile—they are from the same family. You do need to make sure you brew it properly to get the sleepy-sleepy effect. Use two to three tea bags and put a cover over the pot or your cup so all of the good oils don't escape in the steam.

Banana peels are not just brilliant in your compost pile (or fed directly to your rose bushes), you can make an amazing tea out of them—and bananas also contain L-Tryptophan. Cut off the stems and use them fresh, baggy them and freeze them to use frozen, or dehydrate them out to use later. One fresh peel is equal to about 2 tablespoons of dried peel, all of which is equal to one cup of tea. Boil water, throw in the peel, then cover and reduce the heat to let it simmer for about ten minutes. You can add cinnamon and vanilla if you dig, as well. Bananas (including the peels) are a good source of magnesium and potassium, which are both things bodies need anyway and something many people tend to not have enough of.

Substances to Avoid

Alcohol can help you pass out, but it's not going to give you the sleep you need. A study just published in the medical journal The Lancet determined that any health benefits of alcohol (like the classic "red wine is good for your heart!") are far outweighed by the risks. Essentially, the study authors found, there is no such thing as a safe amount of alcohol and it is the leading risk factor for death-and-disability-adjusted life years for those of us ages 15 to 49.

It also doesn't help that drinking makes you have to get up and pee more (because alcohol is a diuretic). It over-relaxes your muscles, even in your throat, making it more likely that you will snore. It disrupts your circadian rhythm, it amps up your alpha brain waves which then compete with your delta brain waves making the restorative sleep less effective, and it blocks REM sleep like a motherfucker.

So seriously. No drankin'. Or at least reduce your amount of alcohol way down. You're tracking your sleep now, so look at the differences on drinking and non-drinking nights. Even better, give it up for a month and track your sleep. If you aren't sure if there is an improvement, add it back in and notice the difference, just like you would with a food detox.

Also, avoid caffeine and nicotine before bedtime. Both are stimulants, right? We all have different rates of metabolism for these substances so pay attention to when you use either and how it affects your sleep. Some people can have coffee after dinner and be fine, while others of us need to cut out caffeine mid-afternoon or earlier.

Cannabis and kratom are two more substances that people often use to help them sleep, but that can have counterproductive effects. The research on both is limited, I realize. Most cannabis and sleep research comes from the 70s, though with it being legal in more states, we will see better studies and confirmatory studies over the next few years, I hope.

Kratom (the tropical tree leaf that has stimulant and opioid properties) is legal in most states but new to the US in general so also has limited studies to back it up.

I know that a lot of people use cannabis (CBD or THC) or kratom to help them manage their symptoms of anxiety, depression, PTSD, and chronic pain. However, the research that is out there does show that both disrupt sleep quality, specifically reducing REM sleep (which we now know is kinda sorta really fucking important). Sleep problems on kratom are an oft-reported side effect. With cannabis, it's slightly more complicated. Deep sleep is enhanced with initial use, but the cannabis-helping-you-sleep effect fades away pretty quickly the more often you use it. The "why" part of that is still unknown.

Because all of these fun herbs can disrupt REM sleep, it also lessens night terrors, and is used by folks with PTSD and the like. But then you also lose all the things REM sleep gives the human body, so not a good trade-off. There is a prescription option that may work better.

For those of you who are using cannabis and/or kratom to help you manage other symptoms, I feel you. I know many people consider them an absolute lifesaver. The lesser the dose, the less impact it has on your sleep. Monitor your dosing along with monitoring your sleep and work to figure out your sweet spot for the amount you take and time(s) of day you take it.

And if you smoke your THC? Consider using another method of ingestion. Smoking increases your risk of breathing issues (asthma, COPD), which will also fuck with your sleep.

Cognitive Behavior Therapy for Insomnia (CBT-I)

Therapy, or at least some forms of it, can also help you sleep. The Chronic Insomnia Task Force of the American Academy of Sleep Medicine has recommended CBT-I as the first professional intervention that someone should undertake for insomnia (assuming apnea, restless leg syndrome, and other medical conditions have been ruled out). CBT-I is a short-term therapy (4–8 sessions, generally) that pairs the principles of cognitive behavior therapy with specific sleep hygiene protocols and relaxation techniques to assist people in untangling the emotional distress that is the general root cause of insomnia.

If you are disrupted consistently by nightmares and night terrors, that means your brain is working hard to make sense of some traumatic shit you have dealt with in the past. CBT-I may be enough to help you through the process, or you may have to do some trauma-informed therapy to work through whatever it is that your brain is trying to figure out. All of the exercises that help you increase vagal tone and widen your window of tolerance will also absolutely help your sleep.

UNFUCK YOUR FOOD

Food and eating have a deep relationship with trauma, inflammation, toxicity, and stress so I would be remiss in not discussing them. However, issues surrounding food and eating can be incredibly emotionally expensive for just about everyone. Eating and dieting disorders exist in people of all shapes, sizes, and genders. Not looking like the media idea of someone with an eating disorder doesn't mean you don't have one. Nor does it mean you are safer from the associated negative health outcomes (eating disorders are the second deadliest mental health disorder, only opioid addiction is higher).

If this is an area in which you are struggling and your inner voice tells you to skip over this chapter, listen to it.

It'll always be here later if you are looking at making some considered food choices from a more stable place. You may find that the chapter on supplements and meds will help in terms of looking at ways of getting some missing nutrients in your body when food is a battleground. And exercise isn't off the table, even if you have used it as a purging mechanism in the past. If you are getting treatment right now, talk to your therapist or group about how strength and muscle building exercise (rather than calorie burning exercise) may be a helpful part of your recovery and get their feedback.

If you are still deciding, please know that this chapter is not at all about weight loss or fitspo or food choice shaming in any way, shape, or form. It's actually pretty political. Shocker coming from me, I know. It's about problems within the food system that are creating problems for our health and the kinds of changes we can make in order to combat these problems. If that's your cup of tea, carry on!

Skinny Doesn't Equal Healthy

One of the most troubling things about food for most of us is its relationship with body weight. We have this cultural myth that fat is unhealthy and skinny is healthy. It's so pervasive, it's everywhere. And it's not true. (Say it out loud for the people in the baaaaaack.) So most people from medical professionals to social media "experts" skip treating real problems and focus on shaming people for the size of their thighs. And we really got to fucking stop.

Fatphobia Is Racist

Centuries ago in Europe, being full figured was synonymous with being healthy and strong (look at Renaissance art work if you want to see the ideal). This carried over to the early days of colonization of Turtle Island (now North and South America).

Because enough food was available, American colonists weren't just heartier, they were much taller than their families back in Europe. By the mid 1800s, there was an eight centimeter height discrepancy between Americans and Europeans. Bigger bodies were considered more beautiful. It was fashionable for women to drink down "weight gain" tonics if they were too skinny to catch a good husband.

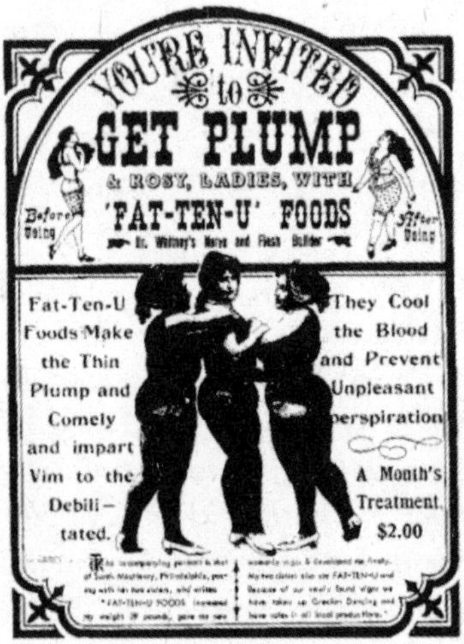

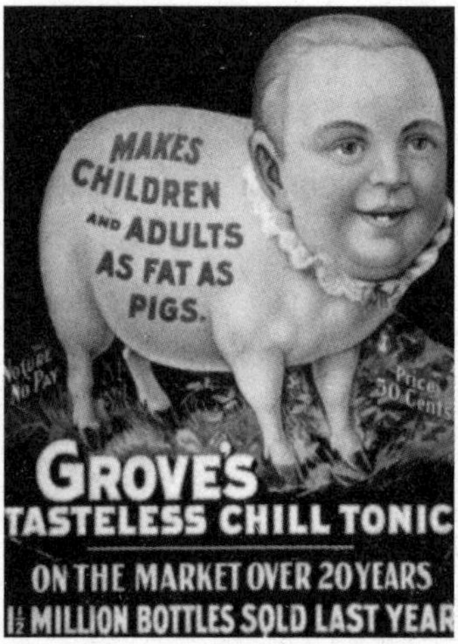

The widespread trade of enslaved people was happening at the same time, and this presented a problem. In order to mentally justify the ownership of some bodies by other bodies, there had to be a mechanism for deciding superiority and inferiority. This was easy at first because of skin tone. But the continued rape by slave owners and interbreeding with enslaved Indigenous peoples (yes that happened, too) meant that future generations had lighter and lighter skin. So the comparison of body types, frame size, and where fat settles on the body became the mechanism for deciding who is superior (see Sabrina Strings's amazing book Fearing the Black Body). White women of a certain class were able to differentiate themselves from enslaved women and poor white women by showing that they didn't have to be solid and strong to get through a day, they could center thinness as an ideal.

A Presbyterian minister by the name of Sylvester Graham (yes, the graham cracker guy) promoted an extremely restrictive lifestyle and diet (the original graham crackers were not yummy, trust). He died in 1851, but his followers remained active through the 1880s.

Tonics meant to put on weight were replaced with ones meant to melt it away.

Lulu Hunt Peters, a young woman who had struggled with "baby fat" into adulthood, earned her MD and translated nutrition research to the public in what became a bestselling book. Diet and Health: With Key to the Calories was released in 1918 and included an extensive list of "100 calorie snacks." Dietary restrictions became the rage. But then the question became, how do we decide what determines an acceptable amount of thin?

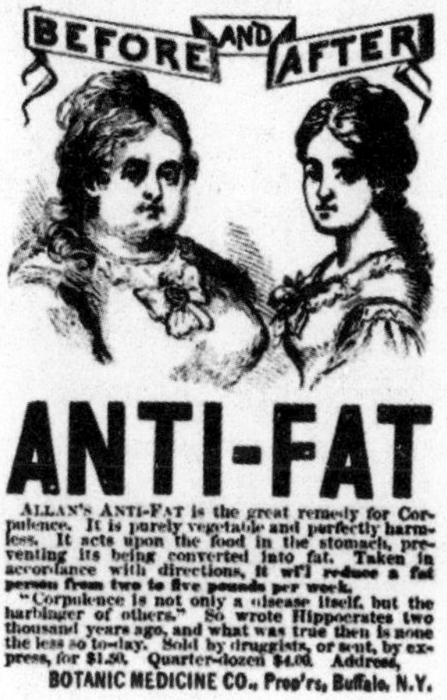

The BMI Is Racist, Sexist, and Transphobic as Fuck

The Body Mass Index (BMI) is the defining metric modern medicine uses to determine if your weight is "healthy." It uses your height in proportion to your weight. Okay, then. As the queen of the "but why" questions, I wanted to know where this came from. The BMI was actually invented 200 years ago. The dude who created it, Adolphe Quetelet, was not a physician, but actually an academic who was super fired up on astronomy, sociology, math, and statistics. A Belgian in the 1800s, he was part of the boom in racist "science"—he is also credited with founding the field of anthropometry, which includes all that phrenology bullshit. He was looking for ways to identify the characteristics of "the average man", thinking that represented the social ideal of manliness.

He believed that someone whose physiology fit the mathematical mean of all people (which for him meant European people, but okay) would be the human ideal, which is bullshit. Based on the measurements of French and Scottish men, he came up with a formula known as Quetelet's Index (now known as the BMI), which ranked people's body size on a curve based on his available study subjects. It was intended as a social tool; he never meant it as a measure of body fat, build, or individual health. By the early 1900s, this index became the mechanism for determining if someone was fit to parent, and as a justification for forced sterilization, or eugenics. And not just against people of color, but also poor people, people with disabilities, and neurodiverse people.

But then, capitalism. US life insurance companies began compiling tables of height and weight to determine what to charge policy holders. The tables were based on the weight and height of the people who could actually afford to purchase life insurance and had the legal means to do so. And the numbers were self-reported. Most tables did not include frame size or factor in age. And all this information was put together by sales agents and actuaries, not medical professionals.

Physicians began using these unscientific tables as a means of evaluating a patient's weight as an indicator of their health. This went on through the 1950s and 60s, until medical science decided to find a more effective measure in the 70s. A research team led by Ancel Keys conducted a study of 7,500 men (yes, only men) from five (yes, only five) different countries, trying to find the most effective measure of body fat that would be easy and cost effective because it could be easily calculated during a regular doctor's office visit. They compared it to the use of skin calipers and water displacement and found that all were weak but the BMI sucked the least.

In this study, Keys found that the BMI diagnosed "obesity"[16] accurately about 50% of the time. Meaning, that half the time individuals are carrying extra weight on their frames, and the other half of the time they just have bigger frames or a lot of dense muscle tissue. This level of "accuracy" has continued to hold at 50%. A 2011 study in the Journal of Obstetrics and Gynecology stated that, yup, it was right half the time. No matter. In 1985, the National Institutes of Health (NIH) redefined obesity in terms of BMI. And that made it literal public policy.

The NIH wasn't done with us though. In 1998, they changed the definitions of both "obese" and "overweight," lowering the threshold of what is medically considered fat. All of a sudden, millions of people became medically (and legally) fat without gaining a pound. And now we can have a good old fashioned public health crisis over our so-called obesity epidemic and blame someone's weight for all of their medical issues.

So now we have a systemic problem that disproportionately affects women, individuals of color, and trans people. There are sex based differences that are not accounted for in the BMI—which was developed measuring only men, remember? But any woman who has ever been heavy at some point in their life has a story of being told by a doctor that their chief complaint will be resolved through weight loss. Many trans individuals are denied surgical gender confirmation interventions

16 According to the modern scale, if a BMI is less than 18.5, it falls within the underweight range, 18.5 to <25, is "normal," 25.0 to <30 is overweight, 30.0 or higher is obese, and 40.0 or higher is morbidly obese.

until they lose weight, even though an 18 year longitudinal study of post-op complications shows this is not the case. A bigger body does not correlate with problems with healing. And according to the World Health Organization (WHO), the BMI overestimates fatness and health risks for Black people while underestimating the health risks for Asian communities.

People are being dismissed, other real illnesses are not being diagnosed and treated, and people are being denied life saving treatments and surgeries based on a two hundred year old tool designed to legitimize ethnic cleansing and cultural genocide.

And I don't think the irony is lost on any of us right now.

A Low BMI Isn't Necessarily Healthy

You can have a low BMI and not be at all healthy. Not just if you have an illness or an eating disorder—some people seem to have these insane metabolisms that keep them slim yet they are not any healthier, or are even far less healthy, than their thicker counterparts. And being actually underweight (BMI less than 18.5) is associated with early death more often with being overweight. As determined in over 50 studies.[17] A friend of mine was bluntly told by her doctor when approaching 40, "Yes, you are tall and slim, but that doesn't mean you aren't rotting on the inside. You gotta take better care of yourself."

The official term for someone with a "normal" or "underweight" BMI who has similar health struggles is metabolically unhealthy non-obese (MUHNO). Just like in the early days of the US when being scrawny was considered problematic, it still is. MUHNO individuals may be eating like crap and not moving their body and can therefore still be insulin resistant and have high triglycerides, high blood pressure, cardiac issues, and high inflammation markers (an indicator we keep returning to again and again). Their body fat patterns are just different, not better. Extreme bodybuilding can also lead to metabolic shut down. I'm not dissing bodybuilding (my son is a weightlifter and it's a huge part of his wellness routine), but all extremes put pressure on our bodies that they aren't equipped to handle, no matter how much we would like to hack the process and live forever. Bodies are all weird and different and each one has its own operating instructions. We can't do a little height and weight algebra equation to know if someone is healthy or not.

But one thing we do know? The greatest indicator of life span is not your mass, it's your class. If I wanted a good test of whether or not

17 I hit the underweight mark some years ago when my iron levels crashed out. I was sick, I felt awful and was shaking with cold all the time, but the number of people who told me "*OMG you are so tiny! You look amazing! You are so cute!*" was freakishly high. When I got treatment and was back at my healthy weight and people commented on that I loved saying "*Right? Thank Buddha, I feel so much better now!*"

you are in good health and will live a long life, I would not look at your BMI, but at your socioeconomic status. This is true for virtually every disease in every industrialized country. And the greater the level of inequality in a country, the greater the health disparities. Your access to care changes, the respect you are given when you do access care changes, and your access to a healthy environment and nutritious food changes. It brings us back to stress, trauma, a toxic environment, and chronically upregulated inflammation once again. If you are interested in reading more about the science of individual weight set-points and the influence of socioeconomic status, read Body Respect by Linda Bacon.

And while suggesting government overthrow just gets NSA agents showing up at my office and scaring my clients, I can suggest potential changes we can make individually to combat the systemic issues we are all dealing with. And fuck if that isn't the narrative arc of all of my books, right?

Our Food System Is Bullshit

So now that we got the "this isn't a chapter about dieting" stuff out of the way, let's talk about our actual diets. Cuz not the same thing, right? And since our diets are not just of the things we like to eat, but are greatly influenced by what's affordable and available, let's talk about why that system is utter trash.

If you have purchased groceries even once in the history of ever, you know that broccoli is way more expensive than a loaf of bread. And if you have ever been on a tight budget, you know that you can get a fast food value meal far cheaper than a healthy meal.

US federal government data states that our primary sources of calories are sweets and simple carbs (stuff like ice cream, pasta, pizza, bread, and sugary drinks). You know what all of these foods have in common besides their carb load? They are produced primarily from the crops and farm foods that are heavily subsidized by the federal government: corn, soybeans, wheat, rice, sorghum, milk, and meat.

Between 1995 and 2010, the government allocated $170 billion in agricultural subsidies to finance the production of these foods. The farm bill is renewed by Congress every five years; the version approved in 2014 called for $956 billion in spending. The farm bill in progress as I write this in 2021 is projected by the Congressional Budget Office (CBO) to total out at $428 billion over the 5-year period 2019-23.

Of course, none of these foods are inherently unhealthy. The problem is not that these foods exist in the world, but only a tiny percent of them are being eaten as is. Most are being converted to additives and cheap products like corn sweeteners, industrially produced oils, refined carbohydrates, and processed meats. They become the building blocks for the ultra processed foods I am going to talk about later in this chapter.

The subsidies program was started with good intentions, as many of our most ridiculous government initiatives are. The idea was to support struggling farmers and strengthen America's food supply. But instead of supporting the small farmers who grow veggies and fruits and nuts and the like (which are formally categorized as "specialty crops" by the government), the money goes to these aforementioned "commodity crops." Ironically, "specialty" farms account for 75% of our farmland in the US but only receive 14% of crop subsidies. And whatever the intentions of the bill, small farmers are not getting the money. Huge industrial agri-business farm-factories are getting half of the subsidies while only representing 7% of US cropland. Some versions of the farm bill even stipulated that you could not grow anything other than commodity foods. Until 2014, you would literally be penalized for growing broccoli. Thanks to advocacy, now a whole 15% of your crop can be "specialty foods" if you receive subsidy funding.

So there are very real reasons that crap foods seem so cheap—but actually, they aren't. You are paying for them out of your tax dollars. But since they are essentially our pre-paid foods, they are the ones that are easiest to access and afford. And they are the ones that even our own government has found to be most likely to cause metabolic distress and chronic inflammation.

Measurable improvements can be made in many health issues by changing how we eat by promoting better well-being, lower health care costs, greater sustainability, reduced disparities among population groups, improved economic competitiveness and greater national security. This means not just changing what we individually put in our mouths every day, but improving how nutrition is supported by the medical establishment and government. And supporting better nutrition is actually cost saving. For example, one program found that a home delivered medically tailored meal program actually saved $9,000 a year in patient health care costs because patients had less health care issues that required medications and other treatments.

What Are "Processed" Foods?

In trying to eat better, you probably keep hearing that we should avoid processed food. But most of our food (no matter what type of diet we subscribe to) is processed in some way, and this isn't necessarily a bad thing. The idea of processed food is super vague. Technically, once we chew our food in order to swallow it without choking, we've processed it. Even putting aside that fact, the US dietary guidelines use a very broad definition of "processed":

> Any raw agricultural commodity [product] that has been subject to processing, such as canning, cooking, freezing, dehydration, or milling. Processing certain foods can make them last longer by killing organisms in the food or slowing their growth.

True all of this: processing foods allowed us to carry harvest through multiple seasons, especially before refrigeration became a widespread thing. Canning, drying, fermenting foods kept us alive after the harvest. Processing can also make foods safer (cooked versus raw chicken, anyone?) and could also create better bioavailability of the nutrition contained within (like the nixtamalization[18] of corn into hominy or the sprouting of grains).

So how do we determine "bad" processing from "good? A team from the Center for Epidemiological Studies in Health and Nutrition at the University of São Paulo in Brazil took on the task of defining food processing as a spectrum. They came up with a scale that helps us determine when we are veering into unhealthy territory. It was published as part of "The UN Decade of Nutrition, the NOVA food classification and the trouble with ultra-processing" and you can find the whole thing online, if that's your kink. But here are their basic classifications:

Unprocessed or Minimally Processed Foods: This includes the edible parts of any foods (plant or animal based) after they have been harvested from their natural source. Minimal processing may include removing parts that are inedible, roasting or broiling, drying, freezing, fermenting without alcohol, or squeezing (like getting juice from fruit).

Processed Culinary Ingredients: This is essentially our oils, fats, salts, and sugars. Like honey removed from a honeycomb, maple syrup extracted from a tree, sugar processed from sugar cane or sugar beets, salt harvested from the sea, or oils extracted from a plant (like olive oil extracted from olives). These ingredients are created by pressing, grinding, crushing, pulverizing, and refining.

Processed Foods: These are foods that are a combination of the first two groups, such as a naturally or minimally processed food that has a processed culinary ingredient added to it. Still not bad, right? Salt cured lemons would be processed while simply dried lemons would not. Toasting a mix of nuts in a little bit of olive oil with salt and spices would be a processed food, while eating them raw or merely sprouting them or toasting them would not. So even at this level, we are seeing that processing isn't bad. This is how we make things taste good.

Ultra-Processed Foods: This is where we get into ingredients that you couldn't replicate at home (think hydrogenated oils, hydrolyzed

---

18 This is when corn is soaked and cooked in an alkaline solution (usually limewater), washed, and hulled to make the body better able to absorb the nutrients within it.

proteins, soy protein isolate, maltodextrin, invert sugar, high fructose corn syrup, dyes, stabilizers, and emulsifiers). These industrialized formulas were synthesized in laboratory settings. They have little (if anything) to do with the first category of foods. Think candy bars, cake mixes, breakfast cereal, instant noodles, and most pre-packaged frozen foods. They taste yummy because they were frankensteined to do so but they aren't food.

So when we are talking about processed foods being a problem, we are talking about these ultra-processed foods. These are the foods that have been correlated with higher risks of cancer, metabolic syndrome, and death from any cause. In the United States, 61% of an adult's total diet comes from ultra-processed foods. We aren't alone though: the proportion in Canada is 62% and in the UK it's 63%.

Awareness makes a huge difference in lessening our ultra-processed food consumption. For example, Finland in the 1980s had the highest rate of cardiovascular disease fatalities. Scientists attributed the high rate to the added sodium in food.

The salt we add to our food to make it taste delicious is composed of sodium and chloride. We generally aren't getting too much salt, but we are often getting too much sodium. Sodium added to food as a preservative includes sodium benzoate, sodium citrate, and sodium sorbate, which is not the same thing as the salt you sprinkled on your tomatoes. Sodium is used to enhance color and give things a firmer texture. More than 75% of the salt in our diet is coming from sodium added to ultra-processed foods as a preservative. When you see "no salt added" on your can of beans, that's the one you want to buy, because it means no added sodium-whatevers. You can salt it to your taste level with real, normal salt when you're cooking at home.

So that's what the Finnish government did. Anything with a high sodium content got a big honking "Don't Buy This Shit" label on it.

Okay, not really. It got a label that said "High Salt Content"—meaning high sodium, but since they get used interchangeably people got the message. So by 2007, sodium consumption had dropped 30% in Finland and that correlated with a 75% decrease in deaths from strokes and heart disease.

Ultra-processed foods have far more inflammatory potential than their whole-food counterparts. For example, one common food additive, tert-Butylhydroquinone, which has been studied fairly extensively at this point, has been demonstrated to hamper the body's immune response. The body treats the buildup of these substances as a toxin, and we develop an inflammatory response.

Ultra-processed foods are also correlated with mental health issues. The journal PLOS ONE published a randomized controlled trial finding that depression, anxiety, and stress symptoms decreased from the "moderate" range to the "normal" range after only three weeks of eating a diet that significantly reduced ultra-processed food consumption. It wasn't a special fancy diet, just a general "Mediterranean-style pattern" according to the study, meaning food instead of crap. The control group continued to eat refined carbs, sugary foods and beverages, and other ultra-processed meals and showed no decrease in their depression scores.

Why do we eat this stuff if it's so bad for us? First of all, it tastes good. Food scientists figured out the ideal level of salt to fat, the right amount of crunch or creaminess, and the general mouthfeel to not only make things taste good, but hijack our brain's ability to signal satiety. Instead of getting the "we're full" we get a "carry on" message. Also? They're cheaper. Cheaper in money and cheaper in labor and time. The processed packaged food industry is extraordinarily efficient at using cheap ingredients to create "meals" to sell. They have also benefited from government subsidies in a way that broccoli farmers have not.

Which makes it make sense that the people most likely to eat ultra-processed foods are young people, poor people, and people who live alone. We all get targeted, but these are the people who are the biggest markets of the industry.

You don't have to go completely off the grid, or give up all of your favorite treats forever, to make big changes. Remember how a 30% reduction in sodium intake alone was correlated with a 75% reduction in cardiovascular death? Start by reading labels. Get the no salt (sodium!) added canned beans and veggies, get the no sugar added fruits. Swap out flour tortillas for corn at the taco stand. If you aren't ready to give up the fast food french fries and chicken nuggets, you can still switch out the soda for an iced tea in your combo meal. If you enjoy cooking (or at least don't absolutely hate it), you'll likely find you really enjoy getting creative with healthier meals. It's not meant to be a punitive plate of steamed broccoli and sadness, right? While it is more expensive to buy quality ingredients than crappy ones, you start to learn how to be clever and budget conscious pretty quickly. Using eggs for protein more than steak, knowing which local farmers you can purchase from directly, etc. It is also 100% true that you will save money in the long run because you absolutely feel better.

Antibiotic Overload

Our systems are overloaded with antibiotics and I don't mean just the ones you are taking for a sinus infection. We've all seen the news articles saying that we overtake antibiotics and we are causing antibiotic resistance because we are whiney babies who demand them from our doctors when all we have is a common cold. But it turns out that's not the full story. We are ingesting most of our antibiotics from our food.

Antibiotics are used to increase the size of animals raised for meat (including cows and chickens). In Vandana Shiva's book Stolen Harvest: The Hijacking of the Global Food Supply, she mentions the use of sulfa drugs (an inexpensive, common antibiotic) in the meat they use at the McDonald's restaurants in India. Sulfa drugs are also commonly fed to conventionally raised animals in the US. The FDA tested sulfa levels and found them at three times the rate allowed by law in the cattle being sold for food. One particular dairy farmer had a cow with 323 times the legal limit. It turns out that 40% of the antibiotics produced in this country go to feedlots, not people. And from there they make their way into our bloodstream. Fairly conservative sources are noting the huge problems with this, from veterinarian programs at the University of Idaho to our own National Institutes for Health.

Our body responds to these drugs as toxins, once again leading to chronic inflammation. Residual drugs have been tied to allergic reactions in the people that consume meat, dairy, and eggs. They've also been tied to increasing instances of cancer in humans. If we eat conventionally-farmed meat, we are at increased risk of developing antibiotic resistance even if we are not taking antibiotics in pill form, and we are also at risk of negative effects if we have an antibiotic allergy, especially to sulfa. The articles about all of this are in my reference section if you want to read along and also throw up a bit in your mouth the way I did.

So what do we do about this? Going organic is more expensive than a lot of us can afford. Fortunately, finding meat that has not been treated with antibiotics is a more cost-effective middle ground. And then we can choose to eat less of it. I'm the queen of making a huge pot of chili with only one pound of actual beef and a ton of lentils to bulk it up. And even though antibiotic-free eggs are more expensive than conventional ones, they are still one of the cheapest non-plant proteins available. All the essential amino acids your body needs are in an egg yolk, which is why a lot of people who follow a plant-based diet will also include unfertilized eggs.

Food Allergies

Food allergies are becoming a larger and larger public health burden. When our body has an immune response to a specific food, like peanuts, we produce antibodies called immunoglobulin E (IgE). These antibodies cause symptoms like swelling, itching, tingling, rashes, wheezing, dizziness, and/or lightheadedness.

Allergic reactions to food itself are actually considered the "second wave" of the allergy epidemic. The recent increase in asthma is thought to be the result of our immune responses to food (not just air quality issues). It's hard to know the exact numbers due to the conflation of allergies with food intolerances (which I'll get into next). Additionally, most sensitized individuals are able to tolerate a food they are allergic to without reaction, which is brilliant for keeping someone from going into anaphylactic shock because someone next to them ate peanut butter, but it makes it harder to test accurately.

Best guess is that one in ten adults have a food allergy (and more than a quarter of them stated that they weren't allergic to foods as children). The rate of food allergies among kids has doubled over the past two decades, and today one in 13 children has a food allergy. If that doesn't seem like a lot, think of it as two kids per classroom in any given K-12 class.

And while allergy rates have increased, so has the range of foods that people are allergic to. Methods of production likely play a role, but so does ancestry. Researchers found that children of African or East Asian descent who were born in a Western environment are at higher risk for food allergies than Caucasian children born in the same environment, which lends support to the idea that there is a genome-environment interaction with food.

There have been several theories that are plausible, but the one that is our current best guess (and fits with many of the other issues described in this book) is the "old friends" theory posited by Graham Rook, an emeritus professor of medical microbiology at the University College of London. Our personal microbiota (the microorganisms within our personal bodies) are changing in ways that don't support our body's capacity to defend itself. Our homes are built of plasterboard and biocide-treated lumber. We're exposed to lots more antibiotics which kill off a portion of everything, not just the bad germs. We're more likely to be born by c-section, and not just for reasons of health and safety of the parent and child. In a multitude of ways we have fewer of the microbes that help our immune system respond to foreign substances (food and other potential allergens). Our struggling microbiome is quite likely the reason that our immune response fails far more often than it used to, leading to a multitude of problems, including an increase in allergic reactions.

Food Sensitivities and Autoimmune Trigger Foods

Another common food problem we're facing more and more is food sensitivities. The American Academy of Allergy, Asthma & Immunology (yes, that's AAAAI, I agree that rebranding would help) defines a food intolerance or a food sensitivity as what occurs when a person has difficulty digesting a particular food, leading to pain, gas, bloating, and/or diarrhea. Unlike allergies, food sensitivities don't cause rashes and restricted airways, but they do cause issues in our gut, leading to leaky gut and chronic inflammation once again.

Figuring out what is an allergy and what is a sensitivity can be difficult. Dairy is the most common food allergy in human beings, and it is also a very common intolerance (most people's bodies turn off the ability to digest the sugars in lactose after age three), leading to chronic inflammation and discomfort.

Some autoimmune diseases, like celiac, are an immune reaction to certain foods. Other autoimmune diseases (there are 150 and still counting) are exacerbated by certain foods. The casein found in milk is a common one and gluten is another. If a person who is sensitive to the food eats it, the resulting inflammation can trigger a nasty flare of Hashimoto's or one of a number of diseases that occur when the body attacks itself, thinking it's an outside invader. So the milk itself isn't a problem, it creates that whole cascade effect of longer term problems in the body.

Going gluten-free has been popular for a minute now, to the point where it's hard to believe it's a real sensitivity and not just a diet fad, but there is merit to the idea that a good number of people struggle to digest gluten properly, even if they don't have celiac. The official term for those people is Non-Celiac Wheat/Gluten Sensitivity (NCWS). There are now a ton of studies where NCWS was tested in people through double-blind methods (meaning the doctors and patients didn't know what had gluten in it and what didn't). And researchers were able to see measurable levels of immune activity in the gut, and irritable bowel symptoms. It's just as measurable as in someone with a real allergy (like I will absolutely get a rash if something has cream cheese in it even if I didn't know it was there). Three out of four people who had been diagnosed with NCWS ate gluten-free at the beginning of a long term study, and had stayed gluten free ten years later. It wasn't a fad for them. And the people in the 75% category had almost total relief from IBS and upregulated inflammation. While the other 25% (unsurprisingly) were still symptomatic. This is all to say that if going gluten free gives you relief, stay gluten free. You aren't alone and it isn't just hype.

Scientists are still trying to figure out the why part with gluten sensitivities, but there are a few good guesses as to what the actual problem is. As I discuss in Unfuck Your Brain, it's partly because the variants of wheat we grow in those subsidized giant farms aren't as wholesome as what our recent ancestors ate. The pesticides used to grow in that quantity don't help either. Which means some people can eat bread baked with organically produced Einkorn wheat, for example, while others have to avoid wheat altogether.

Nightshades are another food sensitivity category for a lot of people that we look at when trying to mitigate inflammation, especially with chronic pain sufferers. Nightshades are a group of plants (think tomatoes, peppers, eggplants, certain spices like paprika and cayenne—

everything delicious) that contain alkaloids. Alkaloids are the plant's way of fending off insects trying to eat them, and for some people with inflammatory conditions like diabetes and arthritis they are disruptive to the body and can create digestive issues.

Taking the time to figure out how your body best functions in regards to food can go a long way to helping your physical and mental health. The standard way to figure out if you have an allergy or sensitivity is through an elimination diet like Whole30 or a low FODMAP diet. If you think a particular type of food might be causing you problems, you can try eliminating the suspect alone but it can be more than one thing and/or a cascade effect. Elimination diets aren't meant to be long term. You generally only need to follow a very restricted diet for a month or so, to give your body a chance to get rid of all traces of the possible offenders. Then after a time you add one food back in every couple of days to see how your body responds and which ones end up getting shown the door with the message "and stay out!"

If you think you might have a bunch of food sensitivities, or if you're dealing with chronic pain, another thing to try is the autoimmune protocol diet (AIP). Some people will just dump out gluten, nightshades, maybe some other common trigger foods like dairy, and feel great. Some people will need to go further and try a complete AIP diet (such as the Wahls Protocol or the Autoimmune Solution). A strict AIP diet isn't a forever thing for most people. After at least a month (and if you are healing gut issues, I would give it a full six months), you can start introducing tomatoes and the like back in and testing your body's reaction. If you aren't chronically inflamed, you will likely not have a spikey reaction to most of these foods.

So What's the Perfect Diet?

The two big universals that we should all do, depending on our financial situation and food availability situation, are to decrease proteins that come from animals that were treated with antibiotics and to decrease ultra-processed foods.

But beyond that, there is no right diet for everyone.

This truth is backed up by science. A large-scale study comparing different weight-loss diets based on different ratios of the three principal dietary macronutrients (fats, carbs, proteins) was sponsored by the NIH and conducted at Brigham and Women's Hospital over a two year period. And they found that everyone is different and there is no one magic diet.

But there are so many options out there and there is always a new diet fad to check out. As a Gen Xer, I came of age in the era of SlimFast and fat-free everything. I remember taking out boxes of Snackwell's cookies with my college roomie while binging on Twin Peaks and wondering why I had horrible sugar headaches. Wasn't this the thing that we were supposed to do? My body needed fat for fuel and was getting none, and it didn't need the amount of ultra processed shelf-stable cookies I was shoving into it.

As you try to figure out the foods that work best for you, one thing to consider is where our ancestors are from and that their bodies evolved while eating the foods that were available in those places. For example, the Tsimané of Bolivia eat far more carbohydrates than the average American (never mind an American on a paleo diet) but researchers found no coronary artery calcium (a significant risk factor for heart disease) among them.

A more ancestral based diet might make far more sense than Slimfast and Snackwells (though both of these brands are still in business so ¯_(:)_/¯), if only for the basic reason that you are eating real foods (which means don't load up on nutrition bars and shakes that are keto and paleo just because they fit your new diet profile) and you are eating the things your body evolved to eat.

But the question is . . . which ancestors? The ancestors of the person who wrote the diet book? Or yours? And why does that matter?

This is the big debate around plant based diets isn't it? People who have a strong value system around eating plant based foods, like His Holiness the Dalai Lama, are being told by their doctors to include some animal based protein back in their diets. Why are some people able to be incredibly healthy on a vegan diet and not others? Although you can get protein from a plant based diet, our ability to convert amino acids is different from person to person. In the book Traditional Foods Are Your Best Medicine (a book that has been around a few decades but was republished in 2015 as Primal Nutrition: Paleolithic and Ancestral Diets for Optimal Health to capitalize on the paleo diet craze), Ronald F. Schmid discusses evidence that shows some people are able to properly convert plant aminos into the essential aminos that the body needs to maintain optimal health. And many people simply can't. So why is that?

The gut microbiome is best conceived of as a holobiont, meaning organisms from different species working and managing challenges together in a way that a singular organism (our human body) cannot do alone. Our gut microbiota range from 100 trillion to 1 quadrillion organisms (best guess) and are a collection of archaea, eukarya, and bacteria that co-evolved with us over time. If you were to compare the amount of microbiota we have versus the number of human cells we have, the microbiota outnumber our human-ness 10 to 1. Our ancestry determines what bacteria we co-evolved with, which plays a big role in what foods our bodies work best with.

While the idea of consuming beneficial bacteria (for example, in the form of fermented foods) isn't new in human history, the Western medicine study of the human microbiome is very new. The term microbiome itself was coined in 2001, and the Human Microbiome project (an NIH funded initiative) wasn't established until 2007. So there is a ton more in the what we don't know category than in the what we know category. But there are a few things that are important.

Half of our current microbiome is shit we have zero control over. For example, our genetics account for about 12% of our microbiome. Then there are factors like how we were born or whether or not we were breastfed and the toxins we were exposed to growing up that we can't control.

The other half of our microbiome is the part we have more control over. We can actively build a good microbiome by reducing antibiotic intake (which will be mostly as consumed in food) and finding the foods that our bodies operate best on. Which brings us back to the idea of food intolerances and doing a time-limited elimination diet to see what you respond poorly to. Your body is always your best intolerance test.

For long-term dietary choices, being super strict about what you eat or avoid almost never makes you healthier. If you are on a medical keto diet to manage seizures, then being super careful with your diet makes sense. But in general? Even for people who are eating a specific diet to manage other health issues like the Auto-Immune Protocol or the Gut and Psychology Syndrome diet, it shouldn't be miserable and all consuming. And as for more conventional diets, counting calories and macros isn't a sustainable or pleasurable way to live. Calories are not created equal (100 calories of soda won't affect your body in at all the same way as 100 calories of almond butter). Ultimately, any diet that you're supposed to stick to indefinitely with strict religious zeal for general health or weight loss is a red flag without an underlying medical reason.

Instead, eat real foods. If you are hungry between meals, try adding more fat, like a dollop of coconut oil in your morning smoothie, or a dollop of almond butter with your banana to get you through to lunch without gnawing on the furniture. If you are working to add muscle, add more protein, like a couple of hard boiled eggs (but not in your smoothie cuz gross). If you don't feel full right after a meal, bulk up on non-starchy veggies like salad greens or carrot sticks. If you are working on healing an inflamed gut, you can add more fiber (like apples or avocados, yum) and anti inflammatory foods like nuts, or fatty fish and herbs like turmeric, green tea, and rosemary.

Shop Like a Lawyer

My motto when I'm reading a food package label is to think like a lawyer.

When buying organic beef recently, I found a package of sausage sitting next to it. Finding sausage that is organic and both pork and dairy-free is a blue moon thing. I was super excited. Then I noticed that while the beef said "Antibiotic Free!" the sausage said "No added antibiotics!"

:::squinty look:::

I put the sausage back. Because no added antibiotics since when? Since they left the farm? All the way through the feedlot? Sorry Charlie, I don't trust your semantics.

If you find yourself reading labels and you spot a loophole in the verbiage, cut and run. Gatrillions of dollars are spent on figuring out how to make things look healthy without them actually being healthy. People who produce legitimately clean food are proud of the fact and say that in straightforward ways.

Farm fresh? All-natural? Mean absolutely nothing. They are advertising buzzwords[19].

No hormones? Important when it comes to cattle. But it doesn't mean anything when it comes to poultry. Poultry isn't treated with hormones in the US anyway, so you may pay more for BS.

Grass fed? Not the same as grass finished. A lot of livestock is started on grass but moved to feedlot corn pretty early, and for most of their lives. But if they ever ate grass at any point, the package is allowed to say "grass fed."

Cage free or free range? Required by law to have some access to the outside. It may be a tiny door at the end of a very long building. Not necessarily animals that are bopping around in the sunlight scratching in the dirt and eating bugs. Lots of egg cartons will claim that the hens are fed a "vegetarian diet" like that's a good thing, but it just means they feed their chickens corn and soy.

Look instead for labels that say antibiotic-free, non-GMO, certified humane, or organic. Though it should be noted that a lot of local farmers use very clean processes that we would consider organic but they haven't gone through the expensive process of organic certification. I always opt for purchasing from someone local without the fancy label who treats their land and the living beings on it with care.

Run across some weird word that you don't know what to do with? Check out the website of an organization called the Lexicon (thelexicon.

19 I fell for this again in the middle of editing this book. My husband bought some salmon that was labeled as "Atlantic Salmon" so I thought it was wild salmon, not farmed. Nope. "Atlantic Salmon" was the name of the company and it was farmed and dyed for color. I could tell it was grody after one bite and looked more carefully at the label. The fuckers.

org), managed by folks who have done a lot of the lawyer-type thinking for us!

Cost Savings Through Being Local, In-Season, and Waste-Free

Does it cost more to eat fresh and local produce? It can. It's really not bad when you shop in season. But health generally does cost more. Because as we talked about, broccoli isn't subsidized by the government. But as someone who was already raised to respect my food, I've noticed that I am even more cognizant of the importance of that respect when I pay for good quality and know where and who it is coming from.

In 2001, when living in the Houston area, I read a book by Barbara Kingsolver called Small Wonder. In this book (which predates Animal, Vegetable, Miracle—another book I highly recommend) she suggests that we spend $20 a month of our grocery budget towards local ingredients. I contacted my local agriculture extension office and was informed by a very nice man that there were no farmer's markets in the Houston area (something that is no longer true). He gave me a list of you-pick farms and I hit up the local blueberry farm and picked berries and bought local honey. I stopped at the local farm stands whenever I saw them. I picked the blackberries in my own backyard. And I generally had a hard time even finding $20 worth of local foods to buy.

Now the majority of my grocery budget each week goes to local goods: meats, cheeses, eggs, and produce. This food comes from sources like local food delivery services, community supported agriculture (CSA—essentially buying a share in a farm's harvests for the season) subscriptions, and local farmer's markets. When shopping at my local produce markets or the grocery store (whether the huge and fancy one or the local, tiny urban farm stand), I look for items marked as local and buy whatever they have, even if just to encourage them to continue to carry local produce. Most local of all, I also have a garden with a pecan tree, citrus trees, lots of herbs, and a few veggies if I think I will be home enough to tend to them. And I also am known to forage things that grow wild in my area. When I was in Houston, I had blackberry brambles on the edge of my property. Here in San Antonio, I can collect cactus fruit and other goodies.

I can and freeze stuff when it is fresh and abundant and inexpensive so I can have delicious things all year. A chest freezer is a healthy-delicious food person's bestest buddy. The strawberries you can buy in the store in November may not taste good, but the ones you buy in May and process and store are going to taste amazing in comparison.

A loaf of bread from the farmer's market will be eaten with dinner and the leftovers will be turned into croutons for next week's salad. Knowing the man who stayed up all night baking those loaves makes me want to respect the work that he did. Besides knowing where my food comes from, and knowing exactly what I'm putting in my body, I'm also directly supporting my local economy instead of a faceless conglomerate.

Looking to buy local? Look for food co-ops, farmer's markets and farms that sell to the public, or CSAs).

Eat Wild (eatwild.com) includes lists of farmers and other purveyors who work to provide foods that have the quality nutrition of the foods that were abundant before we fucked with the system so much. Evidence is growing on an almost daily basis that these wholesome foods give us more of the nutrients we need to fight disease and enjoy optimum health. Additionally, the Eat Well Guide (eatwellguide.org) has information on all kinds of local, sustainable resources including restaurants and stores, not just farms and markets.

I Hate Okra and You Can't Make Me Eat It!

So maybe you are trying to up your inclusion of gut-healing foods. But the foods that have been recommended to you gross you out.

First of all, I totally have tricked a ton of people over the years into eating things like kale, okra, and nopales by tossing them in a big pot of soup. It's rare that I hate a particular ingredient to the point of full melt-down, though getting there took some work. I used to have a serious fight-face about a lot of different things, but challenged myself to look past regular ways of preparing things and trying new ways. So now I'm not a fan of beets, unless you roast them for me. You might surprise yourself or the people you cook for by getting them eating things they would have thrown down about in the past.

I have a "courtesy bite" rule in my house. My family knows I won't force eggplant down their gullets if they really can't stand it. But they have to try it with an open mind. And they, in turn, are excellent about saying "okay, that's delicious, I'll eat it." If you are cooking for kids, it's also helpful to cook with kids. My kids would eat anything they helped cook when they were young. They were the chef, of course they were proud of the meal!

But I also know that everyone is far more likely to eat healthy once they figure out what foods they already like and intentionally eat more of them. If I tell you okra is amazing for you but you hate okra, that isn't going to get us very far. Once you have a good idea of what food components you are looking for (selenium to promote testosterone production, for example) you can check out the World's Healthiest Foods website (whfoods.com) and do a search. For some reason, the site doesn't include nuts and seeds, but you can Google search most anything with "health properties of XYZ" to get a good idea. Try it with whatever foods you love best and see what pops up.

And this is where whole food supplements and herbal supplements can come in handy. Spanish black radish is a fantastic detox but it's hard to find and doesn't taste fabulous (and I generally LIKE roasted radishes). So I take it as a whole food supplement. And that handily leads us to our next chapter. Go take a stretch break, drink a nice glass of water, and meet me over there in a few, ok?

Supplements and Medications

Medications, supplements, vitamins—there are a lot of pills and doses out there that can have a pretty profound impact on how our bodies function (or don't). I'm going to focus in this chapter on supplements that we can use to support our overall health, because they are widely available, often much cheaper than drugs, and there isn't a lot of good information about them out there.

I am not anti-medication. Not even a little bit. I am, however, anti over-medication. For one thing, we have a toxic history with using medications as mechanisms of chemical restraint (disproportionately so within institutional settings and child-serving systems like foster care, and disproportionately of individuals of color within these settings and systems) which many of y'all who are reading this may have been subjected to.

But even for the rest of us, medications are often the first and only line of defense. And they are typically not considered within the context of other treatment interventions. One of my clinical nutrition professors offered this hierarchy as the ideal alternative to over-medication and I'm all for it. When there's a problem, we should start at the top of this list and work our way down (just the way we have in the structure of this book):

Hierarchy of Interventions

1. Lifestyle
2. Food
3. Supplements
4. Drugs
5. Surgery

See how far down that list supplements and drugs come? I worry about the fact that those of us in the US are on a lot of medications. 50% of US adults take at least one prescription drug every month, and one in four of us are taking three or more. 73.9% of doctor's visits end with a prescription being written and 80.4% of hospital visits end with a prescription being written. From 2008 to 2018 the use of opioids went up 22%, but antidepressants went up 97% and anti-anxiety and antiepilepsy meds went up 661%. (Not a typo. Six hundred. And sixty-one.) Medication being the first thing we go to is a really worrisome habit.

And the medicines we're given generally do not work as universally as we are led to believe. Nor are they typically designed for longer term use. Pain medications are a good example. The two medications we use most for chronic pain are opioids (and the opioid crisis is something we all know about) and over the counter NSAIDs (nonsteroidal anti-inflammatory drugs). These include aspirin, ibuprofen, and naproxen. Opioids do block pain, but only for about a month, then your body reacts by increasing the number of receptors to allow the pain signal to get through again. Additionally, they reduce the body's ability to release endorphins, which help us manage pain independently. And opioid use reduces gut motility and interferes with the secretion of digestive enzymes from the gallbladder and pancreas resulting in impaired nutrient absorption.

But over the counter (OTC) pain medications aren't a real, long term pain solution either. NSAIDs (like ibuprofen) account for 3200 deaths per year, and 32,000 hospitalizations. An OTC drug doesn't mean it's a benign drug, and these can cause hypertension, heart disease, kidney damage, and gastrointestinal bleeding. Even more common is that NSAIDs inflame the intestinal tract, which can lead to leaky gut. The intestinal lining is repaired and replaced every 3-5 days, and NSAIDs interrupt and block that process. Intestinal permeability occurs within 24 hours for 60-80% of the people who take an NSAID. With long term use, 50-70% of people develop chronic intestinal inflammation. NSAIDs reduce pain but prevent healing.

Almost all analgesics (Tylenol as well as the NSAIDs) cause hypersensitization to our pain receptors, just like opioids. We end up with increased pain over time by using them. A study of people with episodic migraines who took NSAIDs 10-15 times a month found that many of them ended up having chronic daily headaches. Our own pain relief system (endorphins) shuts down when we take pain medicine, and it takes time to get that system to kick back in.

I have had significant success helping clients avoid needing prescription medications or minimize the number of prescriptions they need to use (under their prescriber's watchful eye—I always work in conjunction with the prescriber!). I've also had clients increase their prescription medication usage, just like I did in 2020, to better manage their symptoms during an unprecedented crisis. Doing so isn't a sign of failure or an over-reliance, so long as it is done thoughtfully and with an eye to the other mechanisms of supporting a healthy body.

I'm saying all this because I am passionate about finding alternative methods to support health beyond the current medical model. Whether we are talking about penicillin or lavender oil, anything we use should be used thoughtfully and holistically (using the true sense of the word). And if you do take allopathic drugs, they'll be most effective when supported with everything else further up the hierarchy.

All that being said, let's talk about how using supplements to support your health might benefit you.

What Are Supplements?

A supplement is something that completes or enhances something else when added to it. The idea is that there is something missing from our bodies and we are trying to complete or enhance our intake of food and prescription medications with other nutrients and bodily support.

According to the World Health Organization, 80% of the medications taken world-wide are naturally derived formulations rather than things grown in a lab. Our history of medication is based on the natural world. Animal, mineral, and herbal products have been used for over 5000 years. As late as the 1890s, 59% of the products in the US Pharmacopoeia were based on herbs or herbal combinations. The WHO reports that in the United States, a third of people are taking some form of supplements. And interestingly, the higher someone's level of education, the more likely they are to use a supplement. (And that one-third number doesn't include individuals taking something like Lovaza, which is a prescription formulary of fish oil).

A lot of times you will see the word "vitamins," which I tend to shy away from since most vitamin products on the market are synthetic isolates and that's exactly the thing we are trying to avoid. Instead, I recommend in my practice (and use in my personal life) a variety of whole food supplements and good quality herbs.

Whole food supplements are literally just food. Or rather, they're pills, but pills that are condensed versions of food, like vitamin C where the C comes from constituted buckwheat juice, not ascorbic acid. You're piling on the nutrition you need for healing. My motto is, you have to either eat it or take it. And honestly, getting enough of the nutrients we need through diet alone is nearly impossible. For example, depleted soil means we may not be getting enough trace minerals in our diet from the veggies we eat, even if they are local and organically raised. And there's less and less biodiversity available in supermarket produce. So we supplement. While I already cook with garlic, I still add a whole food garlic supplement to support my immune system during flu season. And since finding spanish black radish in a grocery store is pretty impossible, I take it as a whole food supplement to help support my digestion as well. Whole food supplements can help bridge that gap without the side effects of the synthetic isolates found in allopathic meds and most over-the-counter vitamins.

Herbal supplements work far more like medications do, but also more like whole food supplements than you would first guess. Instead of treating a symptom, they are also operating to promote the body's own healing and ability to balance itself. That's why so many of the herbal remedies that are most effective for mood disorders are adaptogenic ones, meaning that instead of being just an upper or downer, they function as all-arounders. They're like the thermostat on the wall that is going to kick on the heat when it's cold or the a/c when it's hot as balls. They work by promoting the stabilization of physiological processes.

Do I Need Supplements?

Maybe you don't need to supplement your diet. Maybe you are getting all you need through your food—especially if you are getting organically grown veggies, eggs and meat from pasture raised chickens, beef from grass-fed and grass-finished cattle, on land that has been tended carefully for generations.

I'm not saying all this to be snarky or up-sell you on nutritional support but to point out that almost everyone in this day and age is dealing with numerous barriers to getting adequate nutrition from the foods they eat.

And speaking of that toxic environment? I know, we already did because I am such a joyful person to hang out with. But we have been absorbing way more crap into our systems since WWII. We come into contact with products and byproducts every day that are inflammatory, cancer-causing and the like.

And if we are taking prescription medications? There are side effects to those. Medications can disrupt our nutrient absorption in a multitude of ways. A 2018 study published in the Journal of The American Medical Association found that one-third of U.S. Americans are taking a prescription medication that can cause a mood disorder, stating there are over 200 different prescription medications that can have this effect, including super common medications like proton pump inhibitors that treat acid reflux and beta-blockers that treat hypertension. Anything we put in our body affects the whole system, something that helps our blood pressure may decrease absorption of other nutrients which cause a biochemical issue that presents as depression, anxiety, and the like. And the more of them we are taking, the higher our risk: going from one medication to three more than doubles our risk of developing clinical depression.

This is true of physical health as well—our prescription meds can cause a multitude of long term issues. For example, someone on corticosteroids for rheumatoid arthritis will need calcium supplementation to manage the decrease in calcium absorption. And an individual on angiotensin converting enzyme (ACE) inhibitors for more than 3 months will likely need zinc supplementation.

How Do I Know What Supplements to Take?

So how do we figure out what supplements would benefit us most? Lab work is ideal, so we can look at what your white blood cell count and the like are actually doing, and also look for patterns of issues. You may not be completely out of range by lab standards, but have decreased levels in a few areas that bear looking at. Alternatively, looking at clusters of the symptoms you are experiencing can help find patterns of bodily responses. Nutritionists and functional medicine docs will ask about all the weird symptoms you might be experiencing (not just the ones you came in with) with some kind of questionnaire, and many more traditional MDs are starting to do the same. I do love the smell of a good paradigm shift in the morning, don't you?

If you are on prescription medications, look at what you are taking, check out the pharmacy fact sheet on side effects (or if you are like me and throw those away pretty quickly, log onto drugs.com) and see if any of your current health complaints overlap with the side effects listed. There is tons of information online about which medications and classes of medications can cause issues.

Watch carefully with new meds. Doctors and pharmacists are way overworked in our healthcare system, but they do give a shit and do know these are issues to watch out for so request a consult with them. It is also really helpful to do a "brown-bag" yearly update on your medications. Bring in everything you are taking to your annual check up to review with your doctor or their clinic staff. I have clients who keep spreadsheets of what they are on, what they have been on and when they stopped, etc. It's a ton of work on their part but it makes it way easier to review and go "Oh! This might be the problem!"

Another way to figure out what supplements might help is to keep track of your health and habits daily. If you are trying to figure out how your body responds to all of the input it receives, a health journal is your best tool. Now that there is an app for everything, you can make this as easy and digitized as possible if that is your preference. If you are old school, you can just jot down the following every day:

- The meds you are taking, the dosage, and the time (both prescription and OTC).
- Same for any supplements.
- What you ate.
- What you drank.
- Other substances ingested (ahem).

- Vaccines received.
- Exercise/movement engaged in.
- Any physical ailments and whatever you used to manage them (asthma attack, back pain).
- Any accidents or injuries.

A lot of docs love if your health journal includes your medical history and your family history as well, so if you are sharing it with them you have it all in one place.

There are a lot of benefits to keeping a health journal. You'll be more organized and streamlined for doctor's appointments and your own personal tracking. You'll save money because you can see your history of treatment at a glance. For example, you can go "oh yeah tried that two years ago and it gave me a horrible headache, no thanks." You'll be more likely to figure out food triggers. You'll notice how stressors (lack of sleep, crappy work schedule, people around you being all people-y) are influencing symptoms. And you'll be more likely to figure out what meds/supplements are helping or hindering.

Supplement Safety

You may have heard something along the lines of "supplements don't work," or "supplements are dangerous." It's true that a lot of them are crap.

Part of the reason that dietary supplements get a bad rap is because many of the ones on the market are just bullshit in a bottle. The New York Attorney General did some testing and sent a multitude of cease and desist letters to herbal supplement companies based on the fact that much of what they tested had no active ingredient. University of Guelph in Canada studied a bunch of supplements and found many unlisted ingredients within them, including things that could encourage an allergic response in someone taking them. And synthetic versions of the product, rather than the actual extracted herb or whole food, are generally going to have more side effects because the human body struggles to recognize them for what they are.

So we read about the amazingness of using St. John's Wort for depression, then we feel stupid and/or ripped off when it doesn't work for us. I had that experience with a cheap kava I tried years ago. It made me seriously irritable and more than a little batshit. I was afraid to try kava again until I learned more about finding and using quality products. I was great about educating myself on prescription meds, but it somehow never occurred to me that I should treat supplements just as seriously.

Additionally, supplements aren't magical fixes any more than an allopathic medication is. Nothing is a magical remedy, but you can't convince social media of that. While I was writing this chapter, I saw a well-known herbal store post wild claims about bay leaves. Including the claim that if you have bay leaf (which they sell!) you have no need for a pharmacy. That a bay leaf added to your meat will convert triglycerides to monounsaturated fats and allows the body to produce insulin (among many other magical things).

This particular meme has been going around since 2019 and is easily fact checked. But this company didn't bother to do so. While I am the queen of ignoring stupidity on the internet because it's bad for my mental health, this is the kind of thing that gets my nutritionist knickers riled up. So I did the research and found out that bay leaf impacts circulating blood lipids, metabolism, and glucose by the same mechanisms that certain forms of cinnamon do. Meaning both are helpful in promoting and managing metabolic stability. One leaf added to your pot of beans doesn't do anything but flavor the beans. But in supplement form (which this company did not sell), it works great. Fresh bay leaves can be encapsulated to about 500 mcg per capsule. Two to six of those (3mg total) taken daily for thirty days has been shown to reduce blood glucose by 20%. And yes, that is phenomenal. Especially considering that there would be no accompanying side effects (unless you are allergic). This could be used in conjunction with other treatments and lifestyle changes to help manage blood sugar. And maybe help minimize the amount of insulin or metformin someone needs to take. But telling people adding a leaf to their food means they can throw away their meds? Those are the types of "alternative facts" that kill people.

A new supplement also has to be the right thing for your specific circumstances. I have colleagues message me on the regular because they have a client who wants to try supplementation for their depression and what should they take? I'm not being snarky when I say I have no idea. I don't know their history, their other medications, all their symptoms, I haven't seen their lab work etc. An ethical nutritionist is going to be as careful and considered as an ethical allopathic doc. If you tell an MD buddy you've been moody lately, and ask what would be helpful, they aren't gonna say "Abilify, LMAO, bet," they are gonna tell you to go get a workup. (At least they should. Run like the wind if they throw pills at you like confetti.)

So, takeaway? There is no magical plant to chew on, research matters as much as anything else you are putting in your body. If the claims seem over the top they probably are.

(And the particular company I argued with on the internet gets props for taking down the post rather than just blocking the angry nutritionist who called them out. And here's hoping they won't share dumb shit in the future.)

If you are using supplements (either herbal or whole food), research as much as you can. ConsumerLab.com is a third party lab that rates for purity and truth for labeling. Look for brands that go through third party testing (NSF International, NSF GMP, US Pharmacopeia (USP), TGA, IFOS & IKOS, Consumer Lab . . . my favorite brand is TGA tested and approved) or if it's a cottage industry maker, ask them about how they source, process, store, and the like. You're looking for them having mechanisms in place to make sure you are getting quality product in the dosage amount it claims on the bottle.

If you can afford to, work with a provider who knows their shit, like an herbalist, Chinese medicine practitioner, or clinical nutrition professional. Most of those who do work with supplements professionally are brand-loyal based on experiences, but will also discuss different brand options with you. I always give people a couple of brand recommendations and discuss what to look for if they are exploring other brands (e.g., you want a kava that has been water extracted and you want a fish oil that hasn't been sitting on a pallet in an unheated storage facility behind a club warehouse).

But most important? Trust your body more than you trust me. A whole food supplement or herb will likely have fewer side effects for you than a prescription medication (and research continues to back this up). If your body recognizes something as food, it will metabolize it differently. But not all bodies respond the same way to food, right? Even healthy foods.

Every body is different and your body will be the best tell of whether or not something is helpful. If you start a new supplement, and have a poor reaction to it, believe your reaction. Stop taking it for a few days then try again. Same reaction? That's a nope from the judges. If you notice any weird "new" problem after a period of time, take a "supplement holiday" and see how you feel. Gradually add them back in one at a time and see what happens. FWIW, this can also be a good idea for some prescription medications, but those can come with serious side effects from withdrawal, so only do so with your doc knowing what's going on.

The Obligatory Disclaimer About Supplements

I am about to talk about some specific supplements. But please don't just go out and try them on your own. It is super important to discuss these things with your treatment provider before embarking on any of them. I have a postdoc in clinical nutrition, but if I have a client on prescription meds I always talk to their prescriber before adding anything else. Interactions are no joke and it's important to be careful. Anything you take can also be of concern if you are pregnant, if you are drinking, or if you are using drugs or even over the counter medications. A prime example? I went to a tea making class last year and the person teaching it, a very skilled herbalist, discussed a calming blend that contained St. John's Wort. She failed to mention that St. John's Wort can interact badly with antidepressant medications and HIV medications.

You also need to consider the following statement to hold true to everything I'm discussing in terms of supplemental treatments:

> "This statement has not been evaluated by the Food and Drug Administration. This product is not intended to diagnose, treat, cure, or prevent any disease."

The FDA does not review claims related to the structure and function of supplements, which is what we are discussing here. I'm going to discuss the structure of different supplements and what research is out there regarding how they function in the human body to help it gain equilibrium. And that's not the same as a treatment, right? We are all smart cookies and we got that. I've cited my ass off in terms of the studies related to structure and function but also encourage you to do your own reading and thinking and talking to your treatment peeps before you start mixing the red and blue pills.

Some Supplements to Consider

Ok, I know I just spent pages flapping around saying don't pop supplements like they're Pez because you will kill youself dead. While that's overall true, there are some generally safe things that are helpful for most people. So here is my top 5 for most-everybody list (though keep in mind that if your tummy doesn't like it, your tummy is in charge).

And, as always, a supplement is not intended (nor FDA approved) to diagnose, treat, cure or prevent any disease. Supplements are designed to support your body's best health and functioning. Even with the most generally safe stuff, your doc may have concerns about what you're taking and at what dosage. Consult the nice person who is trying to keep you healthy, yeah?

Probiotics

Our chronic exposure to toxins and our overexposure to antibiotics has done a lot of damage to our gut microbiome. There is a lot of promising research out there that probiotics can help heal gut lining damage and rebalance that biome.

Probiotics are just beneficial bacterial cultures that research demonstrates reduce the severity and the incidence of gut infections (both chronic and acute) thereby reducing inflammation in the body.

Other research has found them to be of benefit to managing cancer and allergies as well.

We don't know the magical cocktail to use (and indeed, how it would vary from person to person), so you may need to experiment with different formulations and brands. A brand with a higher count of strains is generally a good bet.

Something it might be helpful to take along with probiotics is prebiotics, which are a type of indigestible fiber that operates as food for the probiotics. Their job is to keep the good bacteria active in your system. And then, you may also find it helpful to add digestive enzymes which are the proteins that speed up the chemical soup reaction in our body allowing our food to be broken into substances that our digestive tract can absorb. I say all this within the probiotics section because you can get probiotic supplements that also have prebiotics and digestive enzymes in the same compound.

There aren't any contraindications for probiotics. You might get a little gassy from them, but that is about the extent of side effects.

Omega 3s

Omega 3s are on the list of supplements everyone should take because of how efficiently they decrease inflammation and oxidation that is associated with so much disease, from heart disease to depression.

Omega 3 fatty acids consist of alpha-linolenic acid (ALA), eicosapentaenoic acid (EPA), and docosahexaenoic acid (DHA). Most fatty acids are produced within the body. ALA is not, so we must get it from food or food-based supplements. ALA combines with enzymes to create EPA and DHA.

You can get Omega 3s from foods like fatty fish, flax seed, chia seed, and walnuts. Or you can take them in supplement form as fish oil, plant-based blue-green algae, or ahiflower oil. I take cod liver oil because it also has vitamins D and A. Fun fact, cod liver oil was given to children regularly to fight rickets and obviously had a lot of other health benefits we weren't aware of. I know there's a lot of info out there about Omega 6 and Omega 3 ratios. We don't know what is optimal, but all the research shows that focusing on raising Omega 3s is plenty beneficial rather than worrying about lowering Omega 6s or monitoring them in accordance with each other.

Omega 3s can be contraindicated with a host of bowel conditions, as well as liver conditions, appendicitis, and schizophrenia. Check with your doctor first if any of these apply to you.

L-Tryptophan

You read about this one in the Sleep chapter. L-Tryptophan is the sole precursor of serotonin, and experimental research has shown that L-Tryptophan's role in brain serotonin synthesis is an important factor involved in mood, behavior, and cognition. Tryptophan also increases serum melatonin levels and decreases cytokine production. It's kinda a 20 dollar wonder drug. While L-Tryptophan is in food, we don't absorb it as well because of amino acid competition in the transport system, so taking it as a pill will get you more benefit than eating a lot of turkey will. If quality sleep is an ongoing issue, take it at night as one larger dose instead of throughout the day.

L-Tryptophan is contraindicated with eosinophilia myalgia syndrome. It's also something to discuss with your doctor if you are taking an antidepressant. While there is less interaction between antidepressants and L-Tryptophan versus a strong nervine herb like St. John's Wort, there can still be an issue if you are taking a prescription antidepressant.

Magnesium

Odds are literally even that you are magnesium deficient. 50% of Americans (and up to 80% of older Americans) are. Magnesium is the fourth most abundant mineral and the second most abundant positively charged ion in a human cell. It's fundamental to human wellness for a multitude of reasons, including being responsible for cellular function (the importance of which we talked about earlier in the book) and has been shown to directly impact depression in human beings (with demonstrable difference in symptoms in as little as one week).

Fun fact? Because magnesium is so good at preventing lactic acid build up, I like to suggest taking it before and after a workout or a massage (it also increases the available glucose to energize your muscles)!

Contraindications for magnesium include renal disease (big one!) but you should also check with your doctor if you have heart disease, intestinal issues, or diabetes.

Zinc

One-third of the population worldwide is zinc deficient (and deficiency rates are even higher in low- and lower-middle-income countries). Zinc is an essential nutrient for humans. It is extensively involved in pretty much every groovy thing the body does and is therefore considered an antioxidant. Its ability to alleviate depression is related to many mechanisms in the body (supporting immunity, decreasing inflammation, helping manage oxidative/nitrosative stress, mitigating the stress response, supporting recovery from neurotrophic deficits, and regulating transcriptional/epigenetic neural networks).

The body needs to take in zinc regularly, since it doesn't have a way to store zinc "for later." It's found in multiple food groups, like shellfish, legumes, seeds, and nuts, so malnutrition can lead to decreased zinc intake. Zinc deficiency can also be inherited—some people just don't absorb it well.

Zinc deficiency is identified through lab work, though research shows that a zinc assay test (which you can purchase online for like fifteen bucks) is about 70% accurate if you are looking for a cheaper option.

Zinc may be contraindicated if you have a disorder that leaves you with an inadequate amount of copper in your system.

Conclusion

Was this book as hard to read as it was to write? If my editorial team is any indication, it was. So first of all, so many gold stars for tackling something really complex. Between you and me? Mind-body science is so complicated that it still isn't being taught in graduate programs for therapists, at least where I live. It is also a topic that can veer quite easily into depression-inducing overwhelm. I mean, if shit is this fucked then why bother?

Okay, it is fucked. I get that. I agree. But not hopelessly. I don't believe in doomwriting, handwringing, and hopelessness. I do believe we have enormous capacity to heal, both our bodies and the world they reside in. I've been in this field a super long time now, and see over and over the astonishing capacity we all have for healing, even when we know what the fuck we are actually up against.

I've had many people tell me over the years that my book Unfuck Your Brain gave them a different perspective on how to approach their healing. And taught them to not beat themselves up for doing something really fucking difficult. And I hope this book did the same thing for your relationship with your body. And many of the books that I most love that explore these topics in even more depth are listed in the recommended resources section of this book for your next steps forward.

You don't need me telling you how strong and capable you are, do you? You know. You're already doing it. Here's to more support on the journey.

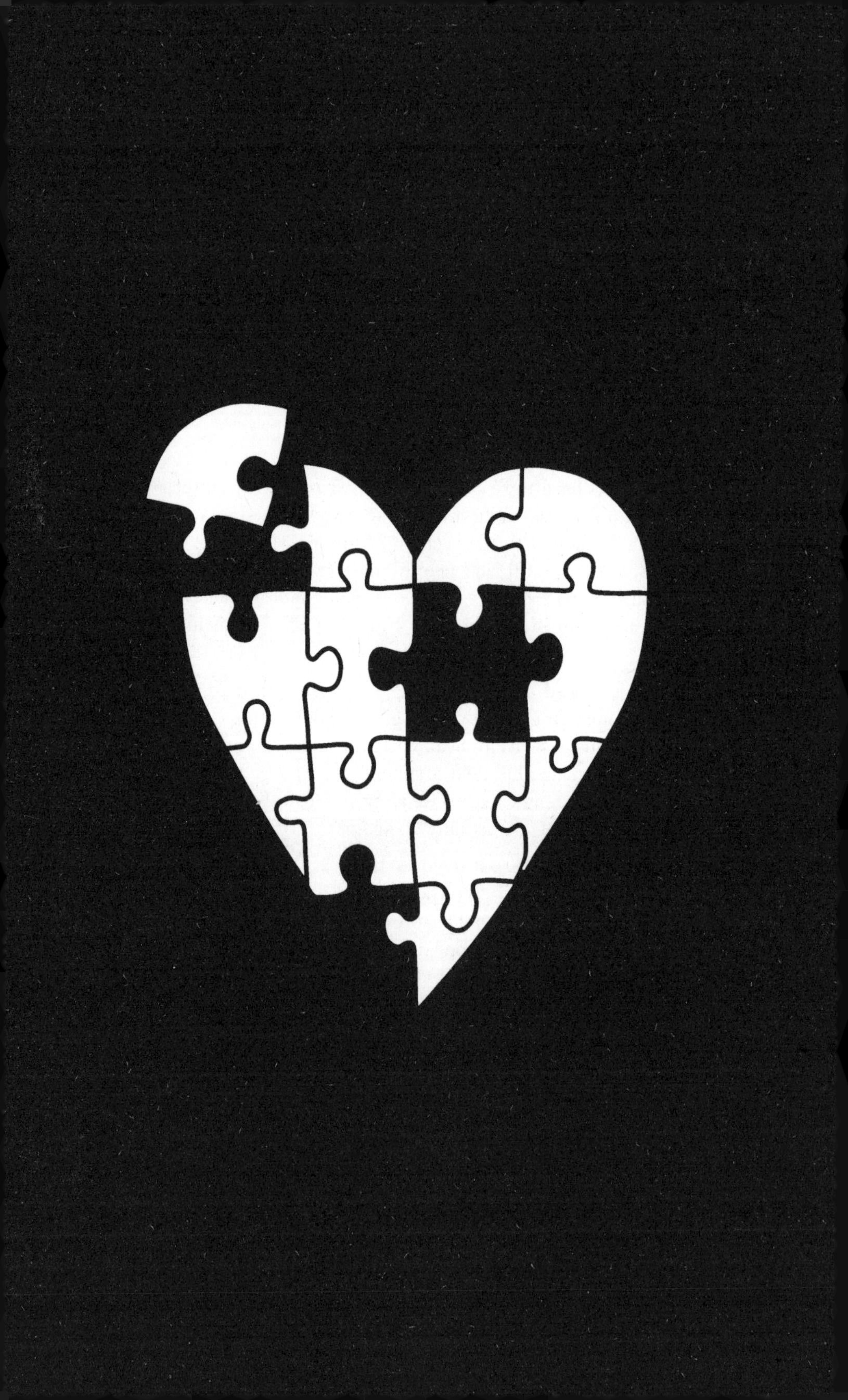

Unfuck Your Intimacy: Relationships, Sex, & Dating

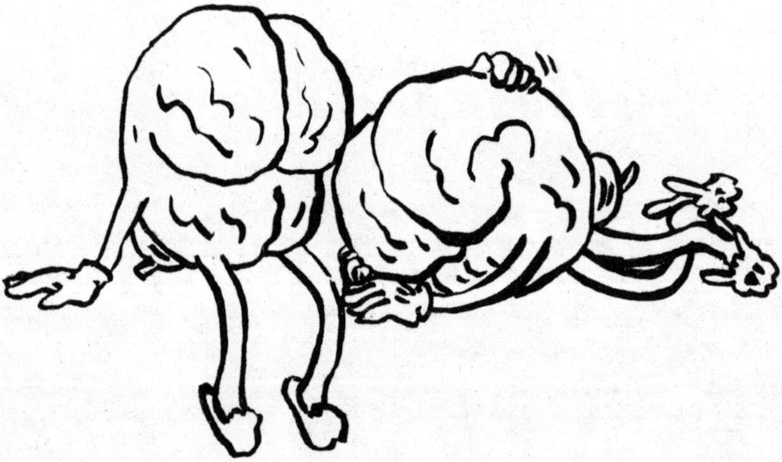

INTRODUCTION

OK, intimacy. What the fuck do I mean by that? I mean, it's more than "just sex," right? In a nutshell, intimacy is our human expression of our most important interpersonal (and yes, intrapersonal) connections.

There are so many cultural messages about the "right" ways to experience intimacy and what is wrong, evil, sinful, or toxic. And about 99.44% of those messages are complete bullshit. Like, such down-to-the-brain-science-of-the-human-experience utter bullshit that I knew this was a topic I really needed to write about.

And creating and maintaining healthy relationships isn't easy. If it was, I wouldn't have a job, after all. We're all trying to figure this shit out. And the market bears that out, right? There are already tons of books out there about sex and relationships. My office and house are stacked to the brim with them. But most fall into one of two categories. They are either super straight-laced (presuming everyone is heterosexual, cisgender, married, Christian, middle-class, etc.) or they focus deeply on a very specific, niche topic like kink or polyamory.

And hey, a book specifically on sexual needle play does have its own target audience. But where are the books for the rest of us? I wrote this for people who don't fit the stereotype on either end. For those of us who are sex-positive (or are really trying to unpack our upbringing so we can be), open-minded (or want to be), non-traditional (no matter how we have tried to fit in with society's expectations), and seeking good information on the variety of issues that come up in our intimate lives.

Where is the inclusivity in mainstream relationship literature? The books that embrace all genders, all sexual orientations, all different kinds of relationship configurations, and all kinds of sexual interests? Seeing ourselves reflected in what we read is FUCKING IMPORTANT. Because we all have unanswered questions. Who and what do we like? How does trauma affect our relationships? What about our religious and spiritual upbringings? How do we unpack our own shit? How do we connect better with our partners? No matter your circumstances, you deserve a happy, healthy, active sex life if you want one.

My background is as a trauma therapist. In my work I've realized that one place trauma tends to show up is in intimate relationships. These are the relationships that require the most vulnerability and where we have the most to gain . . . therefore the most to lose. There are so many ways that sexual intimacy can get fucked up in, and because of, our current culture. I couldn't be a trauma therapist and NOT be a sex therapist. I've found myself working with people on issues surrounding their sexual relationships, so I started studying a lot. Enough, finally, to earn a postdoc in sexology.

Yes, this literally makes me a sexologist. My life does not suck with that as a job title. At my local coffee place my cup usually has "Dr. Perv" scribbled on it by the baristas.

As a sexologist, I think I have two main jobs. The first is coach: I help you figure out how to improve your performance. By performance, I mean reconnecting on an intimate level with yourself and your partners, present or future. Figuring out what is negotiable and what is not. Figuring out what you want your relationships to look like, and then starting to build in that direction.

The second job is intimately (see what I did there?) tied to the first: permission giver. I so often give people permission to start or stop doing things that can immediately impact their intimate relationships. If something is a problem, I give you permission to take it off the table; we can renegotiate it later. If there is something you want to explore, I give you permission to try it.

You are allowed to use a vibrator. You are allowed to stop intercourse if it hurts. You are allowed to schedule an actual date with your partner and enjoy each other's company. You are allowed to not go home for the holidays if sharing a bedroom with your partner is a point of contention with your family.

You can do the thing or not do the thing. My job is to help you figure out what the thing is and encourage you to get back out there and be in charge of your life.

I'll be right here, rooting for you!

What is this book about?

This book is about building intimacy, with or without a partner, through personal and sexual expression. Especially through shit like consent, boundaries, and communication—which we don't talk about on the regular, although we really fucking should.

And this book is also about sex.

For most of us (and yes, I know this doesn't include my ace people . . . more on that later), sex is a big part of our lives and romantic relationships. It's not the foundation of a long term partnership, but it is that super-important spray insulation foam that fills in all the cracks and gaps, keeping the foundation airtight.

We can't separate the relationship stuff from the sex stuff, because they are not separate issues. Sex is generally an instrumental part of connection and communication between partners. So information on building, or rebuilding, that connection is here as well.

But wait! That's not all!!!! I'm not including a free set of Ginsu knives, but this book will also . . .

- Ask a lot of questions. It is surprising what we learn about ourselves when the right questions are asked.
- Apply to all types of relationships, not just heteronormative pairs. Many kinds of relationship configurations exist. Here is to honoring all of them.
- Acknowledge the impacts our upbringing, education, and sexual history have on our current intimate relationships.
- Address the impacts of all traumas in relationships: Everything I have created over the years is intended to work with trauma recovery, rather than accidentally trigger more trauma reactions.
- Address all the ways having a normal, human body can affect our sex lives. Medical problems, aging, having kids. All that normal, human stuff. Many of my referrals come from medical doctors, and I know these issues can be a big deal.
- Include some shorter-term strategies and tips for all the communication shenanigans and other everyday relationship shit that seems to, again and again, impact our sexual intimacy.
- Discuss all the ways we express sexual intimacy. Who we are attracted to and what we like to do with them when we get them naked.
- Attend to the really difficult work of repairing a relationship after there has been a break in trust.
- Help you realize that intimacy is serious business, without discussing it in a painfully serious manner. Life is tough enough, right?

Intimacy is one of the most fundamental expressions of who we are, because we define ourselves in relation to others. But life in general is better handled with as much humor as grace, and hopefully this book reflects that. Some of the stuff we do is empirically funny. And that is a damn good thing! I want to provide you a prescription to improve how you navigate intimacy and relationships. And I want you to giggle some while we do it.

There are some exercises in the book. Y'all have told me you really enjoy trying out the exercises I've included in previous books. Because once the science makes sense, the follow-up exercises don't seem like another dumb waste of time. We are going to just try some new stuff, if you are willing. This is a book of "let's try to figure out what's going on" and "here's some stuff that may help deal with it."

There is no 16-week plan here with steps and readings and assignments and all that jazz. This book is not a heavy, strategic relationship guide: Those already exist and there are plenty that are really good. If you're looking for a book like that, I work from and recommend a mash-up of relationship-specific therapies in my practice on any given day, and invoke strategies from Gary Chapman's 5 Love Languages, Sue Johnson's Attachment Theory, and John and Julie Gottman's Sound Relationship House Theory, though I tend to queer them the fuck up (color you completely unsurprised).

This also is not a guide for either remaining in or leaving an abusive relationship: That is a whole other complicated endeavor that is way out of the scope of this book. If you are turning to this book because you are trying to figure out if your particular relationship may be abusive, listen to your gut and seek some active help. There is no shame in therapy and other mental health support when you are going through some shit. So find someone with some training and perspective who can help you navigate your unique situation. It's really hard to see the forest when your face is pressed up against the tree's bark, right? I've included resources for people in abusive relationships in the appendix.

So just how is the knowledge here going to make your life better? Here's the plan: you are going to read this book and then go try some new stuff. At least, if this approach resonates with you. It's all up to you. These are just tools. You're the one who's gonna do the hard work. One of my favorite jokes is an old standard:

"How many therapists does it take to change a light bulb?" "None! We encourage the light bulbs to change themselves!"

I know, groaner. But seriously, true. Have you ever tried to make a toddler who hates Brussels sprouts eat them? Not without sheer force, and the pushback ain't pretty. I can't make you do anything you don't want to do. Aren't you relieved?

But I do know a lot about sexuality and intimacy work, and have found many common themes over the years. Many of these sections are based on columns written for different publications or my own blog, usually responding to questions people asked me. And if one person asks, they are probably not the only one wondering.

This book is divided into three parts.

Section One: How Our Intimacy Gets Fucked

Human beings are epically skilled at fucking up a good thing. How many bizarre messages have you received about sex and love over the years that really crimped your game? We've got shame issues, abuse issues, religious messages. That's a lot of shit to navigate.

Section Two: Unfucking Our Relationship with Ourselves
Have you never had a handle on what you want and who you are? Or did you once, and then everything changed because you changed? We certainly can't have the deep, interpersonal connections we want if we don't know what we actually, really want. That doesn't make us shitty human beings. It makes us products of a society that tells us how to be, what to be, and who to be. Which means many of us have work to do. What's our identity? How do we communicate with others? How can we interact with our own selves in order to be authentic, connected human beings?

Section Three: Unfucking Our Relationships with Others
Once we get a better handle on who we are, then we have to figure out who we are in connection with other people. And we need to learn to express that honestly, vulnerably, and all that horribly difficult shit. Remember, intimacy is interpersonal. Very few people are an island unto themselves. So how do we do this well in a world that is designed for us to fuck it up?

Getting Started

Sometimes (ok, a lot of times) we have stuff from our history that affects our current life and relationships. And sometimes (a lot of times) we aren't even aware of what that stuff is and where it comes from.

If you're experiencing challenges in your sexual relationships, many medical and therapeutic professionals will work with you on piecing together a "sexual history" of everything you've learned about sex and the kinds of sex you have engaged in. Originally this book was going to include a pretty intensive sexual history questionnaire. There was only one problem with that: it's a pretty intensive questionnaire. Completing such a form on your own has the potential of just being too much.

So instead, there are questions for reflection scattered throughout this book. But even scaled down, these might be anxiety-provoking. You do not have to answer anything that you are not comfortable exploring. You are not graded on completion here. It's totally and completely okay.

However, consider that any question that triggers a strong emotional response may be tied to issues in your current intimate relationships. And if things are getting stirred up, consider investing in your own self-care by working with someone who specializes in these issues. Yeah, I totally mean finding a therapist who specializes in this work. Ugh, I know. Not everyone needs to be in therapy, and it definitely doesn't need to be a long-term thing. But you deserve to be well and happy. And if you aren't getting there on your own, working with someone one-on-one is a worthwhile investment.

One of my favorite sayings is, "Crazy means doing the same thing over and over and expecting different results." So, let's try some different shit, okay?

Questions to Get You Started

- What was your reason for picking up this book? What's the one thing (or the main thing, or the biggest thing) you're hoping to get out of reading it?
- What negative experiences have you had regarding sex and intimacy? You don't have to write out a whole trauma narrative. Maybe just a word or phrase (e.g., "my chronic pain") or an identifier like "the abuse" for more intense experiences. It can be a good way to honor an experience without digging up everything about it in an untethered way.
- What messages have you received about sex in the past? Positive, negative, or neutral? Many people didn't receive negative messages per se, but it was simply omitted from conversations in your household growing up. Was sex discussed at all? If so, how?
- How was sex presented in the media you were exposed to when you were growing up? What kinds of stuff did you discuss with your friends and peers? With people you had romantic relationships with? How about now? Any differences?
- If you could tell your younger self one thing about all these messages and experiences, what would it be?

Section One: How Our Intimacy Gets Fucked

Intimacy is supposed to be easy, right? I mean, neuroscience demonstrates that we are hardwired to connect to others. This is how we are supposed to be.

So if it's all so natural, why do we make such a fucking mess of it all the time? First of all, we're human and make mistakes because that's just part of the process. And it's an ever-changing process. We may have a handle on something and then, boom! Life thought it would be amusing to smash everything to smithereens. And as if that shit wasn't enough, there are so many toxic messages and mainstream bullshit shooting into our ear canals and eyeballs that we can't help but find our authenticity subverted on the regular.

There are a ton of issues that get in the way of fulfilling and healthy intimacy. I could write a fancy multi-volume leather-bound encyclopedia just on that. But for the purposes of this book, I'm gonna focus on the three that I see over and over again. The stuff that most of us bump into in some way, shape, or form in our lives. First up is trauma. Because trauma is a motherfucker that gloms its way into fucking up everything good we experience. Second is religion and spirituality. Connecting to something greater than ourselves is hugely important for a lot of people, but we can get inundated with interpretations and cross-talk that shame our experience rather than enhance it. And finally, we all struggle with bodies that age and change and sometimes require a new set of operating instructions. An aging body beats the alternative . . . but that doesn't mean we pay attention to our emerging needs the way we should!

All our emotional work should start with figuring out what created the problem to begin with. I know that in my own life, understanding how I got somewhere is an essential part of getting out of it. I'm guessing you are also like that. I mean you're reading this right now, when you could be doing so many other things with your time, right?

Reading this book and doing the work serves two purposes. One is to become aware of the pitfalls that lead to your relational fuckery. But also, and I heard this over and over and over again from people who read my book Unfuck Your Brain, it's so helpful to know you aren't just fucking crazy. Or fundamentally broken. Or any of those things we tend to tell ourselves. Relationships get fucked-up because they are hard. Intimacy isn't easy shit to navigate. And everything we have ever been through (and that our partner(s) has been through) has been added to the mix. There is often a bunch of shit that has to be looked at and dealt with so we can get to the good stuff.

So let's start looking and dealing.

FIVE MYTHS ABOUT INTIMACY

I wanna start with the basics. There is so much cultural mythology about what sex is and isn't that I'm going to be addressing over and over and over again within this book. But I bump into these five myths over and over again. I swear, if I could just banish these myths, everything else would fall into place. But then I wouldn't have a job and I'm not sure what else I would be capable of doing to save the world . . . I'll have to marinate on that one.

Myth One: Only Certain Types of Sex Are Real Sex

There is a ridiculous idea that certain types of sex are real. Or, at least, more valid and preferable to others. When we think of "real sex" we usually think partnered penetrative intercourse. But do you know how many people have active and fulfilling sex lives and do not engage in partnered penetrative intercourse? Or, for that matter, how many people have a lot of partnered, penetrative intercourse and still have epically miserable sex lives?

What actually is sex?

- A consensual act
- Between one or more people
- Involving the stimulation of the vagina, vulva, clitoris, penis, testicles, or anus
- For the purpose of pleasure and/or emotional or social connectedness.

Oral sex? Still sex. Solo sex? Still sex. There are no categories of sex that are superior to others. Unless the categories are good sex and bad sex. And you get to define those for yourself.

Myth Two: Sex is Intuitive and Natural

We have this idea that sex should be spontaneous. And that we just sort of "get" what our partner wants. That we are going to run across a field of flowers in slow motion to each other. That everything should be free-flowing. And it will be amazing all the time forever with the right person.

Oh, please. What complete bullshit.

I can vouch with all my years of clinical experience (never mind all my years of, um, experience) that this kind of sex generally happens with people who are the worst possible matches, and in relationships that are completely unsustainable. Insecure attachments with ill-suited people cause a big chemical rush that's fun for a minute. But as most of us have learned the hard way, relationships like these mean you are hanging on for the ride as long as you can, but this ain't someone you bring home to momma.

Sustaining an enjoyable and long-lasting sex life with long term partners takes fucking work, y'all. And communication. And effort. And yes, calendar management. You don't pull together a huge Thanksgiving dinner for 20 people without any forethought, right? You make a plan. Making space for sexual intimacy is often also going to require some planning. Not having a slow-motion field of daisies experience doesn't mean your relationship is a sexual failure.

When I did my TedXSanAntonio talk "Sex, Shame, and Silence" back in 2013 (and go Google that shit if you haven't seen it, I'm still proud as fuck of it!) someone complained on Twitter that my definition of sex (the same one I used above) didn't include the word "natural." Now, sexual interest may be natural (unless you're asexual, demisexual, or graysexual, in which case it would be unnatural), but how we have sex? Not that natural. We are constantly inventing ways to make it weird, interesting, complicated, and technologically advanced. Even professional pervs like the famous sex researcher Alfred Kinsey (who was known for tying up his nut sack with a cord and jamming a toothbrush up his dick) would be all, "Damn, y'all," if he saw what we were up to now.

Sexual desire may be natural. But expecting sex itself to fit some category of natural means we are setting ourselves up for a lot of stigma and shame. Ain't nobody got time for that.

Myth Three: Sex Education Isn't a Universal Necessity

The US is the most sex-obsessed country that never talks about sex in pragmatic ways. It's everywhere. Every car ad is pervy AF. Your steak dinner? Sex was used to sell it in some way, shape or form. But sex education itself? Not acceptable. Just writing a sex column in the newspaper for the past three years has gotten me in hella trouble with the academic establishment. But if there is so much out there that isn't so natural and isn't so intuitive, then we need to have these conversations.

And you know who we need to have these conversations with? Every-fucking-one. Kids. Parents. People with intellectual disabilities. People with physical disabilities. People with severe chronic mental illness. Older people with changing bodies. LGB people. Trans folx. Poly peeps. Kinksters. We all need access to information about safe, healthy, and fun sex that meets our needs and desires.

Myth Four: Sex Is Not That Important In the Grand Scheme of Things

Ok, actually it isn't, if everything is going well.

If the sex is good, it's 10% of your relationship. If it's bad, it's like 90%. Is sex the most important thing in the world? Of course not. But people fighting for fundamental needs like clean water generally also still care about their sex lives and don't like it when things aren't going well.

Sex is important to most people. It's an important part of how we connect and communicate. And it often operates as the sparkly glitter-glue that helps keep relationships together.

If it's important to you, it's important. Don't let anyone diminish that.

Myth Five: Certain People Are Fundamentally Undesirable (and You Are Probably One of Them)

Thank you, media, for continuing to perpetuate the myth that there is only one kind of attractiveness and everyone else is just destined for misery and solitude.

Unless you're an epically unbearable asshole, there's someone out there for you. Your quirks and flaws (whether real or perceived) do not make you unworthy of great sex and wonderful love affairs.

I don't care how long you have been under the impression that you are an ugly duckling. I promise you that there are a decent number of people out there with a duck fetish. And there is nothing sexier than someone who loves their life and is out there enjoying it. That's how all us regular, flawed people find our partners. (Or on OKCupid. Semantics.)

My mission in life is to battle these myths in all the ways they show up in my clients' lives and in society. Kinsey was with me. We may have differing opinions about where a toothbrush goes (FFS dude, in one's mouth) but whatever. Opinions differ. Sex lives differ. And that's what makes it all so fascinating and fun. Everything contained in this book is a means to that end.

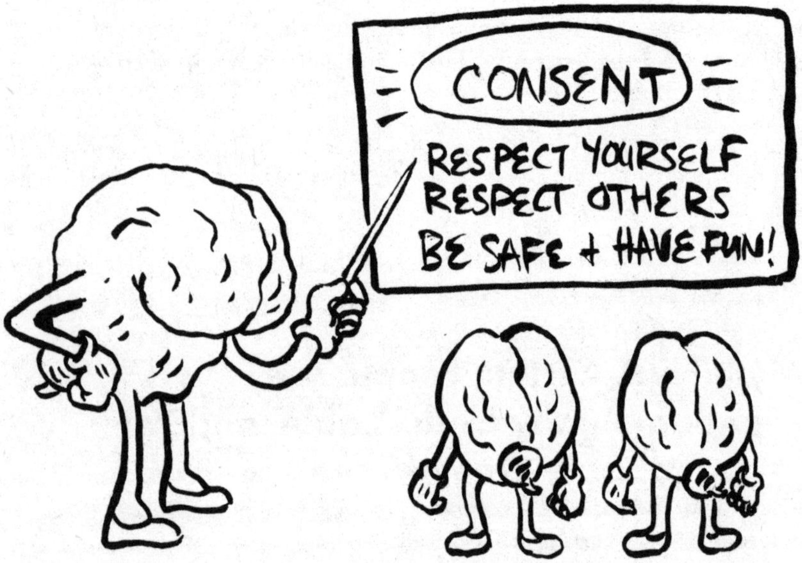
CONSENT
RESPECT YOURSELF
RESPECT OTHERS
BE SAFE + HAVE FUN!

HOW TRAUMA FUCKS US UP

Trauma is an emotional response to a terrible event like an accident, rape or natural disaster. Immediately after the event, shock and denial are typical. Longer-term reactions include unpredictable emotions, flashbacks, strained relationships and even physical symptoms like headaches or nausea. – American Psychological Association

First of all, I go deep into trauma and the neuroscience behind it in Unfuck Your Brain. If you want to catch up on that background, go ahead and do that before you read this chapter.

So why are we talking about trauma again in this book? Besides the fact that, hi, I'm the one stomping around banging pots and pans to get attention paid to trauma in relation to everything?

Actually, it's just that. Trauma does impact everything.

That's the reason I became increasingly interested in sexology as a field of study: The impact of trauma on people's intimate relationships was coming up over and over again and was often the impetus for people seeking support.

A lot of times my clients are super aware that their trauma history is impacting their current relationships. They know there is work to be done and are actively doing that work.

Sometimes, however, we have no clue what's going on inside us and how it is affecting our relationships.

Story time, bear with me. I love a good metaphor. My first car was a tiny, tin can of a thing with great gas mileage and crappy wiring. The taillight would go out on a regular basis, whenever a passenger accidentally kicked the wiring box. I was bopping along, thinking I had no problems when I was causing issues in traffic all around me. Fortunately, I lived in a small college town and knew most everyone. Someone would beep at me and yell "Hey, Faith, light is out again! Almost rear ended you!" And I'd pull over, wiggle the switch, and get it working again.

Why did I never know the brake light wire had been kicked out again? Well, I was in the car, driving the thing around. It seemed okay from my perspective—it was the people trying to navigate around me in our shared space on the road who saw the problem.

Fortunately, I never caused a horrible accident (or even a non-horrible one). Also, fortunately, other people were available to help me to recognize the problem and alert me to it.

Of course, trauma is rarely simple. Most people with a burned-out taillight aren't going to yell and argue, "There is nothing wrong with my car! Go away!" or even minimize, "Yeah, whatever, I'll fix it later, it's not a big deal," as we are apt to do with an unrecognized trauma.

But this is a fantastic analogy about perspective. When we are going about our daily lives, we often don't see the broken bits that are so obvious to those around us. We are navigating our world, thinking everything is status quo until something or someone points it out to us. Or we crash.

Trauma and Intimacy

Intimacy, whether sexual or emotional, may trigger an unwanted response based on past traumas. You want to create a deeper connection with your partner and feel good inside your body, when something that you maybe didn't even realize was there becomes activated.

When I use the word trigger, I'm using it clinically. Meaning you stepped outside the present moment because something from your past made your brain say, "Danger Will Robinson" and freak out. The brain presumes that your past will be your future and goes into survival mode. Maybe you get flooded with memories. Maybe you freeze up and shut down. Maybe you completely disconnect. Your response is not about the present moment, instead your past experiences have gotten reactivated.

The thing I like best about the APA definition of trauma that opens this chapter is that it honors the fact that all types of traumas have the potential to affect our intimate relationships.

When I address the impact of trauma on intimacy, most of the individuals I work with are sexual abuse survivors. But not everyone. All kinds of trauma can create a barrier to the intimacy we want and crave. This barrier can look like struggling to be in the present moment without being triggered, being unable to trust someone enough to be vulnerable, not knowing how to connect with a partner, not being able to identify and articulate boundaries, and feeling disconnected from your own body. Trauma is also associated with many other co-occurring issues including depression, anxiety, and addiction. Any or all of these things can also present obstacles to intimacy. Anyone who has ever been here is head-nodding right now.

What If There Was No Problem Before But It's Hitting Me Now. Why Now????

Congratulations, your brain feels safe enough to let you know that there is a problem and some work to be done. Doesn't that suck?

I have had many people tell me that their sex life with their partner was amazing at first. But as it grew deeper and more connected, they started having more issues. That sounds counterintuitive—the safer you are, the safer you should feel, right?

The more connected and emotionally attached you are to your partner, the scarier it can get. Being close to someone requires a level of vulnerability that you may fear will be taken advantage of. Trust is one of the hardest things for a trauma survivor to experience. But learning to trust again is an enormous sign of strength. Continuing to deepen your trust and connection can help you find the strength you need to continue your healing process.

Other life events can operate as a secondary trauma trigger, dragging you back to the initial unresolved event. Having a child together (whether through pregnancy, adoption, or fostering), or even just thinking about having a child together, can be a trigger. Moving away from a former circle of support can be another. Other big life changes, like in jobs, schools, or the relationship itself—living together, getting engaged, getting married—can also feel destabilizing, even when they are really good changes.

When someone comes to see me for trauma-related intimacy concerns that were not present earlier in the relationship, we usually find there is a fairly recent trigger that makes soooo much sense once we identify it. Oftentimes, just figuring that out is a huge part of moving forward. Because we all need to hear that what we are going through, and our reaction to it, is reasonable.

How Do I Unfuck My Trauma?

The excellent news is this: PTSD (and trauma reactions that don't meet PTSD diagnosis criteria) have the highest "cure" rate of any mental health diagnosis. Even complex traumas with messy co-occurring diagnoses are very, very treatable. The vast majority of people are able to recover from the symptoms they experience related to their trauma. Therapy works. I have zero problem saying in my out-loud voice that I go to therapy. There is zero shame in fighting for your own emotional health.

The important thing is recognizing that the trauma is the root of the other stuff going on, and will be the initial focus of treatment, providing what we now term trauma-informed care. Treatment is grounded in managing the trauma in a safe, structured way. If you are thinking about starting some therapeutic work related to a past trauma, consider finding a therapist trained in an evidence-based, trauma-informed care modality. But of course, different types of treatment are more effective based on your particular situation.

Use the types of interventions you feel comfortable with. I've had lots of patients who've announced, after being dragged to my office by a parent or family member, "I'm not talking about that shit and you can't make me!" And fair enough, getting better doesn't require you to unpack a trauma narrative. The important thing is to look for someone whose approach works for you. Ask them about their theoretical orientation, meaning how they approach healing, and find someone whose worldview aligns with your own.

I'm not referring just to traditional talk therapy. There is a ton of research behind somatic-based treatments like yoga, acupuncture, hypnotherapy, and the like. I recommend doing both somatic and talk therapy at once, but start with what feels safest for you and take it from there. There is no wrong way to start.

When considering what kind of treatment will work best for you, the question to ask yourself is "What do I most need right now?" No one knows more about what it is like to live inside your body and mind than you. What does your inner self say it needs? It could be "I really need to tell this story," or it could be "I don't even know how to be safe in my daily life right now."

Listen to that voice. It's your survivor's voice, the one that has kept you safe during your trauma experience. It knows what you need to heal and move forward.

There are many ways to feel in charge of our lives again after our sense of safety has been violated. Self-compassion is a powerful way to take back your power after a trauma. I've included some self-compassion exercises at the beginning of Section Two of this book for you to check out. I have worked with people who became politically involved after a tragedy in an effort to change the social structures that allowed for the traumatic events to occur, people who began volunteering to work with others who have suffered similarly, and people who began engaging in new activities (such as boxing classes) and self-care (such as body work) in order to feel in control again. And one of the best tools I've found for helping people reconnect to intimacy after trauma is using sensate focus exercises with a partner, like the ones in Section Three.

Everyone's path to healing is different, but the common theme is a return to empowerment and healthy coping in the present moment. Figuring out what that might look like for you is the first step.

Some Questions to Ask Yourself

Empowerment

- What does empowerment look like to you? Feel like?
- How does empowerment connect to safety for you? Recovery?
- What are some ways you have experienced empowerment in the past?
- What are some activities you are interested in exploring to feel more empowered?
- What would be the first steps you'd need to take to explore these options?
- Is that something you are interested in doing right now? Why or why not?

Healthy Coping in the Present Moment

- What signs do you notice in yourself when you are triggered or activated, and not reacting to the present moment? What do you feel emotionally? Think? Feel in your body?
- When it comes to coping skills, we often already know what works for us, but it is difficult to remember to use those skills in the moment when we are distressed. What coping skills have worked for you in the past? What has been working lately? Which others are you willing to try?
- What can you do to help remember to use these skills? Are there individuals who can support you? Are there items you can have available (or items you need to get rid of!) in order to remain safe?
- What positive qualities did you develop in response to having to manage a traumatic life event? How could these skills help you in the future? This isn't an encouragement to gaslight yourself, by any means. While it is one of the hardest ways to learn a life lesson, many people have reported that dealing with a trauma did help them develop life skills that they didn't have before. Even if it was a lesson they never wanted to have to learn.

Creating a Trauma Response Safety Plan

Some individuals feel much safer if they have a very specific safety plan in place in the event of a trauma response. One of the most difficult things about being triggered is feeling so overwhelmed by the experience that making any decision about what to do in the heat of that moment feels impossible. Your brain isn't working the way it normally does, so having a plan to fall back on can be very helpful to both you and any partner with whom you feel safe in sharing that plan. Sharing your plan does not mean you need to share the entirety of your trauma history.

When we are sexually intimate, we are at our most vulnerable. Even if everything is going well, we can feel that we are stepping outside of our comfort zone. But this is the most important time for us to open lines of communication, especially if we feel unsafe. Many people create an effective verbal plan with their partner, meaning they just discuss what works for them via a conversation; others prefer the safety net of a more formal plan, like something written down, that you would refer to as needed.

You can use the following questions to outline a safety plan and open up the discussion with your partners.

- When you are feeling the most healthy, happy, joyful, and well what does life look like? How do you feel? How do you interact with others?
- What things do you do, or are you willing to start doing, as part of your daily wellness plan? What things have you noticed help you manage your triggers more effectively in a general sense? For example, many people have noticed that getting a certain amount of sleep and/or exercise is very beneficial to them. Some people feel better when they eat a certain way, meditate, pray, spend time with people they care about, or take time to enjoy hobbies that are meaningful to them. What activities do you think will work best in your wellness toolbox?
- What are some of the situations that you have come to realize are triggers for you? These are less the big catastrophic things that we sometimes worry about, but the smaller things that can happen on a more regular basis. For many people, this can be certain situations (like being in a crowded room or not doing well on a project), specific dates (like a holiday or birthday), or something they connect to in a very sensory way (like a certain smell or tone of voice). We often don't know what all of our triggers are, and may sometimes get triggered without any idea what caused it. But if we start keeping notes when it does happen, we can start to figure them out. So you may consider this list a work in progress that you keep adding to over time.
- What are your early warning signs that you may be getting triggered? What kinds of thoughts do you have? What emotions arise? What kind of behaviors do you engage in that you don't typically do?
- If you are triggered, what are the things you can do for yourself to help you manage your response? These are often things that you already do for your general wellness that become especially

important in these situations. But they may also be coping skills or activities that you use when you are in especially tough situations.

- While there are a lot of things that you are able to do for yourself, there may be times you need help from others, especially if you are working on your intimate relationships. What do you need from others? Who do you trust to provide that support? How will you ask them about it?
- How will you know that you have been triggered past a point that you, and the individuals who typically support you, can handle?
- If you are at a point where you are not able to manage these triggers on your own, or with the assistance of the people who usually support you, what is the next step for you?
- Once your crisis has been managed, how will you know when you are feeling safe and secure again?

Once you try out your safety plan, jot down any notes about what worked and what didn't and make adjustments as needed.

Healing in Relationships

Whether you are just starting to explore a new relationship with someone or have been with your partner for a very long time, it is important to consider that they may be coping with an unresolved trauma. My late husband and I were married for ten years before he told me about his history of being sexually abused. It took him that long to feel safe with his story, and he was married to a therapist. It also made so many things that we struggled with make sense.

More often than not, statistically, any given person has experienced some kind of trauma. Cindy Crabb, who writes the beautiful and thoughtful Doris zines, suggests that you always assume anyone in your life has a sexual abuse history. This holds true for other traumas, as well. Cindy writes about how difficult it can be to discuss sex as a trauma survivor, especially if the trauma had sexual content. It isn't something we give much voice to in our society.

If you know or suspect your partner is coping with a trauma response, initiating the conversation rather than waiting for them to do so may be a very liberating experience. Of course, that doesn't mean forcing someone into a conversation, but offering it as an option can help you both walk through a door they didn't even know how to open.

Some things to try, or think about, if your partner has experienced a trauma or you think they may have:

- Expect them to not be present sometimes. Either during sex or just in general. If you get a sense that they are checked out, ask them if they are present. Ask if they need space to be alone, or if your presence helps. Ask what you can do to help if they are struggling. ("I think I lost you back there. Are you okay? Is there anything I can do to help?")
- Create a safe word. "No" is a crappy safe word, especially if you are into BDSM or edge play. Your word can be something silly that lightens the mood ("cheese doodles!"), or something that speaks to the experience ("darkness") but decide on this ahead of time with an action plan of what you will both do if the safe word is used during intimacy.
- If your partner needs space in the heat of the moment, offer them a chance to discuss it during a less stressful time within the next day or two. ("I know last night really triggered you, is there anything that you'd like to talk about now that you've had some time to think about it? Anything else that would help?")
- It's okay to ask. Did you fail your mind reading classes? I did. It's OK to say something like "I get a sense that your mood shifted all of a sudden/It feels like you just shut down/Is something going on, I can't tell." Try to do so in the most non-accusatory way possible, of course. But only ask once. A power struggle of "I'm fine!" versus "No, you are not!" is a terrible one that nobody wins.
- Be patient and understand that the sensations in a trauma survivor's body can be very contradictory. And the partner working through a trauma has to choose what sensations to focus on at each moment. That can be a complicated process for you to be present for. Sometimes your partner is doing everything possible to be okay. Maybe part of their healing experience is working through the issue in the moment and it's best to keep doing exactly what you were doing.
- Some things you can say include, "I'm not sure if you liked that. I was hoping that you did and you said that you were okay, but I felt that maybe you were struggling. I want this to be good for you, so it won't hurt my feelings if there is something else you need or something you want me to do differently. And if you insist you really were okay, I promise to believe you until you tell me otherwise!"

Remember that if your partner has a trauma history, they are the one who is responsible for themselves in the end. You can't rescue them or fix them. You can be part of their journey rather than an obstacle, but only if they let you and only if what they need is something you are able to give. This may be a continuing conversation throughout your relationship.

If you choose to be with them on their journey, don't forget your own wants, needs, and desires. Take responsibility for your self-care throughout the process, as well!

Grounding Exercises

Adding to your toolbox the coping skills that work best for you is good, proactive medicine. I've written a book entirely on coping skills (creatively titled: Coping Skills), which you can use to find a ton of ideas. The go-to skill I encourage everyone to learn is grounding exercises. I go into detail on these in Unfuck Your Brain, so make sure to check that out.

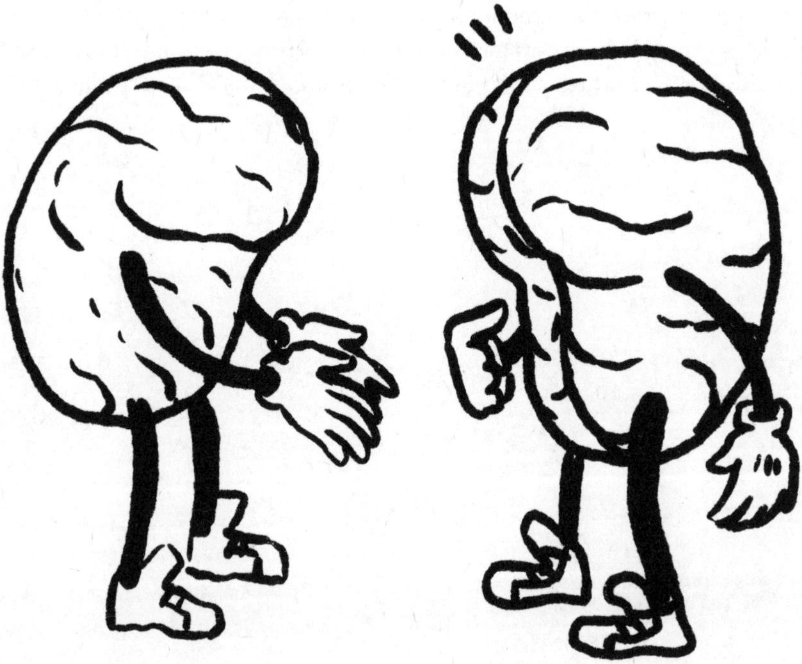

SEXUALITY, RELIGION, AND SPIRITUALITY

They try to say what you are, spiritual or sexual?
They wonder about Solomon and all his wives.
In the body of the world, they say, there is a soul
and you are that.
But we have ways within each other
that will never be said by anyone.
–Rumi

Religion and spirituality are a big part of most people's lives. Even if they aren't part of your life now, chances are still pretty good that they played a huge part in the messages you got growing up, whether you wanted it or not.

I define spirituality as a larger experience of purposeful belonging. It can provide hope, healing, and connection to something larger than ourselves. Religion, at its best, is the organized expression of our spiritual selves. Just as we are hardwired for connection, intimacy, and touch, we are hardwired for ritual. For many people, religious practice fulfills their human need for the ritual expression of spirit.

The practice of spirituality, generally interpreted and defined within the scope of religion, has a history of seriously fucking people up. On one hand, we are told we are a beloved child of God (or another deity), and on the other we are told we are sinful and broken . . . that our thoughts, feelings, and behaviors bring shame to ourselves and those who love us. That's a good way to keep people in line, but it's a shitty way to help people create an authentic spiritual connection.

Being a spiritual person and expressing it through religious practice isn't wrong or unnecessary. But problems arise when aspects of that practice conflict with something fundamental about who we are as people. Religion is totally boss when it reminds us to be good, and kind, and patient. To care for others who need caring for. But it's a huge fucking problem when it tells us our mere existence requires redemption.

I don't know anyone who hasn't had religious values from their past create some kind of internal conflict in how they express themselves as sexual beings. The first instance we generally think of is when individuals have a sexual orientation or gender identity that their religious practice deems sinful. And yeah, those are big ones. But in reality, conflicts between religion and sexuality occur in almost all of our interactions all of the time. What level of commitment should we have with another person before engaging in sexual activity—marriage only? Is solo sex acceptable or is that cheating on a partner? Is porn usage sinful? What about BDSM? Polyamory? Fetish play?

While I was raised in a deeply religious home, I was also fortunate enough to be raised by parents who attached no shame or restrictions to sex. Not everyone has had that experience, and many individuals struggle because of it. Most worrisome to me is the enormous sense of shame that many people experience due to these conflicts. Brené Brown, the well-known shame researcher, notes that there is a fundamental difference between guilt and shame. Guilt implies that you made a mistake, shame implies that you are a mistake. Religious doctrine regularly invokes shame around sex and intimacy, with deliverance from this shame tethered to renunciation and confined behavior.

The general message you may have heard from sex-positive, affirming people is along the lines of well then, fuck religion. But not everyone wants to give up something that has grounded their identity in so many ways throughout their lives. It's akin to saying "Fuck your mom, she's an abusive asshole," and you're thinking, "Yeah, but she's still my mom. I dunno about that . . . "

The intent of unpacking your religious messages is not to dissuade you from any of them, but to help you recognize them and evaluate whether or not they make sense for your authentic self. Finding people you trust to help you work through the process as you reflect on these questions can be invaluable. Reading books by people who have dedicated their lives to resolving this conflict may also help . . . and if you are looking for good recommendations for books, check out the recommended resources at the end!

Your mission here is to figure out what your unique experiences are in this domain and how they have been impacting your intimate relationships. Sometimes just asking the right question helps us go "oh, yeah . . . I didn't even think about how that's a thing in my life." So here's some shit to start asking yourself.

Some Questions to Ask Yourself

What is your spiritual and religious background?

- How have your spiritual or religious beliefs and practices changed through childhood, adolescence, and adulthood?
- Are your current religious or spiritual beliefs and practices different from many of the individuals who share your faith tradition?

- How do the teachings of your spiritual beliefs/practices address sexual intimacy? What role has it played in your spiritual development?
- Have you undergone any body modifications as a consequence of your religious beliefs that affect your sexual identity and practices (e.g., circumcision, castration, tattooing, piercing, or other body art)? If so, how have these changed your self-image? Your ability to engage in sexual intimacy?

How do you navigate your sexuality and spirituality now?

- How do you view the integration between your spiritual self and sexual self?
- Do your spiritual or religious beliefs and practices have any suggestions or rules about sex and intimacy? If so, what are your thoughts and feelings about these suggestions or rules?
- Do you engage in any sexual activities that are in conflict with these rules? If so, what are your thoughts and feelings about these conflicts?
- According to your spiritual or religious beliefs, what are the consequences of engaging in activities that are in conflict with this belief system? What are your thoughts and feelings about these possible consequences?
- Have you, or someone you know, experienced negative consequences from a conflict between your religious beliefs and your sexual practices (e.g. judgment, criticism, exclusion from certain events or membership in general, corporal punishment, etc.)? How has that affected you?

How do you negotiate spirituality in your relationships and community?

- If you are partnered, do you and your partner practice the same faith tradition? If not, how is your spirituality similar? How is it different?
- If you are partnered, do you or your partner experience any conflict between sexual expression and religious beliefs and practices? If so, how have these conflicts been negotiated? Have they been navigated successfully or are there still areas of tension?
- Have you received any guidance from a spiritual or religious leader about these conflicts? How about from a mental health or medical professional? What about family or peers? What was their advice or feedback? If you consulted with more than one person, did you receive conflicting feedback?

- Are there any areas that you and/or your partner feel are non-negotiable? Are there any avenues of compromise that you and/or your partner are willing to consider?
- What are your thoughts and feelings about the intersection of spirituality and sexuality at this time? Have they changed from the past? Do you think they are likely to change over time?
- What would allow you to be both a spiritual and sexual individual?

CHANGING BODIES AND OTHER FUCKITUDE

Oh hey, there. I have a normal human body, capable of misfires and weirdness and continuing issues regarding its maintenance and functioning. I bet you do, too. In fact, I have a sneaking suspicion that we all do.

So why don't we talk about how this whole business of walking around in a wonky meatsuit affects our sexual intimacy? Because shame. Because embarrassment. Because not even realizing the connection between the two. Because not knowing what to say.

Trauma and societal messages aren't the only things that get in the way of having the sex life we desire. Maybe you struggle with chronic pain. Or you're otherwise healthy but broke your damn leg recently. Maybe you had a baby. Or you're just getting older, which does strange-ass shit to the body. It's time to start thinking and talking about these things in a better way.

Sexual Disorders

Keeping your sex life fully charged can be like tending a hothouse orchid. So many little things can go wrong and knock things off course. At some point in our lives for most everyone, we'll experience a sexual disorder.

The word "disorder" is a clinical term. A crappy one, I know. But it really only means that things are not working in an orderly way. And of course "orderly" is one of those consensus statements reflecting the general, cultural expectation of how things work, right? A disorder is not emblematic of being fundamentally broken or wrong or fucked up. It's just how it is sometimes. Which can add a layer of complication to our sexual intimacy. But we can totally work around all that stuff.

So let's start off by talking about the different categories of sexual "disorders" before we go into managing them, okay? We tend to think first of erectile dysfunction (because that's where the pharmaceutical dollars are), but there are actually four different types of sexual disorders.

- Desire disorders occur when there is no desire or interest in sex (this is not the same thing as being asexual . . . which we'll talk about in Section Two).
- Arousal disorders happen when the mind is ready and willing (which doesn't happen in desire disorders) but the body isn't

up to the task. This is the category for erectile dysfunction, though of course you don't have to have a penis to experience an arousal disorder.

- Orgasm disorders are what we call it when someone either cannot orgasm or it takes way longer and extra effort. This is also the category where "premature ejaculation" falls.
- Pain disorders are when intercourse literally hurts (this generally affects individuals with vaginas more than individuals with penises).

These issues may manifest in relation to other bodily changes, or they may present themselves just because they do. We are often so wrapped up in treating the symptoms by taking a pill (like the ones in commercials that involve some dude throwing a football through a tire swing) that we don't look at the underlying issues in a holistic way. Sex therapist and author Marty Klein states that this kind of work requires a different level of sexual intelligence. So let's ensmarten ourselves more on the topic.

Aging

Being in an aging body isn't anyone's idea of fun, but we all agree it beats the alternative. No matter how healthy we are, we all can benefit from attending to certain things in order to maintain a body that enjoys sexual intimacy.

The biggest sexual change most of us face as we age is hormonal. Testosterone and estrogen levels generally drop as we get older.

For cis men, this can mean erectile dysfunction or even just full arousal being more difficult to gain and maintain (read: a chubby instead of a stiffy). And when you do get the blood flowing, completing to orgasm doesn't always happen. Thanks, wang.

For cis women, the reduction in estrogen can lead to vaginal dryness as well as emotional and bodily changes that increase stress levels and decrease sexual desire.

There isn't a ton of research for non-cis folx on how any hormone therapy is affected by aging, but it is definitely something to take into consideration and chat with your doc about.

Disabilities and Chronic Disease

Of all the ways someone can achieve a "minority" status in the world, disability is the category where any of us can end up at any time. Whether you have a disability you've lived with your whole life or you entered this category later due to an accident or illness, it doesn't take a rocket scientist to realize that this can mean huge adjustments in all aspects of your life, including your sex life.

Some of the stuff that may come up around disabilities includes:

- Body image issues (your body may look and work differently than it has in the past, or than other people's around you)
- Anxiety about things changing or about things differing from what partners are used to or expect
- Anger at having a disability or chronic disease
- Feelings of guilt, as if the disease or disability is punishment for past actions
- Worry about a partner's unhappiness or dissatisfaction
- Worry about your partner being unfaithful or leaving you
- Frustration that your desire doesn't match your current access or ability
- Anger that your partner is healthy and you aren't

Possible issues for partners can include:

- Frustration with the limitations put upon your sex life because of the disability
- Feeling deprived. And angry about it. And then maybe guilty for being angry
- Resenting being in a caretaker role
- Guilty that you are not sick
- Challenged by your partner's changing body and struggling with physical attraction
- Worrying about hurting them

Of course, these kinds of feelings can come up for many other reasons too, but they are generally most prevalent when individuals are dealing with a chronic condition that seriously impacts their physical health and ability to express themselves sexually.

Childbirth

The general media portrayal is that birth is a mystical experience from which your body bounces back immediately. Hah. My kids are adults and I haven't gotten my body back.

Even if you had the most glorious pregnancy ever, with no morning sickness, stretch marks, or cramps. Even if you had the easiest birth experience ever, with no C-section, or episiotomy, or tearing, or hemorrhoids, and your body bounced right back? Childbirth still changes us. It changes our relationship with our body because we used it to grow another human. So many people have told me that during pregnancy and after birth their body simply didn't feel like theirs anymore, and it was a disconcerting realization.

And if you are breast or chest feeding? The whole matter of sustaining a small, dependent living thing with your body lives on. With chapped nipples, leaks, clogged ducts, and all that other fun stuff. And hey, even if you aren't, you still have a tiny, fully dependent, and wildly fragile human attached to you on a regular basis. Your sleep is fucked. You are completely done with being touched by other humans by the end of the day. Talk about a disruption of an orderly sex life!

Other Mental and Physical Health Stuff

You might be thinking, "Doc. I'm not in a wheelchair and I'm not 97 years old. This whole section doesn't apply to me." But hey. We are all living in an increasingly toxic world and issues around sexual functioning are so damn commonplace for everyone that it merits discussion.

Mental and physical health diagnoses that do not directly affect sexual functioning can still indirectly affect it. Meaning, problems can occur because of something else you are living with. For example, over 100 million people in the United States have a diabetes diagnosis. Research shows that 50% of men and 35% of women with diabetes experience sexual dysfunction as a result. The good news is that if their diabetes is well controlled, those numbers drop quite a bit. The bad news is literally millions of people are struggling in this way and we aren't talking about it.

Cancer treatment, high blood pressure, heart disease, and just good ol' common stress can all impact our interest in sex and/or our ability to engage in the types of sex we want. And lest we forget, mental health also has a huge impact on the physical body. We talked about PTSD earlier, but all mental health issues impact our sense of self and our place in the world and that will absolutely affect how we connect to others. For example, if you are experiencing a depressive episode so bad you haven't had a shower in three days, the chance of you being interested in sex is probably about nil.

Long term medication use can also affect sexual functioning. This is by far not an exhaustive list, but just to give you an idea: hormones can cause desire disorders, anti-hypertensive (blood pressure) medications can cause arousal disorders, many antidepressants and some mood stabilizers can cause desire and arousal disorders. Even just plain old over the counter decongestants and antihistamines can cause arousal and ejaculation disorders.

So What Do We Do?

Everyone's experience is really unique, so I can't hook you up with a specific plan to have the best sex possible while dealing with physical changes, challenges, ailments, and disabilities. But I can help you look at some good general solutions, give you a list of questions to bring to your doctor's office, and then give you a few more things to think about and talk to your partner about while you do this work.

Back in 2003 the medical journal American Family Physician published a piece on sexual functioning and chronic illness that had some pragmatic general advice about optimizing sexual functioning as much as possible for individuals with chronic issues. Here's the breakdown of what the authors of that article suggest, along with a few ideas from me. You'll notice that these are organized by intervention instead of by disorder. Disorders are just how issues manifest. They aren't causal in and of themselves. So any interventions we try should be about being as healthy as possible, not just popping one of those damn tire-swing pills.

Dietary Interventions

- No tobacco. No matter how you are getting it in your body. No smoking, vaping, chewing, etc.
- Limit your alcohol intake (if you're a drinker) and consider a no-drinking experiment to see if it makes a difference for you.
- Wait two hours after eating or drinking alcohol before engaging in sexual activity
- Eat as cleanly as possible. The fewer additives and toxins you consume, the better you'll feel in general. Cleaning up your diet isn't easy and it is expensive. I totally get that. But any small changes you can afford to make may have a huge impact on your wellbeing
- Consider whole food supplements to help you get the nutrients you are missing out on. For example, soil depletion means we have far less trace minerals in our fruits and vegetables than we did 100 years ago
- Talk to your doctor about what types of exercise you can tolerate physically. Match that list against your list of the types of exercise you can tolerate emotionally. Gentle movement that actually feels good can be incredibly beneficial in building strength and flexibility . . . or at least slowing the loss of strength and flexibility

Medication Interventions

- If you have chronic pain, take your pain medications 30 minutes before starting sexual activity

- Talk to your prescriber about which of your medications may have sexual side effects and discuss replacing them with something you tolerate better or finding ways to manage those side effects
- Consider complementary therapies like acupuncture, neurofeedback, biofeedback, and the like to help manage pain
- If your diagnosis has caused an onset of depression (which is entirely probable and makes a ton of sense), make sure you get that depression treated

Environmental Interventions

- Keep your home at a comfortable temperature. If you need it warmer to help your pain, do that. If you need it cooler to help your breathing, do that. Figure out your best operational setting for sexual intimacy and adjust as needed
- Plan sexual activity for the times you know you have gotten the most rest and your energy levels are good. This may be time of day, time of week, or time of month. For example, many people on chemotherapy get breaks in the cycles and know their energy levels are the best near the end of the break
- Be flexible with types of sex as well as bodily positions. Use pillows, wedges, or other supports if they help
- Consider using sexual aids (sex toys!) to augment your experience

Emotional Interventions

- Communicate openly and honestly with your partners about your needs, wants, likes, and dislikes
- Explore your own body through solo sex. It's easier to communicate what works for you if you've already figured it out for yourself. Plus regular orgasms may help you feel better physically and emotionally
- Use intimate touching that isn't designed to lead directly to sex every time
- Use all of your senses to focus on the parts of your body where you enjoy stimulation the most, even if they aren't traditional erogenous zones. A friend of mine sustained a nasty spinal injury. He recovered fully, except afterwards he realized that he had more sensation above the point of injury than below. While he is still able to maintain an erection, his neck being stroked was the best way to encourage his arousal.

Questions for Your Doctor

In a perfect world, your doctors would be the ones opening up conversations about sex, saying something like, "It's pretty common for people with this condition to notice that it's affected their sex lives in some way. Have you noticed anything we need to address?" This opens the door for you to bring up any questions you have. However, a lot of doctors are uncomfortable bringing up the topic of sex, even if they are comfortable discussing it. For example, many docs could tell you that kegel exercises can help you better control your PC muscles, which can help with bladder control, premature ejaculation, and pain associated with penetration. But they'll only talk about this if you bring it up.

So you may have to be the person to say you have questions. And if they can't answer the questions, tell them to refer you to someone who can.

Not sure what to ask? Here are some questions to start with:

- Are certain kinds of sexual activity off limits? Which ones?
- What is the safest kind of sexual activity for me right now?
- What should I do if I have pain or medical issues during sexual activity?
- Will my meds affect my sex life (libido/desire/ability to perform)?
- If so, do I have other medication options? Other ways of managing these effects?
- Are there any circumstances under which I should avoid sexual activity?
- Will I ever be able to ________________ again? What are the best case, worst case, and most likely scenarios?
- Is it possible I could regain the ability to engage in some sexual activity that I can't do now? What would help me be able to do that?
- Are there any resources that are specific to my situation that you recommend?
- Are there any other treatment professionals you recommend working with that may help with this issue?

Questions for Yourself

When it comes down to it, self-reflection and partner communication may help far more than any doctor or sex therapist. Here are some things to think and talk about.

- What was the quality of the sexual relationship before the illness/injury if you had one? Sometimes if things were already not going well, a new health issue can become the excuse to just stop trying altogether.
- What makes something "sex?" Has that changed? Could it change to encompass more activities than you've done in the past?
- Where do you feel sensation and pleasure?
- What do you miss most?
- What does your partner say that they miss most?
- What things are working well?
- What do you most want to communicate to your partner?
- What are your fears in doing so?

Kegel Exercises

Being healthy is far easier if we exercise, right? Sexual health has its own exercise . . . the Kegel. Obviously, Kegels aren't magically curative for all kinds of sexual disorders but they are one of the go-to exercises that really help a lot of people! Kegel exercises are designed to strengthen the pelvic floor muscles, focusing specifically on the "PC" (pubococcygeus) muscles. Kegels have tons of practical use for all kinds of issues, whether you have a vagina or penis.

Dr. Arnold Kegel was a gynecologist who developed these exercises for women who had pelvic floor weakening post childbirth. He found another interesting side benefit: His patients who were doing kegels regularly were achieving orgasm with greater ease and frequency, and had a more intense experience, showing that kegels have an additional benefit to sexual intimacy. They have been found to help both women and men better achieve orgasm, and can help both sexes feel more in control of their sexual experience for a few reasons:

- Kegels help control urinary incontinence, so many individuals feel more secure during sexual activity and less likely to leak urine.
- Kegels help give the individual on the receiving end of penetrative intercourse more control over the experience and more intense orgasms. They also create a tighter vagina or anus, therefore increasing the pleasure of the penetrating partner as well.
- Kegels help bring more blood flow to the pelvic region in women and the perineum region in men, potentially intensifying arousal.

Kegels can be done with or without an aid (such as a dildo, vibrator, or tool designed specifically for kegel mastery like Betty Dodson's kegelcizer). They can be done solo (which is usually a good place to start) as well as during penetrative intercourse (which can be a lot of fun for both partners).

Here's how to do them:

- Locate the muscle group in question by squeezing the muscles you use to stop your urine flow. If you are urinating and are able to halt the flow, you have the right muscle group. Your stomach and buttock muscles should not tighten in the process. You also don't want to do your kegel exercises when emptying your bladder on a regular basis. That can lead to weakening the pelvic floor muscles which can prevent you from fully emptying your bladder (which, in turn, can lead to an increase in urinary tract infections).
- If you are using a kegel aid, lubricate the aid before insertion and practice kegels lying down. If you are not using an aid, it may be of benefit at first to practice lying down.
- Squeeze the muscle group for three seconds, then release for three seconds. Complete 10 to 15 cycles of squeeze and release.
- Try to do this at least three times a day. The more regularly you perform the exercise, the better results you will get (just like any exercise).

As you get more comfortable doing this, you will find that you don't have to set aside "kegel time" to be effective. You can do them while engaging in other activities since no one will know what you are up to—unless of course you are doing them during sex, in which case your partner will know and appreciate it!

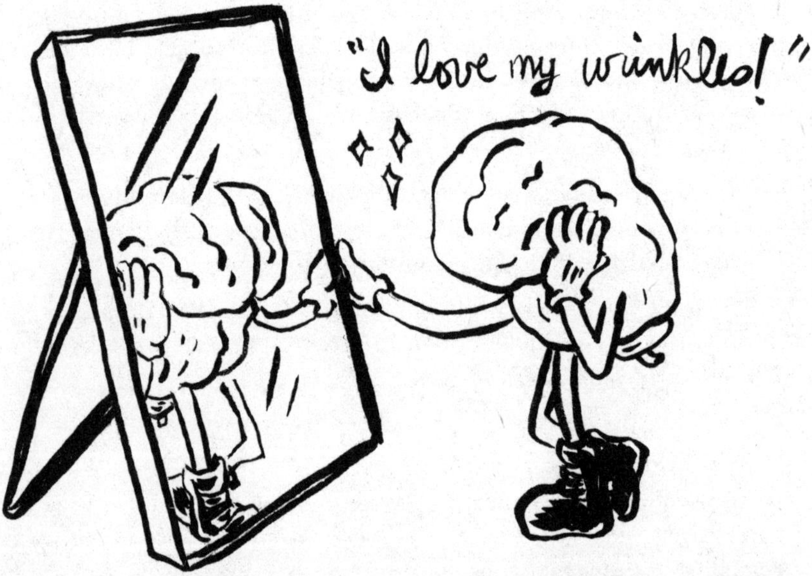
"I love my wrinkles!"

Section Two: Unfuck Your Relationship with Yourself

If you are reading this right now, you are a grown-ass human (either officially grown or grown enough to know what you're reading) who understands that the only person you have any real power over is yourself. Sucks, doesn't it?

That's why we are starting by dealing with our own shit first. After we get a better handle on where some of our more fucked up messages about intimacy come from, the best place to get to work is with the person we know the best, have known the longest, and are gonna be stuck with forever. Which is to say, our own damn selves. When we do our own work, understand our own responses, and stay truly connected to our own bodies, we are far better able to connect with others.

Much of this part of the book is focused on your experience of your body. Super weird in a book about relationships with others, right? Why don't we just move on to the partner stuff, FFS? Because our relationship to our own bodies is an essential starting place. How can we know who we are in relation to others if we have no idea what's going on within ourselves? We really can't separate the body and mind, though we sure as fuck keep getting that as a message!

We'll start with the ways we relate to our bodies emotionally, like being self-compassionate and figuring out our boundaries. Then we'll move on to how we live in them physically. Which means, yes, totally going to talk about body image and masturbation.

It's entirely okay (and really very normal) if everything you read in this section is super new to you. Or if it's stuff you've tried but felt like you failed at accomplishing. You may be fighting years of conditioning around sexual expression, and that may take awhile. Keep fighting for yourself. You have every right to be empowered, comfortable in your skin, and deeply satisfied with yourself!

SELF-COMPASSION

I went over self-compassion in Unfuck Your Brain, and I'm going to talk more about it here because it's so important to intimate relationships.

Self-compassion is inclusive instead of competitive. It is always available to us, even when we are not our best selves or successful by the standards we have established. And it's pretty much impossible to connect with others intimately if we don't have some level of comfort with our own flawed existence.

I think of self-compassion as a gift of desperation. Meaning, it's something that we come to when we are desperate enough to stop trying to do things the way we always have and try something completely different. Self-compassion was a huge struggle for me when I first learned about it in my mid-30s. Beating myself up wasn't working. Willing my self-esteem to be magically better didn't work either. Finally, I was desperate and exhausted enough to just try loving myself instead. And my whole fucking world changed.

Why is self-compassion so hard? We are raised with the socio-cultural message that we are responsible for our own actions. That's not a bad thing, and to a certain extent I'd say it's an empirical truth. However, tied to that idea is a belief that you should never let yourself off the hook for failings and bad behavior. And because we all fail frequently, repeatedly, and epically, because we are imperfect, we are always bashing ourselves against the metaphorical rocks.

That voice inside your head? The one that tells you that you must be perfect?

That voice is setting you up for failure.

As human beings, we are flawed and fault-filled. We also have the ability to accomplish amazing things and have deep, fulfilling relationships. When we view ourselves with compassion, we see the truest picture of both our flaws and our capacity for transcendence. And when we value ourselves for our efforts, we learn to confront, forgive, and transform our shortcomings.

Intimacy work can be fun, but it is quite often difficult and requires confronting issues and having conversations that we are not used to. Our ability to face many of the barriers to intimacy requires a great deal of self-compassion: it is the currency we need for change. One of the truest forms of emotional intelligence, it means we are both mindful of and engaged with our thoughts and feelings. Life, in general, requires a great deal of self-compassion. And the more we connect to our own failings, the more we are able to empathize with the failings of those around us. Compassion starts at home then radiates outwards, right? Holy shit, that sounded woo-woo as fuck. Truth, tho.

Kristin Neff, who literally wrote the book Self-Compassion, breaks this sort of work down into three parts. My version adds a fourth component (self-empathy) as a way of focusing on your core experience during the process. My hacked model is as follows:

- Mindfulness – Here, this simply means awareness of our current experience. Literally what is going on inside you in the present moment—all of your thoughts, feelings, and physical sensations. Without trying to suppress it or control it or judge it. Just saying "Oh hey. There you are."
- Self-Empathy – Self-empathy is thoughtful and active listening to our feelings, thoughts, and sensations. The same way you would listen to a friend. This term comes from psychologist and mediator Marshall Rosenberg's work on non-violent communication. With mindfulness, we are tuning in to all of our internal experiences. Self-empathy, per Rosenberg, is an inner questioning of the core inner experience to which we are the most attuned. What do you notice most? What is most important to you?
- Self-Kindness – This means being tender with ourselves rather than shitty and judgmental about our failings. Similar to the practice of loving-kindness, which is a consideration of and tenderness toward others, compassionate self-kindness means actively giving ourselves care and comfort in the presence of our own pain. If you cut your hand, even doing something dumb, you would go clean it off and bandage it, right? We do this with our physical selves, but rarely with our emotional selves. Self-kindness is the cleaning and caring of the wound, so it can heal.
- Common Humanity – Recognizing our common humanity means simply recognizing "wow yeah, I'm human, and I'm hurting, and other people feel this way too . . . we're all part of it." It's the realization that I am not alone in my pain and imperfection, and do not have to isolate myself while going through it. I am experiencing something that all human beings experience because we are all fucking human.

Self-compassion is something I hope you will explore holding for yourself throughout this unfuckening process. Intimacy is so very raw and reaches into the core components of who we are individually and in connection. This process is replete with opportunities to practice self-compassion. And, honestly, will probably be the thing that most helps you through it.

As you move forward through this book, you are going to bump into all your intimacy hobgoblins. These are the perfect times to practice self-compassion. Body issues? Bullshit religious messages? A history of fucked up relationships? Are you used to beating yourself up, and then beating yourself up for beating yourself up? Aren't you really fucking sick of it? Gift of desperation time.

Questions to ask yourself

- How do you deal with making mistakes? With "failing" or being "a failure?" How badly does it fuck you up? Do you ruminate and perseverate and tell yourself horrible fucking things?
- How does your self-criticism impact your internal life and choices? How does it affect your relationships with others?
- Where is your best opportunity for growth right now in your relationship with yourself? What do you want to change? What scares the fuck out of you about trying to do so?

Some self-compassion exercises to try:

- Approach your emotions with curiosity rather than judgment. Just notice them instead of labeling them in a positive or negative category. As in "Oh, I'm feeling . . . I wonder where that is coming from? I wonder what that's about? Is that emotion connected to something I need that I'm not getting?"
- Reflect back on a time when someone you cared about was going through a difficult experience. How did you support them? They may have fucked up royally, but you still recognized their personhood, right? Now, how can you use those same skills for yourself?
- Picture someone who is a kind and encouraging motivator for you. If you don't have any ideas on deck, picture me. I totally want you out there doing awesome shit and having a fulfilling life. What motivation strategies would this person use to help you move toward change? How would they approach you? Guess what: now you have to do this for yourself!

BOUNDARIES

Nutshell definition? Boundaries are the everyday expression of consent.

Of course, I wrote a whole book on this topic called Unfuck Your Boundaries, so definitely check that out for a deeper dive. But here, we're going to focus on boundaries in your intimate relationships.

Boundaries within an intimate relationship can take many forms. They range from sexual boundaries ("No butt stuff, stop pressuring me!") to privacy boundaries ("Stay out of my journal, FFS!") to just everyday interactions ("I don't like to be touched when I'm cooking" or "I need 20 minutes to decompress when I get home from work").

Boundaries are necessary in all of our relationships, but they are the most important in our intimate relationships. And it's one of the great ironies of the human condition that our closest relationships are the ones in which our boundaries are often the least respected.

What Are Your Boundaries?

Understanding your boundaries is the first step in communicating them. And hey, don't forget there is a whole chapter on unfucking your communication later on in this book. But you gotta know what to communicate first, right?

Here are some essential questions to consider for yourself within your intimate relationships.

- What's your deal breaker?
- What is the absolute no fly zone in your intimate life?
- When do you know you are done with an intimate partner or situation for good?

  Okay, do you have an answer? Now it's gut check time.

- When you read those questions, what was your emotional response? Not what you think you should have answered, not what you know the intellectual answer to be, but what your body tells you the answer actually is.

The Consent Commandments

Consent is an active process of communication. It's not just the "can I ________________ this part of your body with ________________ part of my body" that we see repeated ad nauseum in mainstream media. It's just as much my cat flattening her ears when she doesn't want pickieuppies. Or my husband scrunching his face when I even think about putting onions in whatever I'm cooking.

At its core, consent is simply permission for something to happen. Consent defines our rules of engagement, the ones we express through boundaries.

We have all had experiences where our boundaries were violated and others did not request permission to interact with us, especially in regard to sex and intimacy. I am continuously surprised/not surprised by how often my fellow clinicians in the field, even, misunderstand the need for active consent in relationships. We presume that permission for one activity implies permission for others.

Consent provides a safe framework for interactions. For those of us with trauma histories, a safe framework can be a very healing experience. And, equally important, it allows us to experience our own desires in a sex-positive way. In an ideal situation, you aren't having to be convinced, you're saying yes!

These 10 commandments came from a class I was teaching a few years ago for clinicians working with teens. We walked through group activities they could use to teach consent and boundaries and work with issues related to boundary violations. When it comes down to the basics, however, there are some fundamentals that apply universally. And as a good preacher's kid, I dug the idea of some basic commandments. Just like the OG commandments that Moses lugged down on stone tablets, they operate as a guide for our relational interactions, without weighing near as much, thankfully.

1. Consent for sex (and any other behaviors you are asking someone to engage in) cannot be given by people who are drunk. Or under the influence of drugs. Or hardcore medications. People under the influence are already doing seriously dumb stuff, like craving those two-for-a-dollar tacos from Jack in the Box. So don't add something to their regret list that has large, long-term consequences.
2. Going through a lot of emotional stuff can be just as bad for your decision-making process as being drunk. If someone is stressed out or dealing with a lot, they may be seeking comfort and connection, and we often equate that with sex. If you think someone isn't making a good decision, put sex on hold and be there for them in other ways—like ones that won't embarrass them a week from now.
3. Consent isn't static. Agreeing to something on one occasion does not mean agreeing to it forever. So I let you borrow my car last week. Maybe you brought it back with the gas tank empty and full of used Starbucks cups and candy wrappers and I don't

want you using it again. Maybe you took fantastic care of it, but I still don't want you using it again. Either way, it's still my car, not yours. You don't just march into my house, grab the keys off the counter, and take off in my car because I let you do it last week. A lack of consent equals grand theft auto, right?

4. Consent for one thing isn't consent for another. Someone gets naked in front of you? This is an excellent sign, yes. Is it consent for any specific sexual activity? No. Agreeing to one kind of activity isn't agreeing to all of them. Making out doesn't mean oral sex is cool. And yes to oral sex doesn't mean yes to penetrative sex. Our interactions are a salad bar, not a casserole. Wanting croutons doesn't mean you also have to have bell peppers, yanno?

5. Silence isn't consent. Someone may not actively say no, but being passive isn't a yes. Many times individuals don't speak up because they are freaked out or don't know how to. They could be quietly unhappy or quietly enjoying themselves. You don't know if you don't ask.

6. Consent needs to be informed. Are you sleeping with other people? That's ok—it's called dating, not getting married, for a reason. Have a sexually transmitted infection? That happens, too. Moving out of state in a week? That can impact future plans a bit. Potential partners need to know all of the above and any other information that may inform their decision about sexual activity. Be grown-up enough to have the awkward conversations.

7. Consent is a community obligation, not just a personal one. We need to help support each other with gray areas of consent. Speak up if you see someone in an uncomfortable situation and back up their right to say no. Friends don't let friends listen to Nickelback, and they don't let them get into situations where they are not really giving consent or not really getting consent. If you see someone at a party getting into a danger zone, then be the protective wingperson. And if the DJ plays Nickelback, it's time to leave altogether.

8. Having to convince someone is not consent. You aren't trying to win a court case by wooing a jury member. You're awesome, right? If they aren't into you enough to realize that and you have to convince them, then they don't deserve your awesomeness. If you get a "Welllllllll, I don't knowwwwww," respond with, "That's cool, let me know if you change your mind" and then step away from the sex.

9. Consent doesn't just mean the right to say no; it also means the right to say yes. Shaming people because they choose to engage in sexual activity makes active, enthusiastic consent way more complicated. Affirmative consent is difficult for many people (usually women) because they think that an enthusiastic yes means they are slutty, and that they are supposed to pretend they don't want sex and must be "convinced." This sends mixed messages to their partners. When are we supposed to "convince" and when are we supposed to just stop? If everyone is sexually empowered, no one ever has to be "convinced."

10. Consent is about more than just sex, it's about boundaries in general. You should get people's permission to touch them for any reason (e.g., "You look like you could use a hug right now, would you like one?"). Consent extends past physical boundaries, as well. You should never force your will on others. Don't share others' information, experiences, images, or things without their permission. Don't make plans on their behalf without their permission. Don't force them to share information with you or anyone else if they are uncomfortable doing so. No matter what you think is in their best interest, unless you are their legal guardian, let them make their own decisions. You do you and let them be them.

While accountability is one of those terms that has been overused and weaponized to emotionally beat the fuck out of people, it's useful in the context of consent and boundaries. Since almost none of us were raised with these kinds of consent expectations, we've likely all had boundaries violated by others and done some boundary violating ourselves. Now, I'm not talking about clearly awful and unlawful shit. I'm talking about the more sneaky gray areas. Places where we could have done so much better in terms of autonomy and respecting others. In Unfuck Your Boundaries, I go deep into how to take accountability for boundary violations, so be sure to check that out.

Questions for Reflection

- How were boundaries presented to you when you were younger? How has that informed the ways you treat others now and expect to be treated?
- If someone hurt you in the past, how do you need to better understand and stand your ground regarding your boundaries?
- If you hurt someone in the past, what amends can you make and how can you act differently from here on out?

EXPLORING YOUR SEXUAL IDENTITY

We have recently seen great progress in the acceptance of how truly diverse, fluid, and interesting sexual orientation is. But we have also seen continuous pushback from those who want to erase identities that they don't understand or that are not able to be neatly categorized.

Maybe you're trying to figure out your own sexual identity, or maybe you want to better understand a loved one's experience. All the competing messages out there make it difficult for many people to figure out who they really are. Since I haven't found a way to envelop everyone in a judgment-free zone bubble while they explore their sexual identity, I figure I can provide the best factual, evidence-based information about sexual identity I can find in order to support your process.

Sexuality is Fluid

We're queer AF, y'all.

There was a big kerfuffle in 2016 when the trend forecasting agency J. Walter Thompson Innovation Group put out the following survey results. Only 48 percent of Gen Zs (people born from 1995 to 2010) identified as exclusively heterosexual. Less than half. But it's not like we suddenly queered-out in one generational shift. Their survey of millennials (ages 21 to 34 at the time of the survey) showed that only 65% considered themselves exclusively heterosexual. That's still pretty damn queer.

Why this shift? What's causing it? Environmental toxins? Impending armageddon? The musical stylings of Miley Cyrus? Hillary Clinton's emails?

Or maybe we've just always been this way. After all, fluid sexual orientation (and gender identity) existed without rancor in many places before colonialism. Alfred Kinsey (toothbrush dude, yes) realized back in the 40s that sexuality exists on a spectrum . . . hence the creation of his famous Kinsey Scale. The Kinsey Scale was the attempt to rate and quantify where people fall on the spectrum of heterosexual (a zero) to homosexual (a six). Kinsey also found people who didn't fit anywhere on that scale—more on that later.

Sexuality is fluid. It's also fluid across our lifespan. Where you land on the Kinsey Scale today is not necessarily where you will be in a decade. Or where you were a decade ago. Per research, women are more likely to change their sexual orientation over time than men. But a lot of us have the capacity to have our head turned by someone we never expected. I'm a sexologist with short hair who teaches yoga. It's a common assumption that my partner would be a woman. My response when people ask is, "Nope, but the day ain't over."

In 1948, Kinsey wrote "The living world is a continuum in each and every one of its aspects." Queer is just how we roll. There is literally nothing new here.

Except for the first time since the industrial revolution, we've opened the door to better exploring the experience of human attraction. This means creating the language we need to support our experiences. Language informs our thoughts which informs our identity.

Many people do not need a language label (like gay, queer, straight, or pan) to validate their existence. Which I totally appreciate. But for many others, realizing that something exists, that it has a word, means that they can claim it. That they exist. And others like them exist who they can connect to. And that's powerful shit. So let's talk language.

Monosexuality means you have one category of attraction. You are either hetero or homosexual. Monosexuality is widely presumed to be how all of us roll, but clearly it ain't. In fact when you look at the LGBT stats, the majority of folx are not monosexual.

Polysexuality is the opposite of monsexuality. It just means that you are attracted to more than one gender. This doesn't necessarily mean all genders, just more than one. It's different from early exploration or hesitation before fully coming out. And it's not just a porn trope. There are millions of people who experience sexual attraction that doesn't confine itself to a singular gender identity. There are far more polysexual people than there are gay or lesbian people.

One reason that this is all important to talk about is that individuals who are non-monosexual face greater discrimination than their gay and lesbian counterparts within the LGBT+ community in regards to medical care, mental health care, and employment. Bi women are twice as likely to be assaulted as other women and bi men also have an increased risk.

We can use polysexual as an umbrella term. It used to be that the only polysexual label was "bisexual" (which is why toothbrush guy's scale is now pretty outdated). There are plenty of people who find that bisexual doesn't fit their sexual orientation, and the term pansexual has gained more attention in the process. And, also thanks to Deadpool. Bisexuality implies a binary attraction, at least in definition, while individuals who embrace pansexuality as their identity generally express that they can experience attraction to individuals with a wide variety of gender identities, not just men or women.

Though it should not be left unsaid that plenty of people who embrace the term bi also express attraction across the gender spectrum. I've found it tends to be more a generational term than anything else. People of my generation (Xers) and older (Boomers) are more likely to use the term bisexual without necessarily differentiating it from pansexuality.

Other terms include queer (which is an umbrella term for people who identify outside the presumed norm), sapiosexual (attracted to homosapiens in many shapes and forms), or humasexual ("I am attracted to humans. But of course, not many." – Morrissey). I'm attracted to an intellectual type more than a physical one—should we add the term intellectasexual to the list? I kinda dig it.

Just because you're polysexual, doesn't mean you are open to getting busy with literally everyone (though no shade thrown from me if you are!). Just like Morrissey, we all have certain types of people we gravitate toward. Sometimes we just gotta smell right to each other, yanno?

Orientation Is Not the Same Thing as Gender, but It Is Informed by Gender

Where does gender identity come into all this, you may ask? Here's some super-basic definitions:

Gender Identity: This is who you know yourself to be. You are assigned a sex at birth which may or may not reflect your actual gender. Whatever your gender identity, it's valid and true. You are exactly who you are supposed to be and I'm really glad you share the planet with me.

Sexual Orientation: This is who you are oriented toward, in terms of romantic and sexual attraction. It is not the same thing as sexual preference. Preference is what you like to do in bed. Orientation is who you like to do it with. Your sexual orientation is a vital part of who you are. Whatever yours is, you are not broken, you don't need correction, and I'm really glad you share the planet with me.

Gender is not sexual orientation, though your gender identity may direct the label of your sexual orientation. If for example, you are a trans woman and are attracted to men, you are a straight woman. If you had been attracted to men pre-transition, you may have been labeled (or identified) as a gay man.

If you are in a partnership with someone who is transitioning or has transitioned from the gender identity you initially understood them to have, it may or may not affect your perception of your own sexual orientation. It may feel more fluid at this point. Or it may simply be that your orientation hasn't changed, but you continue to be in love with the person you fell in love with, since their fundamental selfhood has not changed.

And if you don't have a binary gender identity (that is, neither male nor female), then how you describe your attraction alignment can get even more complicated. If you're non-binary or agender and you like women, does that make you straight or a lesbian? Neither, right? We don't have great language for these cases, so saying, "I'm genderqueer and I date women" is a mouthful but might be the most accurate.

Obviously, there is a shit-ton of additional information about gender identity that we aren't getting into here. But the important takeaway? If your identity isn't easily explained or understood by others, the reality is that you don't owe an explanation to anyone who is not living in your relationship at this moment. Fuck 'em if they don't get it.

Asexuality

Asexuality is a sexual orientation characterized by a persistent lack of sexual attraction toward any gender. –Asexuality Archive

So we got all that fluid polysexual info down. But, hah, we ain't done yet. Guess what? Even with all those categories, we still have a group of people who will step up and say "hell, naw" to all of them.

All the asexuals quietly minding their business, preferring chocolate cake to sex, are now thinking, "Oh, shit, she's bringing us into the equation?" Yes, my ace buddies, you deserve a place in the conversation, too. So let's tackle some ace fundamentals.

Asexuality is sort of the forgotten orientation. It's been referred to as the third orientation in a lot of literature, but of course that presumes that the other two are gay or straight.

According to a 2004 study, at least 1% of people qualify for this orientation. UCLA's Williams Institute published a study in 202 (as part of the NIH Generations project) found a slight increase in that number, to 1.7%. Though, as researchers note that if you aren't interested in sex, you probably aren't interested in surveys about sex, so it might be higher). But don't forget, this isn't new data. Kinsey had a Category X in his research: About 1.5% of his respondents weren't interested in sex with anyone, and therefore didn't fit on his scale. So the asexual (ace) identity isn't a newfangled thing that kids these days invented on Tumblr.

Ace people are not fundamentally broken or mentally ill. It's all about our level of attraction. If there is such a huge variety of ways to feel attraction, doesn't it make sense that some people have a none of the above button?

If you're asexual, you might choose to never have sex. But it's not the same as celibacy or abstinence. Celibacy and abstinence are about action, not attraction. If you choose not to engage in sexual activity because of religious values, a trauma history, or other life circumstances, that's a choice you make. It's not about to whom you are attracted, but your behavior around your attraction. Asexuality, on the other hand, is about your actual level of attraction. Not everyone who is ace never has sex. You might choose to have sex because a partner desires that connection, or to conceive, or for a multitude of other reasons. But the sex itself? A means to an end, not something you are interested in for its own sake.

Being ace doesn't mean you don't experience love. Although you may be aromantic (aro), meaning that you don't experience romantic attraction any more than you experience sexual attraction. But there are plenty of ace people who are heteroromantic (experiencing romantic attraction to people of the opposite sex), homoromantic, biromantic, or panromantic. Sexual attraction and romantic attraction are two different ways of relating to other people. You can absolutely be aromantic without being asexual. And being aromantic doesn't mean you don't experience love at all, just not romantic love. Aro people can still experience intense love for friends, family, the world around them, and those adorable dogs that look like tiny Chewbaccas.

If you are ace and romantically inclined, dating another romantically-inclined person who is also ace might be ideal, though life rarely works that way. Being with someone who does experience sexual attraction doesn't mean the relationship is doomed, though it may mean more work and communication between you to find a middle ground that everyone is comfortable with.

A related pair of identities: Demisexuals and graysexuals fall under the ace umbrella but have a few differences. To invoke huge generalities, demisexual individuals usually only experience sexual attraction when they feel a strong emotional connection to someone. Graysexual individuals only feel sexual attraction to someone under certain circumstances, which may or may not correlate with their level of emotional intimacy.

Of the individuals I have worked with over the years, more identify as demisexual than graysexual or ace. They often seek help because they are struggling to maintain the level of sexual intimacy that their partner desires. It's something they are just not wired to have on the forefront of their minds, so we work on building the emotional attachment that helps them feel more secure and invested.

One more: Some people are not ace/gray/or demi and still love partnered sex, but their pleasure comes from pleasing a partner. The term you will generally see for this is stone, coming from Les Feinberg's novel Stone Butch Blues. And I have found that many different people identify as or experience their sexuality as stone.

Exploring Your Orientation

There may have been zero new words or concepts in this chapter for you. Which probably means you have already done a lot of work around understanding identity. But for a lot of folx, this may be seriously new information which means some new shit to think about.

This is where I remind you that all of this is fluid. Questions arise all throughout our lifespan about our attraction to others. My youngest client currently grappling with this issue is in junior high and the oldest is in their 60s. Fluidity in orientation is a normal, healthy, good thing. And embracing who you have been, who you are now, and possibilities for the future is what helps us grow as human beings.

Some questions to consider about your sexual orientation:

- What kinds of thoughts do you have regarding sexual attraction? Who do you find yourself noticing? What piques your interest? What kinds of fantasies have you had? (Fantasies don't always equate to things you are actually interested in, but can sometimes provide a good clue.) What do you find erotic? What do you find yourself craving?
- To whom do you find yourself emotionally attached, and under what circumstances? What do you look for in terms of emotional closeness? In what ways have you experienced emotional attraction to someone?
- What types of sexual experiences have you had? Not just sex but also foreplay. Kissing. Even non-sexual touch that ended up being a turn on for you. What did you enjoy? What did you not enjoy?
- Have you ever experienced internal conflict regarding your attractions or lack thereof? What was the source of the conflict? What steps have you taken to address that?
- Have you ever experienced external conflict or erasure based on your attractions or lack thereof? Or been told that your identity is not valid? What steps have you taken to address that?
- What is your current relationship configuration, if any? (Example: Maybe you're pansexual but currently in a heterosexual relationship.) Have people tried to define or label you based on that relationship, therefore disregarding the complexity of who you are? What steps have you taken to address that?

RECONNECTING WITH YOUR BODY

Having the words to better describe who we are can be powerful magic. But do you know what's even more bad-ass? Feeling comfortable in your skin and accepting your perfectly imperfect self.

I know how fucking difficult this is. It's a complicated, ongoing process that is often deeply uncomfortable. And that's exactly what makes it all the more necessary to do. This chapter is going to look at how these issues get their hooks into us, plus exercises to help us come back home to our bodies.

One major trigger for disconnecting from our physical selves is trauma. Another is just plain being unhappy with our bodies. Self-image related to physical appearance is one of the biggest barriers I have seen individuals and couples work to overcome in their quest for healthy intimacy. I've provided more context on each of these issues, and exercises designed to help in each situation (but all the exercises will help, no matter the reason for your mind-body disconnection).

Trauma, Disconnect, and Dissociation

How often are we really in our bodies? Rarely. And for some people, literally never.

At a fairly young age we realize that our bodies can be in one place, while our minds can wander somewhere else entirely. If third grade science was boring, our minds could already be out on the playground monkey bars. Once we learn this skill, it becomes increasingly difficult to keep our minds grounded to the present and connected to our bodies. We are always off on the proverbial monkey bars instead of being where we actually, physically are.

When we are trying to increase our intimacy with another person, reconnecting our minds and bodies to be present can be intensely difficult. To say it as simply as I do to my clients on the regular, your partner (hopefully) wants to have sex with you, not on you. This means you have to be engaged, not just with their experience and pleasure, but with your own.

As I discuss in Unfuck Your Body, interoception is the fancy clinical term used to describe our awareness of our body's reactions. If perception is how we know what is going on around us, interoception is how we know what is going on inside us.

This is often a super foreign concept, especially for people with trauma histories. Dissociation from our experiences is a form of protection in fucked-up situations. If someone is harming us and we can't escape physically, we escape mentally. But getting back into our bodies when we are safe to do so can seem impossible. Research demonstrates that people with severe trauma histories often have significant differences in the areas of their brains mapped as interoceptive pathways.

A lot of us without trauma histories still struggle with interoception. Trauma reactions aren't the only cause of body disconnect. Body image bullshit is nearly universal. All kinds of shame issues can trigger disassociation. And that means we aren't connected to how our body is reacting, so we are not connected to how it is affecting our emotions, and do not have a conscious awareness of our behaviors. When we don't practice interoception, we struggle to act with purpose. Including in regard to healthy sexual intimacy. In Unfuck Your Body, I include instructions for an interoception exercise. Below is another exercise you can try.

Progressive Muscle Relaxation

The purpose of this exercise is to gain awareness of how our body is operating from the inside. You know, that interoception thing I was yammering on about. Actively engaging in progressive muscle relaxation effectively loosens and relaxes the muscles. By tightening a muscle and then releasing it, you can feel the difference between tense and relaxed.

Make sure not to do any movements that cause pain. If any of these exercises cause discomfort, ease up or stop. Sometimes if you are very tense already, actively tensing your muscles with a progressive muscle relaxation exercise will not be helpful. If this is the case, you may want to try passive progressive muscle relaxation exercises instead (focus on relaxing parts of your body, rather than tensing and then relaxing to feel the difference).

Here is a script for the guided progressive muscle relaxation exercise. You can read it as you go or have someone read it to you:

Find a comfortable position sitting, standing, or lying down. You can change positions at any time during the exercise.

Breathe in forcefully and deeply, and hold this breath. Hold it . . . hold it . . . and now release. Let all the air go out slowly, and release all the tension.

Take another deep breath in. Hold it . . . and then exhale slowly, allowing the tension to leave your body with the air.

Now breathe even more slowly and gently . . . breathe in . . . hold . . . out . . . breathe in . . . hold . . . out . . .

Continue to breathe slowly and gently. Allow your breathing to relax you.

Focus on the large muscles of your legs. Tighten all your leg muscles. Now tense them even further. Hold on to this tension. Feel how tight and tense the muscles in your legs are right now. Squeeze the muscles harder, tighter . . . Continue to hold this tension. Feel the muscles wanting to give up this tension. Hold it for a few moments more . . . and now relax. Let all the tension go. Feel the muscles in your legs going limp, loose, and relaxed. Notice how relaxed the muscles feel now. Feel the difference between tension and relaxation. Enjoy the pleasant feeling of relaxation in your legs.

Now focus on the muscles in your arms. Tighten your shoulders, upper arms, lower arms, and hands. Squeeze your hands into tight fists. Tense the muscles in your arms and hands as tightly as you can. Squeeze harder . . . harder . . . hold the tension in your arms, shoulders, and hands. Feel the tension in these muscles. Hold it for a few moments more . . . and now release.

Let the muscles of your shoulders, arms, and hands relax and go limp.

Feel the relaxation as your shoulders lower into a comfortable position and your hands relax at your sides. Allow the muscles in your arms to relax completely.

Focus again on your breathing. Slow, even, regular breaths. Breathe in relaxation . . . and breathe out tension . . . in relaxation . . . and out tension . . . Continue to breathe slowly and rhythmically.

Now focus on the muscles of your buttocks. Tighten these muscles as much as you can.

Hold this tension . . . and then release.

Relax your muscles.

Tighten the muscles of your back now. Feel your back tightening, pulling your shoulders back and tensing the muscles along your spine. Arch your back slightly as you tighten these muscles. Hold . . . and relax. Let all the tension go. Feel your back comfortably relaxing into a good and healthy posture.

Turn your attention now to the muscles of your chest and stomach. Tighten and tense these muscles. Tighten them further . . . hold this tension . . . and release. Relax the muscles of your trunk.

Finally, tighten the muscles of your face. Scrunch your eyes shut tightly, wrinkle your nose, and tighten your cheeks and chin. Hold this tension in your face . . . and relax.

Release all the tension. Feel how relaxed your face is.

Notice all of the muscles in your body . . . notice how relaxed your muscles feel. Allow any last bits of tension to drain away. Enjoy the relaxation you are experiencing. Notice your calm breathing . . . your relaxed muscles . . . Enjoy the relaxation for a few moments . . .

When you are ready to return to your usual level of alertness and awareness, slowly begin to re-awaken your body. Wiggle your toes and fingers. Swing your arms gently. Shrug your shoulders. Stretch if you like.

You may now end this progressive muscle relaxation exercise feeling calm and refreshed.

Body Image

Body image issues can arise for a billion different reasons. All of us eventually experience some kind of unwanted body changes due to accident, injury, giving birth, or just getting older. Other people struggle with their overall size, height, hair or lack of it, or how certain parts of their bodies stack up to traditional beauty standards. Folx with gender dysphoria may struggle greatly with a body that has features out of alignment with their true gender. Most everyone struggles with some aspect of the skin suit they wear around during their time on the planet.

Anxious and negative thoughts about our bodies are so commonplace they have become the new normal. Fun fact: approximately 80% of women report feeling dissatisfied with their bodies. A Glamour study found that the average woman says 13 negative statements about her body to herself on a given day (one per hour of being awake, on average). 97% had at least one negative statement in a day.

But body image issues are no longer primarily the domain of women, if they ever were. A UK study looked at body image among women and men and found that 75% of women and almost 81% of men experience anxiety related to their body. The number of men struggling with body image is starting to match, and in some places, surpass that of women. No one is safe from the self-destruction we impose on ourselves with negative body image self-talk. Male body issues are something we talk about quite rarely. In trying to do something about that, my friend Aaron Sapp and I wrote a zine specifically about male body image issues. It's called Unfuck Your Masculinity, if you are looking for more resources and ideas.

So how do you unfuck your body image? Studies of individuals who have positive images of their bodies show an interesting trend. The majority of people with a positive image of their physical self had actively done work to combat a negative body image at some point in their lives. They had developed an awareness of the issue and worked on changing it in a conscious way, rather than hitting the gym, going on the latest on-trend diet, or investing in tons of plastic surgery. Doing things to feel healthy and good about yourself is awesome, but if you don't do the inside work the outside work doesn't truly fix anything.

As is true about most research, these studies didn't look at the lived experience of non-cis people, so I can only speak from my practice as a therapist in this regard. Gender dysphoria (for those who experience it . . . and you can absolutely have a non-cis identity without experiencing dysphoria) is a very real struggle that I would never discount by saying "let's work on a more positive body image!"

I have found it most helpful to partner with my non-cis clients on how to care for the body they have now, so they are the healthiest they can be when they do receive gender congruence treatments (e.g., managing hormone side effects, preparing for surgeries). The focus of the internal work is on validating their authentic identity, not just finding peace with the body they currently have. I've used the phrase "Despite others' perceptions or opinions about me, I know who I am" as a hypnotherapy affirmation. It's a small shift in thinking that has given many people the support they truly needed.

The exercises in this chapter are designed to help with the inside work, both as an individual and with a romantic partner. If you do not have active body issues (and if so, congratulations you rare gem, you!) you may still benefit from these exercises. Connecting to your body through awareness exercises can promote increased intimacy, even for people who are already generally body-confident.

You can complete these exercises by yourself or with a partner. It can be helpful, in partnered relationships, to have the person who is most comfortable with their body complete and share the exercises first. This can create a safe zone for the less comfortable partner to do the same. Or if you're anxious about sharing, it might be more helpful for you to try the exercises on your own first. If you are doing these exercises by yourself, you can then consider which aspects of the experience you are willing to share with a current or future partner.

Also, keep in mind that there are trained body workers (in all their shapes and forms) available in many communities to help guide you through these exercises, which can be helpful for people who struggle with following along in a workbook and who can benefit from a more direct teaching experience. Check out the Institute for Mind Body Therapy as a good starting point to find a body worker who matches with your particular needs. Body work can encompass a lot of different things, including surrogate partner therapy, massage therapy, therapeutic touch work, somatic experiencing, and a host of other interventions that involve working with a hands-on practitioner.

The goals of these exercises are:

- To feel more connected to and comfortable with your physical body

- To feel more connected to and comfortable with your partner's physical body
- To gain empathy for your partner's body image issues, if present
- To identify any body image issues you may be experiencing
- To build respect and appreciation for the strength and functionality of your body
- To cultivate persistent, gentle curiosity about the experience of being human

Clothed Body Work

This is another activity designed to help you build your interoception and enhance your comfort and acceptance of your external, physical self.

If you are working with a partner during this activity, discuss in advance their role in the process. The important thing is that they listen to your words rather than correct anything you say, especially your thoughts and feelings. We often want to tell our partners how we perceive them, and we often see them with much less criticism than they see themselves. It's hard not to say something akin to "No! I love your neck!" The point of the exercise is to share our own internal experience without fear of argument or correction.

It is also not your partner's job to ask questions or give feedback about your experience. The partner's job is to provide a supportive presence, then complete the activity with your support as well. It's amazing what you will learn about each other, if you are in a place where you feel safe enough to do this activity together.

Stand in front of a full-length mirror, wearing whatever clothing feels comfortable (as much or as little as you'd like). Take a deep breath and look at your body in its entirety for a few minutes. If this isn't something you often do, give yourself time to become accustomed to the experience.

Starting at the top of your head and moving downward, describe out loud each part of your body and the feelings you have about each part. If you are doing this activity alone, still say everything you are thinking out loud. It is amazing how much we say to ourselves that we are not aware of, because we don't give literal voice to those thoughts and feelings. When you're done, ask yourself some of these questions:

- What did you notice about yourself? Did anything surprise you? Did anything you found yourself saying out loud surprise you?

- If you were to pick out one or two body parts/areas that you most dislike, what would these be and why? You can be present for these feelings, acknowledge them, and work to generate self-compassion for your experience.
- If you were to pick out one or two body parts/areas that are your favorite, what would they be and why?
- Did your perceptions of yourself shift when you moved from looking at your entire body to focusing on parts of it at a time? If so, in what ways?
- If you did this activity with a partner, please ask your partner to answer the following questions: What surprised you about your partner's experience? Did they say anything you didn't expect? Did you notice that they ignored any areas? Express any thoughts or feelings that you weren't aware of?

Nude Body Work

Now, you are going to complete the same exercise, but without clothing.

If you are doing this exercise with a partner, undress, acknowledge the expected nervousness, and give permission to look at one another's bodies. Hold hands and look together for a couple of minutes, then take turns looking at each other's backsides.

If becoming completely nude immediately, whether alone or with a partner, makes you uncomfortable, you can disrobe slowly as you complete the exercise. You can also incorporate softer lighting and soothing music if you find that helpful, but you don't want ambient music to be a distraction or have lighting so low you can't really see yourself.

Repeat the above steps, speaking all your thoughts and feelings about each part of yourself out loud (or writing them down if that feels more comfortable . . . I know this already feels weird!), and consider these questions:

- What did you notice about yourself? Did anything surprise you? Did anything you found yourself saying out loud surprise you? Was there anything different from the clothed version of this exercise?
- If you were to pick out one or two body parts/areas that you most dislike, what would these be and why? Was there anything different from the clothed version of this exercise?
- If you were to pick out one or two body parts/areas that are your favorite, what would they be and why? Was there anything different from the clothed version of this exercise?

- Did your perceptions of yourself shift when you moved from looking at your entire body to focusing on parts of it at a time? If so, in what ways? Was there anything different from the clothed version of this exercise?
- If you did this activity with a partner, please ask your partner to answer the following questions. What surprised you about your partner's experience? Did they say anything you didn't expect? Express any thoughts or feelings that you weren't aware of? Did you notice that they skipped over any areas? Did anything different happen from the clothed version of this exercise?

Some Tips for Being More Accepting of Your Own Body

- Focus on an aspect of yourself that is separate from the destructive body image messages you are combating. Consider this aspect a different dimension from what you are unhappy about. Focus on your strong self, playful self, sensual self, etc. and let that aspect become engaged during sexual intimacy.
- Focus on your body in its entirety, rather than certain parts. Look at yourself and ask your partner to look at you with "soft eyes," or focusing on the entirety of what you, and they, love, appreciate, and respect about you. This may be easier to believe than "I love your eyes" and "I think your butt is sexy."
- Hold space for the possibility that even if you do not accept and love your body right now, it is possible to feel differently in the future. "Not right now" has far less a pervasive hold on us than "never," and allows small shifts to occur that move us in a healthy direction.
- When positivity seems completely impossible, work toward neutrality. Just like "not right now," neutrality is far less damaging self-talk than continued negativity. When you catch yourself saying something negative to yourself and a positive statement seems like unbearable bullshit when you feel awful, try something along the lines of "My body just is. Nothing is empirically good or bad. My body and I are doing the best we can."
- Apologize (as authentically as possible, even if it feels cheesy) to your body for treating it like the enemy. For treating it like it is somehow a separate entity from the rest of you. Tell it you will work on incorporating it back into the whole and appreciate all it has done to keep you moving forward despite your negativity toward it.

Your Sense of Touch

> I have perceiv'd that to be with those I like is enough,
> To stop in company with the rest at evening is enough,
> To be surrounded by beautiful, curious, breathing, laughing flesh is enough,
>
> To pass among them or touch any one, or rest my arm ever so lightly round his or her neck for a moment, what is this then?
> I do not ask any more delight, I swim in it as in a sea.
>
> There is something in staying close to men and women and looking on them, and in the contact and odor of them, that pleases the soul well,
> All things please the soul, but these please the soul well.
>
> –Walt Whitman, from "I Sing the Body Electric" in *Leaves of Grass*

A friend told me recently that he knew his marriage was over when his wife wouldn't let him touch her anymore. He was by no means the first person to tell me that, and unfortunately won't be the last.

The sense of touch is, when you think about it, an exercise in paradox.

Jennifer Kennerk, a Waldorf school educator, wrote how our sense of touch is the way we first learn to differentiate ourselves from the rest of the world. If we touch someone or something, we develop awareness of where we end and the other person or object begins. She states that touch "allows us to understand our own individual place in the world, and also to understand that others have their own individuality as well. The sense of touch provides human beings with the ability to understand their own uniqueness and therefore the uniqueness of others." Touch is the sense that demonstrates the boundaries between our individual bodies and the rest of the universe.

The paradox arises because touch is also our primary means of experiencing intimacy with others. Human beings are hardwired to connect, and the primary mechanism for doing so is through touch. We express closeness through touch. We experience others, gain awareness of their presence, and invite them into our own.

We also need touch to survive. In the thirteenth century, King Frederick II of Germany wanted to study language acquisition. He was curious as to whether children are born with knowledge of language or if it is something they learn from caregivers over time. He's alleged to have set up an experiment to determine if children would speak spontaneously, if they never heard language to begin with. He took 50 babies within his kingdom and assigned them each to foster mothers. The babies had their basic needs met. They were bathed and nursed, but were not held or cuddled or talked to. The experiment failed because all fifty infants died.

In more recent years, the world has learned about the horrific overcrowding and miserable conditions in many orphanages. Harvard Medical School researcher Mary Carlson observed the conditions in a Romanian orphanage, where due to understaffing and overcrowding, babies lay neglected in their cribs and were rarely touched, even during meal times. She observed no engagement, no crying, no babbling, and no whimpering. While their physical needs were being met, in theory, Carlson found that by age two the babies had unusually high amounts of cortisol, a stress hormone known to cause brain damage. Growth was stunted; the children acted half their age.

What conclusions can be drawn from King Frederick's failed experiment and the Romanian orphanage scandal? Lack of touch impedes the human ability to thrive. In some cases it leads to death. Caring for basic physical needs is not enough; we need touch to survive.

Those of us who did not get a lot of touching before age 12 often struggle with touch as adults. Snuggling, cuddling, hugging, and holding hands often makes us uncomfortable. And we thereby lose opportunities for connection. We communicate best through touch, as many of our ancestors did throughout the ages. Touch is universal. Touch, both sexual and non-sexual, is essential for intimacy. Non-sexual touch is an essential building block for physical intimacy.

Touch makes us more relationally honest. Studies of compliance in field settings have shown amazing results when touch was involved. In one study, researchers put a dime in the change box of a public telephone. (This study was clearly conducted in the 70s.) Study participants would go into the phone booth, make a call, and then put their hand in the little coin receiver to see if there was any extra change. As they exited the booth, they were approached and asked, "Did you find any money in the change box in the telephone booth?" 97% lied and said no. But in the same experiment, if the researcher reached out and touched the individual on the shoulder while asking the question, 95% told the truth. They would say they found money there and would offer it to the person who asked.

The famous family therapist Virginia Satir said that we need four hugs a day for survival, eight for maintenance, and twelve for growth.

Do you get the amount of touch that you need in a day? Depending on the country you live in, maybe not.

Psychologist Sidney Journal studied touch by observing couples dining in various countries and counted the number of times they touched each other. On average, in Mexico City, couples touched each other 185 times an hour; in Paris it was 115 times an hour. In London, couples did not touch each other at all and in Gainesville, Florida it was twice an hour.

The couples in Mexico City did not engage in passionate kisses 185 times an hour (no time to eat their dinner!) but they stroked each other's arms, or hair. Leaned into each other. Continued to convey the message that they desired each other. They communicated their connection to each other through different levels of touch.

Understanding What Touch Means to You

The idea that there are different levels of touch is wild to many people. It definitely isn't something that we talk about. The concept of five levels of touch comes from the work of clinical sexologist Dr. Patti Britton, whose work has informed mine for many years now.

Go through these questions and write down your answers. If you are partnered, consider having your partner answer these questions separately from you, then compare your answers:

- The first level of touch is healing. What does that mean to you? What kind of touch do you consider healing? What kind of healing touch do you enjoy receiving? Giving?
- The second level of touch is affectionate. What does that mean to you? What kind of touch do you consider affectionate? What kind of affectionate touch do you enjoy receiving? Giving?
- The third level of touch is sensual. What does that mean to you? What kind of touch do you consider sensual? What kind of sensual touch do you enjoy receiving? Giving?
- The fourth level of touch is erotic. What does that mean to you? What kind of touch do you consider erotic? What kind of erotic touch do you enjoy receiving? Giving?
- The fifth level of touch is sexual. What does that mean to you? What kind of touch do you consider sexual? What kind of sexual touch do you enjoy receiving? Giving?

I've had many people complete this exercise over the years and come back and tell me that it really blew their minds. That, for example, they hadn't considered a difference between sensual and erotic touch, and realized that sensual touch was something they really were missing and craved.

The process is as deeply individual and unique as everything else that we do as people. There is no right or wrong, there are just your definitions. If you do this exercise with a partner and they have wildly different definitions, that's OK, too. You are discovering some really important shit about yourself and them. The point isn't to fit into a box, it's to understand our own experiences and how those impact our connections with others.

More Questions to Consider

- Of the kinds of touch you described above, which do you enjoy most? What makes you feel safe? Desired?
- What kind of touch makes you feel uncomfortable?
- Does your interest in touch, or the different types of touch you typically enjoy, change when you are feeling strong (possibly negative) emotions? How so? Are you aware of these changes at the time or is it something you notice in retrospect?
- If you are partnered, in your experience, what kind of touch does your partner(s) most respond to?
- Have you and your partner(s) experienced any issues or struggles with touch in your relationship(s)? How so?
- If a partner also did some reflecting on the levels of touch, did any of their answers surprise you? What surprised you most? How do you think that knowing different information about them may change your relationship?

SEXING YOURSELF

"Everyone does it, but no one admits it."

This statement almost always refers to one of two human activities. One is eating Jack in the Box egg rolls at 3 a.m. The other is masturbation.

Masturbation is simply the touching of one's genitals for the purpose of sexual pleasure and is part of the normal human expression of sexuality. It is a healthy and empowering practice that leads to better sex lives, and it's just something people do. Like brushing our teeth, baking cookies, or playing board games, it's a normal human behavior.

Historical records and anthropological studies indicate that masturbation has always been a part of human history. In the grand tradition of ruining anything fun, the public tides turned against the art of self-love as society "modernized" and an organized movement against the practice of masturbation began. Religious leaders and medical professionals became outspoken regarding their view that masturbation was dangerous. It led to weakness, disease, and insanity, they said. It was decried as an affront to God.

Only in the past 50 years have researchers like Alfred Kinsey (hey there, toothbrush dude!), William Masters, Virginia Johnson, and Betty Dodson begun confronting these views of masturbation. They all argued that masturbation is a healthy, normal, and valuable part of human development. Dodson specifically encouraged women to masturbate as an act of feminist resistance to negative images of womanhood common in many families, religious organizations, and society in general. Dodson also proposed using masturbation as a way of enhancing self-esteem, and perhaps most importantly, as the best means of becoming orgasmic.

Despite their work, there remains a prevailing attitude about the inherent wrongness of masturbation that we can't seem to shake.

Sigh.

So let me add my voice to the mix.

Masturbation is not a sin. It is not a shameful practice. It is way healthier than fast food at 3 a.m., and it shouldn't be so damn secretive. As Betty Dodson states in her book Sex for One: The Joy of Selfloving: "Our cultural denial of masturbation sustains sexual repression." How else are you going to know what you like and then communicate that to present or future partners?

I endeavored to raise kids who are open and self-confident. The work that I do is embarrassing enough for them, so I won't detail the conversations we have in our home—but I have always normalized masturbation as a way of relieving stress and maintaining control of their sexual selves. Doing so helped them make educated and empowered choices with as much information available to them as possible, with partners as they got older and matured to adulthood.

And masturbation is just as important for us grown people. Whether you're single or partnered, enjoying sexual release through masturbation can be both relaxing and liberating.

I've been asked, Doesn't this make me a total loser? This question somehow implies that masturbation is an inferior form of sex, and what the fuck is up with that? In the age of Craigslist, anyone can find partnered sex; it isn't like you somehow win extra points because someone was willing to fuck you silly. This question also presumes that if you are masturbating, then you don't have someone around who is fucking you silly, which isn't always the case.

Not all sex has to be partnered, and scrounging up a partner-person may not be on your agenda for the afternoon. Why should it be? Taking care of yourself and having a nice orgasm doesn't have to always be a team effort.

When working with single individuals who want to prevent future relationship mistakes, I encourage them to get in touch with their body and find out what they like and don't like. This may include exercise, massage, touch exercises (like the ones in this book!), and/or masturbation. You are far less likely to rush into a poor partner choice if you know what you want in a relationship before you start looking.

For those of us who are already partnered? Just because we are already having sex with someone else doesn't mean we can't also have sex with ourselves—whether to relax, to learn more about ourselves, or just because we want to.

No matter what age you are, and no matter what your relationship status is, if you aren't sure what turns you on, isn't it time to start finding out?

Why Is Masturbation Important?

Sexual expression should be an empowering part of your experience as a human being. We live in a world that is continuously disempowering, and we get all kinds of competing and fucked-up messages about what it means to be a sexual being. The reality is, there are as many answers as there are people on the planet.

Exploring your sexuality with a partner is a wonderful thing, should you have or want to have a partner at the time. But sex with someone else is as much about them and the connection you create by being together as it is about figuring out your own body. Solo sex is just for you and can have an entirely different intent. Such as:

- Figuring out what you like—for yourself, or to share with future partners if you are so inclined to have them
- Reclaiming your sexuality from the fucked-up shit you've dealt with in your past
- Reclaiming your sexuality from the fucked-up messages our culture inundates us with on a constant basis
- Healing from trauma
- Empowering yourself, Betty Dodson style
- Political activism to actively fight sexual repression
- You've got a headache. Or cramps
- You are having trouble falling asleep
- Because orgasms feel good, duh!
- Because WHYTHEFUCKNOT?

What Do I Do, Though?

Turn yourself on: figure out where and how you like to be touched and touch away.

There are lots of places on the human body that are erogenous, meaning they connect you to your sexual self. When erogenous areas are stimulated, you find yourself sexually aroused. So, start touching. Your breasts and nipples and all aspects of your genitalia, your perineum, your anus, your G-spot. Anywhere else you might like to be touched . . . the crease of your left pinky toe, if that does it for ya. Yes, it makes sense to stroke your clitoris if you have one, or your penis if you have one of those (and just so you know, most of the nerve endings in the penis are under the head of it).

The point is to listen to your body while you explore.

Do you like firm touch, light touch, vibrating touch, warm water from the bath faucet? If you discover touch you enjoy, blood will rush to that area (which leads to swollen erectile tissue in the clitoris, penis, or nipples). Lubricants (dry like talc powder or wet like lube or lotion) may help your sensory experience, as can sex toys in general (more on that in a minute).

The Orgasm

Rebecca Chalker writes about this in her book The Clitoral Truth: When we are turned on, sensory messages are sent to the brain and the brain says "woohoo!" and starts increasing the number of nerves in the body that are activated. Once one system is on high alert, it boops the next system in the chain and gets it going. After the whole system is activated, we reach overload. And that energy has to discharge somehow, right?

This whole chain reaction thing works best with certain rhythmic cycles, which are very much linked to our own heartbeats. This is our "excitability cycle." We all have our own rhythm. Which makes sense, because not everyone has the exact same heartbeat cadence, right? You know your own rhythm best, or want to find out. So, explore.

Masturbation lets you figure out your own dance steps without having to dance in sync with someone else. And yay for that.

I realize that not everyone is naturally orgasmic. You may be reading this right now out of frustration about, or fear of, that being true for you. There are a lot of things that can affect our ability to be orgasmic, generally falling under one of the following categories:

- Physical Issues. For example, medical things you have going on or medications you are taking. If you are struggling in that regard, going to a doctor to see if there's a physical cause makes a lot of sense. And it may be an easy fix. For example, if your antidepressant is decreasing your sex drive, your doc can switch it up or add something to mitigate that side effect.
- Emotional Issues. For example, if you have had sexual trauma, that can play a huge role in shutting down your sexual responses. But it doesn't have to be something so big and complicated as that. Some people got so many negative messages about sex growing up that they have become insidious mental blocks to feeling comfortable with being orgasmic. I do a lot of work with people in my private practice on unpacking some of those messages and reclaiming their sexual selves.

And hey, there's good information earlier in this book about both physical and emotional issues and tips on working with those issues. And it is all information that is meant to help with both solo and partnered sex!

The larger point here is that you may be exploring yourself and not getting anywhere. And it's okay to get more help from a professional (doesn't that sound dirty?) to figure out if there are other things going on.

And make sure you read my chapter later on sex toys—ahem—sexual aids. It has lots of good info about using aids for solo sex as well as partnered sex.

What About Us Ace, Grey, Demi, and Stone People?

About 1% (ish) of the world is asexual (or demisexual, graysexual, etc.), which I talked about earlier in this book. Some of y'all have zero interest in orgasms at all. And some of y'all do have interest, just not at the same level. Or not every time a stiff wind blows past your junk.

If orgasms through masturbation are part of your life, that's great. If not, that's great, too. I just don't want anyone thinking they shouldn't masturbate because it somehow makes them a bad person. I have no more patience for shitty societal messages.

Don't masturbate if that's not your thing. But if it is your thing, and other people are telling you it shouldn't be? Who gives a fuck what they think. Get to it.

And for stone folx—people who enjoy their partner's pleasure rather than their own—it's entirely okay to not have interest in solo sex, and still want partnered sex where your sexual satisfaction comes from satisfying your partner.

What About Us Non-Cis People?

A lot of the above stuff totally may apply to you, but it also isn't fair to go, "Here is info for cisfolk. Everyone else? Your mileage may vary." So whether you are trans, nonbinary, agender, bigender, genderqueer, gender nonconforming, or anything other than cisgender, here is some basic information and research that is specific to gender confirmation treatments and the changes that may occur if someone is undergoing these treatments. I mean, I am the science-y, research-y chick and I haven't yet seen any research published around this topic and that makes me grumpy. Because gender confirmation treatments don't mean we have to give up the experience of our sexual selves, right?

Generally speaking, if you are no-hormone and/or no-op, the info for cis people applies, except for the (sometimes huge) added issue of possible dysphoria triggers. And just like any person for any reason having triggers around any kind of sex, the important thing is to find ways to work with that issue. Or around it, if need be.

For instance, you can try sensate focus work (like the exercises in Section Three) that omits areas that trigger dysphoria. Or you can find other ways to create comfort in the experience, such as leaving your binder on during sexual activity (yes, even during solo sex!). You know your body and your comfort level best, and get to set the boundaries around that experience. Especially in solo sex, when your focus is pleasure, exploration, and comfort.

Solo Sex After Starting Feminizing Hormone Therapy

A lot of trans women and transfem* individuals on hormone therapy (HT) who have not had a vaginoplasty note a difference in their sex drive and inclination to masturbate and/or have sex. Notice I said difference? Difference isn't bad or good . . . it's just not the same as before.

You may notice that your ejaculate seems more like pre-cum than a traditional load (but don't take that as me saying you can't get a fertile partner with a uterus pregnant, okay??), and a lot of folx report that it takes far more intellectual and/or emotional stimulation than it did in the past. If physical stimulation isn't enough, consider adding some of these elements before giving up.

There are also some activities you may not have even thought of engaging in before that might be something you want to try. Some no-op trans women and transfem* folx like stimulating the inguinal canals during solo (or partnered) sex as an alternative to penis stimulation. This is better known as muffing, and Mira Bellwether's guide to doing so can be found online if you're intrigued.

Solo Sex After Vaginoplasties

Vaginal care after a vaginoplasty is already going to be something you hear about ad nauseum, which is a good thing because it's really important. Some of the stuff you will hear about is the importance of using lubricant and using a vasodilator for a year or so after surgery to keep your vagina from contracting closed or scarring shut. Solo sex may be a place where you incorporate post-op care for your new vulva and vagina, because you can do so in the context of enjoying yourself as a sexual being.

The best research roundup I have found for individuals who have had vaginoplasties with clitoroplasties was on the now-defunct site transresearch.info. The studies they cite showed that 30% of trans women had difficulty masturbating to orgasm after surgery (but it was doable!) and another 18% couldn't orgasm at all. Interestingly, that number decreased to 14% when all sexual activity was included, not just masturbation. This means, again, that intellectual and emotional stimulation plays a big role in our sexual satisfaction, right?

Orgasms just may take more creativity to accomplish. We've all learned to do complicated things that have become simple with practice, and it's important to use that same mindset when focusing on our sexual pleasure. Surgically speaking, the clitoris is formed from the most sensitive area of the penis, so a clitoral orgasm is entirely possible. But it isn't the only way for a post-op transwoman or transfem* individual (or anyone born with a clitoris for that matter) to have an orgasm. G spot stimulation and anal stimulation thrown into the mix might be really helpful.

Solo Sex After Starting Masculinizing Hormone Treatment

So first off: if you are taking testosterone (T), congrats. If your clitoris doesn't cause dysphoria for you, you are going to reap some fun benefits.

The clitoris has twice the nerve endings as the penis (8000 versus 4000), and your clitoris grows due to the T (probably around an inch or two, although there are reports of up to 3 inches), which means more of it will protrude from the hood, meaning more of those nerve endings are exposed. Which means your orgasms will likely be more intense and happen faster.

More good news: there are sexual aids designed specifically for transmen and transmasc* folx who take T, such as stroker toys and lubricants specifically formulated for the dryness that can occur as a side effect of testosterone therapy.

Solo Sex After Metoidioplasty

Some transmen and transmasc folx opt for a metoidioplasty, which essentially works with the clitoris you already have (and have enlarged somewhat on T). Metoidioplasty takes the clitoris that has already been enlarged from testosterone therapy and repositions it to give additional length and place it in the usual position for a penis. This means your penis will be bioconstructed with your existing erectile tissue. While there may not be enough erectile tissue for you to penetrate a partner without a sexual aid (they exist now! do a Google search if you are interested!), you can definitely still enjoy solo sex quite easily and a sexual aid will still work great.

Solo Sex After Phalloplasty

With a phalloplasty, skin grafts are collected from other places on your body to bio-construct a larger penis. But since erectile tissue can't be constructed, a penile implant will need to be used (just like it would with a cisgender man who has incurable erectile dysfunction). Less erectile tissue is salvaged with this procedure, which can decrease ability to orgasm.

But even with the phalloplasty, most trans men and transmasc folx report having more sex (of all kinds) and more sexual satisfaction. Enjoying and exploring your new penis can be empowering and enjoyable, even if you don't climax. It's another aspect of being authentically who you are, and that's awesome.

My Partner Wants to Watch, the Perv-o. What's Up with That?

Maybe they think it's hot. We are visual creatures after all. Or maybe they want to see how you touch yourself so they can better know how to touch you in the ways you like (which makes for an excellent partner).

It can feel really intimidating and vulnerable, but it can also really enhance partner intimacy. Don't rule it out. Consider how to up your comfort level by changing lighting, maybe staying partially clothed, or having them engage in masturbation at the same time as you.

Sex Toys

Sex toys, aka sexual aids, provide stimulation and sensation: vibration, movement, warmth, etc. All the stuff we create for each other and ourselves for the purpose of sexual pleasure. I wrote a book called Unfuck Your Sex Toys all about sexual aids, how to shop for them, how to take care of them, and all that needful etcetera that you don't generally see.

By far the biggest question I get from people is about whether sex toys will "break" them for other types of sex, therefore ruining their sex lives. Sex toys can provide a more intensive version of sexual sensations. But that isn't gonna break anything.

Think of it this way: you can walk to the store or drive, right? If you walk it might take you a while longer, but you're still gonna get there. Walking has its benefits. You slow down, you connect to the world around you, you enjoy the view. Walking can be a ton of fun. But sometimes you just need to run into the grocery store and grab a bag of chips before the party, you know? Nothing wrong with driving, is there?

So the other question you may have is, "What if walking isn't getting me there and I can only get the chips from the store if I drive?" That totally does not make you broken. It just means you need more stimulation than other people. The toy didn't create that, that's just how you're wired down there.

If that kind of bums you out, the question I would ask is: what exactly does the driving do for you that the walking doesn't? For example, if you are a clitoris-having person, you may have a clitoral hood that blocks a lot of sensation. A toy might provide the extra sensation you need to get the job done. You might be able to get a similar effect if you or your partner push back your clitoral hood during sex. Some people also have that hood pierced, so the piercing provides the stimulation. Some people have a clitoral hood reduction surgery if it's really getting in the way.

So a toy may be solving a problem you didn't really know existed until you investigate a bit further.

So many people born with penises have had circumcisions (or at least gotten decent information about pushing back their foreskin for stimulation) so that muffling of sensation is less of an issue. But missing out on sensation can happen in other ways, too. Maybe your g-spot (which is not limited to vagina-having people, BTW!) is getting stimulated in just the right way by a certain toy, and that can be replicated with your or your partner's fingers. Or maybe it's your perineum (taint, durf, gooch, etc . . . .and yes, the perineum is not limited to penis-having people) that is getting hit the right way.

Pay attention to what the toy is actually doing for you, not just the final outcome. Erm, bag of chips. Whatever.

Toys can be lifesavers for both solo and partnered sex. They are nothing to be ashamed about. Some people have mobility issues that would make masturbation impossible without them. Sometimes toys allow people to participate in sex in a way they couldn't otherwise. Individuals who struggle to maintain an erection might find using a hollow core strap helpful in still allowing them penetrative intercourse with their partner. Or someone who doesn't have a penis but wants to penetrate a partner may use a traditional strap-on. In short? Sex toys are meant to enhance our experience, not replace partners. And technology is letting many of us experience sexual pleasure that we wouldn't have access to otherwise.

Because doesn't everyone deserve to be all that and a bag of chips?

Sex Addiction and Porn Addiction Don't Exist

High sex drive, porn usage, masturbation, cheating, and other behaviors around sex have been increasingly attributed to sex addiction over recent decades. Sex addiction is a multi-billion dollar treatment industry . . . and it's based on something that literally doesn't exist.

I have many people come to see me because their behavior regarding sex or porn is really pissing off their partner. The word "addiction" starts getting thrown around, and the do-er gets an ultimatum that shit's over if they don't get therapy for their "problem."

Can you engage in sex (partnered or solo, porn-enhanced or not) in a way that is problematic? Sure. And we're gonna get into that. But there is one thing that needs to be said first: wanting sex, enjoying sex, and being excited about sex does not make you a sex addict. Having cheated on a partner means you did something shitty to someone you love, but it doesn't make you a sex addict. Wanting porn, enjoying porn, and being excited about porn does not make you a porn addict.

Let me say that one more time for the people in the back: being sex and porn positive does not an addiction make. Alfred Kinsey (hey there again, toothbrush dude!) once remarked, "A nymphomaniac is someone who has more sex than you do."

A therapist shouldn't diagnose you with a sex or porn addiction, because the diagnosis doesn't exist in the DSM. And according to the research, there is simply no such thing.

Generally speaking, an addiction requires some physiological dependence for diagnosis. Problems with sexual activity tend to be labeled as a process addiction, which means there is no involvement of a substance that creates a literal physical dependency (like alcohol, nicotine, and other drugs), but the behavior itself has addictive qualities. When the brain lights up in the process of doing something like shoe shopping or gambling, it's easy to see the reward circuit being activated in a way it doesn't for someone who doesn't share that process addiction.

But sex (solo or partnered) is supposed to light up the reward centers of the brain. Everyone's brains light up that way. So can you safely label it an addiction? No. More research on better mechanisms for diagnosis is needed. But since we don't yet have a sex addiction blood test or brain scan test to rely on, figuring out problematic sexual behavior is individual and contextual. And it's one of those places where a well-trained, sex-positive therapist can be of benefit.

Can someone engage in sexual behaviors that harm their relationships and other life domains? Sure. But it is very important to call it what it really is. Dismissing problematic behaviors as addiction is a denial of responsibility and a declaration of a lack of self-control. And that right there is some fucking bullshit. Anyone who is engaging in problematic behavior around sex is absolutely accountable for their behavior and absolutely able to recognize their urges and consider how acting on them will impact their partners and their lives in general in the long term.

First of all, if you are worried that you may fall into the sex/porn problematic usage category, here are some questions to consider. But don't take your score as immutable evidence of your "addiction," okay? The point here is to discover patterns of behavior in order to create better strategies around the actions that are causing harm.

- Is partnered sexual activity itself more important than the person with whom you are having sex?
- Does sexual activity take the place of true connection?
- Are you experiencing a lot of life stress right now? Or depression or grief or anything else that's really difficult to deal with, and have started using porn and/or sex more than usual as a coping skill?
- Are you skipping out on other important things in your life because of your behavior around sex and porn?
- Are you feeling out of control of your behavior, instead of seeing sex and porn as another way of expressing who you are as a person? Like, is it costing you money you don't have or causing legal or health consequences?

- Is sex or porn something you use for connection and/or fun, or is it a compulsion you fight with every day?
- Is your behavior at odds with what your partner thinks is appropriate? Your church? Your family? Your community? Is this about other people's core values or your own?

Here is the big thing I want you to look at: how sex and porn either hinder or support your relationships. In the end, all addictions are replacement relationships. They become more important than the people we love. They become more important than we are ourselves, and prevent us from being a human out there connecting in the world.

Problematic use of sex, masturbation, and/or porn comes about when the thing we are doing becomes more important than all of our reasons for being, and all of the meaning of our behaviors is drained of context. I don't know anyone who is unhappy with their usage of sex and/or porn who actually likes what they are doing. Not past the immediate moment of engagement, anyway. And they don't like themselves all too much, either. Because their behavior is separating them from all the amazing, messy, authentic, beautiful relationships the world has to offer, it's no longer aligned with their values and keeps them from prioritizing the people they love. That's what defines a problem.

If you are worried that your solo sex activities are problematic to your partnered sex (or if your partner states that they are), it's important to unpack the impetus of the behavior and the effect it's having on your other life domains. Generally speaking, when you are dealing with the other stressors in your life effectively, this "problem" takes care of itself.

If you realize that your current sexual activities are posing a problem for you, then it may be of benefit to get some support. One of the biggest problems in this area is the number of clinicians profiting on the stigma and shame surrounding sex. Which means that doing careful research is really important. Ask any therapists that you are interested in seeing what their stance on sex addiction and porn usage is. If you are dealing with past religious or cultural messages around your sex and pornography usage, ask them if they are comfortable with helping you explore that without adding their own value system to the conversation. I recently read an article by a therapist who views masturbation as a form of spousal abuse. Yes, literally. There is enough shame and stigma around sex out there as it is. You sure as fuck don't need it from your therapist.

Section Three: Unfuck Your Relationships with Others

Is this the part of the book you were most interested in? Did you skip or skim the other stuff because you wanted to get to this stuff? Ok, go ahead and insert a big Kermit yaaaaaaaaayyyyyyyy right here. This is all the dating and relationshipping advice we could squeeze in, plus lots of activities to try. Fair warning though, I'm gonna refer back to the other two sections on occasion. So if you skipped them and emotional stuff comes up, you may have to head on back a few chapters and do some more unpacking!

My therapeutic training is grounded in relational-cultural theory. One of the biggest differences between this treatment orientation and others is that we regard relationships as their own entity. Meaning that in every connection we have with someone else, there is us, there is them, and there is the relationship itself as its own third party. This perspective is a bit of sorcery that can have an amazing impact on your romantic partnership.

So if Section Two of this book was the "you" part, this is the "relationship itself" part. And since you're a smart motherfucker, you noticed that I didn't include a "them" section. Because someone else is not your job, right? You are responsible for you. And you have a joint responsibility to the relationship. So we are focusing on you-in-relation here, not them. That's their job.

So this last part of the book includes far fewer naked shenanigans than you might expect. Because even if you are an exceptional specimen, only a small percentage of your time is actually spent on naked shenanigans. And all this other self-in-relationship stuff, like the communication and healthy boundaries, is the foundation for making that part far better.

DATE LIKE A GROWN UP

Dating. What ever happened to dating? Wooing? Courting? Shaking your plumage and doing the mating dance?

There seems to be zero space these days between hooking up/friends-with-benefits and having the U-Haul number on speed dial. Either we make the beast with two backs and then take off or we move in and adopt a dog together in 3 minutes flat. Let's be honest, neither one is authentic. If sex without feelings has become your long-term solution, then you've fallen into the "it's cooler not to care" trap. It's safer there, you don't get hurt if it wasn't emotional to begin with. But belly flopping into something time after time isn't the more mature response. Then it becomes about being in a relationship, rather than being with a particular person with whom you want to build a relationship. Desperate to connect is no more toxic, in the end, than desperate to stay disconnected.

Fuck. It's all pretty bonkers. The amount of time I have spent with clients and friends discussing the merits of different dating apps, local bars and hangouts, and other minutia of the dating scene is not small. Everything is a question: When do I start opening up about the heavy stuff? What's considered heavy stuff? When is too soon? When is too late? Why am I always friend-zoned? No wonder we end up saying "fuck that noise" and settling in for another round of Candy Crush instead. Or end up spending years with someone who is not right for us, making each other miserable, because someone is better than no one, right? Dating becomes an obstacle course instead of what it is supposed to be, which is something fun.

Are you in that space? Early-stage almost-relationshipping? Considering the FTR (friends to relationship if you aren't fluent in acronym) move? Dating? Thinking about dating? Opening up the OKCupid website then feeling nauseous and closing the browser window immediately? Stressful as balls, isn't it?

I don't know about you, but I'm so over it. It's time for us to reclaim this space from the asshole culture around us. Roll up your sleeves, my blueberry muffins. Let's get to work.

How to Find a Date

It used to be that we met the people we dated at school or church or because our parents arranged everything down to the number of goats everyone got out of the deal. Then the internet happened and shit changed. And generally for the better. Online chat rooms turned into IRL relationships and by 1995, the first official dating website (Match.com if you're interested) went live.

Instead of being limited to being only one or two degrees from Kevin Bacon, the whole world opened up and we connected with people completely outside our small social circles. Researchers from the University of Essex and University of Vienna were able to model the changes created by the advent of online dating. Currently, more than a third of marriages start with online dating. The number of interracial marriages has gone up significantly. Marriages born of meeting online are often stronger than those of people who meet in more traditional ways. The internet is the second most likely way someone who is heterosexual will find a partner, and it is far and away the most likely place for someone who is queer to find someone to date.

That's not to say it's all well and good. Online dating can suck, too. The advent of swipe-apps (starting with Tinder in 2012) has made the process more game-like. You're essentially flipping through a card deck, creating accept and reject piles. And the process has fucked with a lot of people's self-esteem. Research presented at the American Psychological Association conference in 2012 demonstrated that people who used Tinder as a dating app had worse self-esteem than people who used other dating apps (going back to why self-compassion is so important, am I right??) and men specifically reported more negative body image perceptions than their counterparts on other sites.

So what's a modern human to do?

- If you are using a dating site, choose carefully. Think about your end goals (Marriage and all the baby-raising? Netflix and chill?) and pick a site that matches.
- Also, be honest about your end goals. Don't say you are good with keeping things casual when your reality is a ticking biological clock. And if you aren't sure, say that too. Maybe you are open to an LTR but that's not your immediate goal. If people self-select out because they want something different, then fine, that wasn't meant to be your person anyway.
- Be honest about all of it. Don't lie about your age, your weight, your circumstances. Seriously stop with the snap filter enhanced photos and the artful hand-under-the-chin tuck. Look your best, but look yourself. And be yourself. Separated but not yet divorced? Own it. Have four kids? Own it. Polyam? Spill the details on what that means for you, your primary partner, other partners, and anyone you might date. Again, if people self-select out, they weren't meant to be your person anyway.

If online isn't your cup of tea, then you are gonna have to put yourself out there in other ways. Awkward and vulnerable, but far better than staying home and playing video games all weekend if what you actually want to do is meet someone. So you are gonna have to expand your social circle.

- Find people who are doing the interesting shit that you like to do. If tabletop gaming is your thing, join a meetup for gamers rather than just hanging out with your same crew all the time. If you're a jogger, join a running group. If you like movies and popcorn there are totally meetups just for people to get together to go to the movies as a group. You may not meet the love of your life but at least you are doing something you enjoy and getting out of your regular circle. And maybe one of those people will end up introducing you to the love of your life at some point!
- Volunteer. If you are passionate about animal rescue or electing a particular candidate to office or anything else then volunteer to help make that happen. Just like with the above, at least you aren't doing something that feels like a waste of time otherwise (fruitlessly hanging out at a bar, anyone?), you will expand your social network, and you are racking up some bonus world-changing points in the process.
- Ask people who they know. Yeah, awkward. But if you want to go out with someone you gotta meet them first. You don't have to look for the Carrie Fisher in When Harry Met Sally friend who has a dude rolodex or anything, but just put it out there that you have an eye out, what you're looking for, and that you are amenable to an intro. And lest we forget? Carrie Fisher's character ended up marrying Bruno Kirby's character . . . and they met through Harry and Sally!
- Be prepared to approach in a way that is engaging but still authentic. Don't be the person in the coffee shop that interrupts someone who is reading or has headphones in. But if they're standing in line to order and are holding a book maybe try "I keep seeing that book around (or I've never seen that book around, whatever works)—any good?" as an opening line. Do you need a cold open? I have a friend who is not super-hot but has great game because he first approaches with "Are you waiting on anyone?" and if they say no, or say yes, but indicate it's a friend and not a date, he follows up with "Is it cool if I flirt with you for a little while then?" If you don't have the Sergeant Smooth gene, embrace your discomfort. The right person will think that's pretty cute. Maybe "I'm gonna kick myself later if I didn't at least come up and introduce myself. And I'm feeling

super awkward, so here's hoping I don't embarrass myself so badly that I will feel the urge to go walk into traffic. Hi, I'm . . ."

- Make it your mission to start conversations with people in general so that approaching someone you think is super cute will seem less intimidating. Go practice!

Date Like a Therapist

Ok, so you met someone. The best dating advice I've got for ya? Date like a therapist.

I married early in my adult life while others my age were still dating. Then, in my late 30s, my husband died of cancer. Suddenly I was a young widow with two teenagers and a complicated career. The dating world has become a very different world since my years as a teenager. By the time I was ready to date I wasn't sure what awaited me. My specialty in private practice is intimacy and relationships. Would that complicate matters? Would I over-analyze everything and scare my dates away?

Instead, I found that the same qualities that made me a good therapist were of great benefit to dating. I was no longer in my early 20s, but neither were the men I met. Maturity was part of it, but an even more important factor was my therapeutic training. I didn't need to turn that part of myself off to enter the dating world; instead I found it to be very useful.

Eventually, I got married again, something I had no expectation of ever happening. I truly believe that dating like a therapist helped me find the man I am completely crazy about. and I wanted to share the benefit of these experiences with others in the dating market.

Be Present, Engaged, and Authentic

Most individuals give off certain signals demonstrating interest and availability in a dating environment. I was told by more than one person that I didn't send any of them. I didn't twirl my hair, giggle, or make extraneous physical contact on dates. One guy told me that at first he didn't know how to respond to me. He was used to gauging if someone was interested in him by reading these signals, but then he realized that he felt completely comfortable with me because I was focusing all my attention on him.

If I committed to a date with someone, even a meeting for coffee, I was committing my time and attention to that person. Everyone deserves the respect of an engaged and present response. My intent is to get to know the person, not put on a show for them. If someone comes to see me for therapy, they receive my undivided attention whether or not I find them interesting or likable. Dating someone should be the same. If

I was too busy sending out flirty signals, I would miss getting to know someone in a truly authentic way.

Use SMART Goal Setting

When writing a treatment plan for a client, I ask the following questions to help formulate goals. Is the goal: Specific? Measurable? Achievable? Realistic? Time-sensitive?

Dating should be no different. What do you want from your dating experience? How will you know if you are getting that? If you are looking for a life partner how will you know if you are on that path? If you are looking for someone to have fun with, what does fun look like for you?

Don't waste your time or theirs. Know what you want and how you plan on getting there. Consider where you are now and pay attention to any signals that suggest that your goals are changing. Not that wandering aimlessly is always a bad thing, but you are far more likely to get what you want if you know what that actually is.

Realize That Everyone Has Their Own Agenda

Much like someone walking into a therapist's office, anyone you are dating has their own agenda for their dating experience, an agenda that may or may not be congruent with your own. (The word agenda seems like a sinister one, I know. But in reality, it just refers to the motivations and intentions that we all carry into everything we do, including into our dating lives.) They may not even be fully aware of what they want. Not all agendas are explicit. Their hidden agendas may not have anything to do with you. Their motivations are not nearly as much about you as you think they are, so don't take everything personally.

I not only expect people to be guarded starting out in therapy, I respect it. If anything, dating is even more anxiety-provoking than starting therapy. So give both the other people and yourself some space. Be willing to explore, rather than make immediate demands. Relationship-building takes time, so give each potential new one space to grow.

Be Aware of Your Countertransference

Countertransference is a therapeutic word first coined by Freud in correspondence with Jung in 1909. He defined it as the therapist's emotional response to their client based on their own history or issues. Freud conceived of this as a personal problem on the part of the therapist and something that should be guarded against and tamped down at all times.

More than 100 years later, we think about countertransference much differently. I teach my students that countertransference is entirely normal, and can be beneficial (as well as diagnostic) as long as we remain aware of it when it happens. This means parsing out whether other people have a similar response to this person, or just you. Essentially, the question becomes . . . when you have a strong emotional reaction to someone, is it your stuff or theirs?

This is no different when dating someone new. If their behavior is upsetting or anxiety provoking in any way, listen for cues that other people have the same response to that person. This can lend insight into how they interact with others in general, and help you decide whether or not this is a behavior you want to endure.

On the other hand, if it seems to be just your response, then it is important that you do your own work around that, rather than expecting someone else to adapt to your triggers. Chances are, this will be something that will come up for you over and over again, even if you don't end up with this particular person, so you might as well do the work. We all have our own baggage in relationships, and it is important that we take responsibility for carrying it.

Know When to Terminate

"Firing" clients is a tough thing for a therapist to do. We struggle with knowing when it is appropriate and how to do so in the best possible way. This is where the SMART goal setting comes in. Are we progressing along the lines that we should be? Are we progressing at all? Is their agenda becoming more explicit? Can I adapt to the agenda and needs of the person I am seeing? Is the client showing up when they are supposed to and doing the things they said they are going to do?

Can you think of any better analogy for a break-up? I might be biased, but I never could.

The poet Maya Angelou was known for saying, "When someone shows you who they are, believe them." In the end, love is a behavior. Do you feel respected? Is your time valued? Do you feel the relationship is moving forward? If not, have you addressed these issues and asked for change?

I have told clients, "I don't think this is helping you and it is important that I don't waste your time. We either need to find a way to make this work or I can refer you to someone else." I have had similar conversations with people I have dated. Termination doesn't mean someone is a bad person. It means you are ending a bad match.

In the end, all of us deserve relationships that let us be our best possible selves, and support us in that endeavor. We need to know what we want, and give our relationships a chance to meet these desires. We also need to know when to let them go, or change the nature of them to better meet our needs. Therapy, in the end, should model what a healthy relationship can be like.

A therapeutic approach to dating can be a very effective strategy for creating the types of relationships we are seeking. It isn't your typical smoke and mirrors dating advice. Instead of hiding who you are, be exactly who you are—because that is the person you want others to see and know.

More Dating Tips for Grown-Ass People

My date-like-a-therapist advice was originally published by a local news organization and it was a hit. One of my bonus kiddos ended up getting it as a reading assignment in a class at the local community college, which cracked her up mightily. In the ensuing years, I've added other dating tips to the list based on the patterns I see happening with my clients, with my single friends, and even based on the what-the-fucks I think when reading shit online. So here's some more taking the crazy out of dating advice.

Have Fun. Yes. Seriously.

The fun part? That's the number one priority.

That doesn't mean don't be nervous. Because, duh, you likely will be. But at some point, you should be relaxing a bit and having a blast. If you aren't busy picking out the names for your future children in your head, you can actually have fun. If you do an internal fun check and you aren't thinking "I'm digging this person! Woohoo!" then nothing is there for you. That's okay. A date is just a date. Far less serious and heart-wrenching if it ends with just that.

Do a Deep-Down Gut Check

Does something feel off? Unsafe? Listen to that. Listen hard. If your intuition tells you that something is fundamentally wrong at any point, don't ignore it. This is so difficult for people who have spent their lives being silenced and being told that what they think and feel doesn't matter. You may have been told for so many years about the wrongness of your instincts that you have trained yourself to stop listening to them. Dating is the time to listen again. Get down in your gut and see what it's telling you. Like I talk about in Unfuck Your Body, the vagus nerve connects the brain and stomach. We really do, at a literal level, have a second brain in our stomachs. Listen to it.

Beyond the gut check, do the spark check. Do you get the little pitter-patter when you brush someone's arm or during that first kiss? You deserve pitter-patter. Maybe there's no pitter-patter because you are super nervous or maybe it's because you really aren't feeling it. It's okay if you're not. Pay attention to that.

Everyone Deserves to Be Chocolate Cake

I had a client tell me that his partner of 30+ years still makes his heart skip a beat. That's amazing. We all deserve to feel that for someone and be that for someone. If you are dating a person who is amazingly fantastic but doesn't pass the fun check and the spark check, you don't have to keep digging for it. It's okay to think someone is amazing but have zero interest in seeing them naked. They can be a great person, but not a great person for you. The important thing is that you tell them that.

I dated my way to a lot of great friendships. It's not an easy conversation, but it doesn't have to be a complicated one. Be honest. Say something like "This may sound like bullshit but I mean every word when I say I think you're amazing and totally deserve someone who thinks you hung the moon and I'm not going to be that person. I don't want you out of my life, but I respect it if not wanting to date you anymore means you'd rather not see me at all." This is better for everyone in the long run, even if it feels awful in the short run. If they get butthurt at your disinclination to sexitimes with them and don't want to remain friends, that's okay, too.

You also should be aware of your own patterns in this regard. Do you find you always get bored pretty quickly with genuinely nice people who aren't creating a level of chaos energy that keeps things exciting (but still ultimately toxic)? Did all your relationship models function on drama and dysfunction? Do you tend to have three week stands and then wander off to the next big thing? Chocolate cake doesn't require crazy sprinkles to be yummy. If you are realizing that about yourself, maybe it's time to go back to Parts One and Two and do some work on yourself, yeah?

Beware the Oxytocin Trap

Oxytocin is the love drug . . . the neurochemical best known as Wheeeeeeeeeeeeeeeeeee! Oxytocin is released in physical touch (and yes, especially in orgasms). And it's awesome. But it can also be an asshole. We call it the love drug, but it's really the trust drug. It makes us feel like we can trust the person we are with far more than we likely would otherwise. This is why a salesperson will touch your arm when trying to get you to close a deal. This is also why if you go all-in on a new relationship it will burn out fast.

If you are with a new person 24/7, you never get a break from the oxytocin flood to actually do a good gut check. Kinda like Kilgrave's hold on his victims in season one of Jessica Jones. Make space away from them to see how you feel. Are you halfway-relieved when they aren't around? Do you feel better about yourself without them there? Less on guard? Why is that? Do you miss them? What do you actually miss? Are they being shitty about you taking time and space for yourself? Are they pressuring you to be present when you aren't? Does that make you feel controlled? This goes back to the gut check questions. It's important to pay attention to how the trust drug may impact our answers and lead us astray, so you may need to make space for yourself to answer them better.

Don't Make Your Friends and Family Ride Your Drama Llama with You

If you tend to live in the land of one week stands, that's your decision. Dragging everyone along with you is a pretty dick move, however. Even if you don't have a new person in place on the reg, it's important to live your life, not your new relationship.

My general rule of thumb is if you are out with your other people, spend about 25% of your time talking about your new person and 75% of the time talking about all the rest of your life. It's important to remember that you have one and it's important not to irritate the fuck out of the people around you. Your new relationship is important, too. I get it. But is it 100% of everything you say important? Nah, 25% is plenty.

The people who I've seen working out in the long term are the ones that are out living their lives, not dissecting every move every single minute. What is going on that you feel the need to do a critical incident stress debriefing over every text? Is this something about you that you need to work on, or something about the relationship? If you are feeling so unsettled with this new person that you are having to water-cooler quarterback every play? Something is up. Maybe with you, if that's your pattern. And if it is? Work on that shit. But if you are generally Captain Chill? Gut check this thing.

Consider Stepping Back a Bit on Having Your Friends Meet Each New Person

Give it at least a month. My general rule was 3-4 months. And if you have kids? More like 6 months. And if this new person is pressuring you otherwise? Ask them (and yourself) why? If they aren't going anywhere, then they aren't going anywhere. They don't have to be dumped full force into your life to prove anything.

Look for Slippage

There is something about that four-month mark, I swear. We can hold ourselves together and show our best sides for about that long, tops.

Then our authentic self starts leaking out around the edges. Keep an eye out for boo-person's real personality to start showing up. This isn't a bad thing. In fact, a lot of idiosyncrasies can be downright adorable. Like Friday night pancakes for dinner or leaving the Sunday paper on the floor because the cat loves to sleep on it. Some things aren't great but are tolerable, and are important to know about someone, like low blood sugar hanger, irritability in traffic, that kinda thing.

Some things may need to be deeply considered and discussed: Rudeness to waitstaff. Disinterest in voting in elections. A deep and abiding love of Nickelback. You know, seriously important, possibly deal-breaking shit.

When I asked friends for their dating rules, one said "Don't date . . . interrogate." Another said, "Talk to one another until dawn at least three times." Again, no matter how much you think you know this person's soul after a couple of weeks, you don't. And no matter how much you think they know you, they really, really don't. Oxytocin is a fucking liar. Take the time to have those deep conversations and really get to know someone.

Don't Give Your Power Away

A friend of mine said, in regard to dating, "Never treat them like a priority if they only treat you like an option." Another said, "Want what you want for yourself (love, connection, desire) more than you want any one person." This may seem like two separate pieces of advice, but it really isn't. Both people, in their way, are saying, don't give your power away.

Anyone you are with should enhance your life, enhance your hopes and dreams, and enhance your compassion and engagement with yourself and the world around you. Someone who is not excited about you and about what you bring into the world isn't worth your time.

A Rejection May Not Have a Damn Thing to Do with You

If all your relationships end at date number three, it may be time to figure out what is happening there, either in your behavior or in the people you are choosing. But generally speaking? If you are dating someone and you get a big ole swipe left? That is far less about you than you realize. Seriously. Someone you asked out? Or you've been out with them a couple times? They don't know you well enough to reject the actual awesomeness that is you.

They are rejecting your offer for getting to know the real, awesome you. For whatever reason. Maybe their ex called. Maybe they don't like your choice of band t-shirts. Maybe they are oxytocin junkies off in search of their next hit. Maybe they are stupid motherfuckers who don't know a good thing when it is standing right in front of them. But, hey.

You haven't had the deep getting to know each other conversations for you to take this rejection all kinds of personally. Dating doesn't magically lead to relationshipping. It isn't supposed to. It's supposed to be a try out period. Next candidate!

Date Safely and Have a Disclosure Plan

There are all kinds of things we may need to disclose to a new dating partner. Things that are not any of the business of other people in our life but could affect an intimate relationship. That we are unemployed and broke AF. That we have kids. That we are polyam or into kink. That we have an STI. Information about our gender identity or sexual orientation.

If you have something big that can affect relationships, it's really important to have a disclosure plan. And sometimes the information you are disclosing can put you at risk with the other person (and/or anyone they tell). If your truthbomb conversation runs the risk of ending very badly, also have a safety plan: Have the conversation in a public place, have a friend on stand-by, and have an escape plan.

I can tell you as a rule of thumb, I generally go with "lay it all on the table and let people self-select out if it's a problem." If this is presented immediately, there is less need for big disclosure sessions later. And yes, I totally get that people will self-select out that would have been great partners if they had gotten to know you first. But I am not that invested in developing the emotional maturity of people I don't know and may or may not end up liking. And just looking at the number of trans women of color who are victims of intimate partner violence makes me desperate to encourage all y'all to err on the side of caution and keep yourself safe in the long run.

Many of my clients have decided to use dating sites that are specific to their situation for just this reason. There are sites for individuals who have STIs, who are trans, who are poly, who are into BDSM, who are into roleplay. There is legit an app for all the different kinds of ways we can be a human in relationships.

Some things on the "need to disclose" list may have legal consequences if you don't handle them right. For example, knowingly transmitting an STI to a new, uninformed partner could get you into legal trouble. I live in Texas, where some STIs could carry the weight of an assault charge and others (namely, HIV and AIDS) could find you charged with attempted murder or assault with a deadly weapon.

But, hey. I'm not a lawyer. This is not legal advice. And legal shit aside, telling people the truth is just the right fucking thing to do. So disclose. Before you don't-disclose to someone who finds out, freaks out, dumps you, tells the world, and maybe even presses charges.

You Are Allowed to Be Crazy, You Aren't Allowed to Act Crazy

I have said this so many times, I need to get a tattoo at this point. Whatever nutty things are running through your mind? Don't act on them.

Yes, you have baggage. We all do. If you know your past history has messed up your thinking about relationships, then you need to work on that shit and not foist it upon the people you are dating. Emotions are just information from our body—whatever you feel isn't right or wrong. But your actions are your responsibility. If you know that doing something will embarrass you later, do not do the thing.

What's the thing, you ask innocently? Different for different people. But we all have a pair of big, striped crazy pants hidden in the backs of our closets. And we all feel the urge to dig them out, put them on, and act all kinds of stupid over relationship issues. It may be driving by their house to see who is parked there, setting up a fake Facebook account to stalk them, or getting color contacts so your eyes match. Whatever weirdness your brain is telling you is a good idea? Don't do it.

If you know you will look back on the situation and realize you were wearing your big striped crazy pants that day? Do not do the thing. Get a friendtervention. Hide your phone and car keys from yourself. Don't lash out. Don't be reactionary. You are responsible for yourself and whatever baggage you still carry (no matter who packed those bags to begin with). Hold yourself accountable.

Be Wise

This piece of advice was given to me by Joe McBride (yes, of Rock 'n' Roll High School fame). If you haven't read his memoir, The Broken Places, you really should. If you have, you know he has some intense and dark relationships. When I asked him what he meant by "be wise," he responded, "It's like when Gertrude Stein was dying, and Alice B. Toklas said, 'Gertrude, Gertrude, what is the answer?' Gertrude replied, 'What is the question?'"

I know, academics tell the most esoteric jokes. Joe was really saying, be wise in whatever ways make sense for you, your needs, and your relationships. Shift based on what you need to shift. Be aware enough of your own shit to know where you need to be careful. Listen to your instincts. Believe what people show you more than what they tell you. Be thoughtful. Consider all the ways they are communicating with you. People are always telling their stories and sometimes they even use words. This kind of attention to the world around us is how we can be wise.

On The Glories of Not Dating (And Maybe Even Still Having Sex!)

You don't have to be in one of the ace/demi/gray/aro categories to not be interested in dating. After all, you can have plenty of sex, solo or partnered, without ever dating, right?

It usually boils down to a few basic reasons:

1) You've got shit you are actively working on so you can be a good human being in relation to other human beings.

2) You are way too fucking busy with other shit to add more shit to your plate. You can't focus on it, you don't have the time, and you don't want to be dickish to someone else in the process of you finishing school, working crazy hours, raising kids, etc.

3) You just aren't that into it. You're happy and fulfilled and dating doesn't add anything to the mix for you at this time in your life.

All of these reasons are excellent ones. And you are totally entitled to not-date to your single-lovin' heart's content. But hey, if you are not-dating because of anxieties or other reasons when the truth is you really, really actually want to date? It isn't the worst idea in the world to unpack what's holding you back. Therapy can help with that. You deserve to be happy, and if dating will help you get there, let's figure that shit out.

Are you not-dating but still wanting some partnered-sex game? Also totally fine. Despite how progressive culture has gotten in so many ways, we still manage to get our prude on about no-strings sex. There is zero wrong with having an FWB or pick ups and hookups. If that's what works for you, go for it. Just as long as everyone is on the same page about the plan. It should probably go without saying that you need to be careful about preventing STIs and unwanted pregnancies and the like. But you're a responsible person and you know that, right?

You may notice that your level of sexual satisfaction is not as good with partners you don't have an emotional attachment to. Research says that's generally the case. That's not me saying you should be all boo'd up with anyone you have sex with. But there is a reason the expression is friends with benefits. The friends part is legit important for most people. As a general rule, if you wouldn't vote for someone if they were running for public office, letting them have naked sexitimes isn't something you are going to feel great about in the grander scheme.

Of course, all this can lead to the problem of someone in the hook-up relationship catching feelings. It's not a bad thing or an embarrassing thing. But it is something that needs to be discussed and dealt with. Which goes back to the full disclosure dialogue. Not a fun conversation, but a needful one. Even just "I know this is supposed to be low-key, but lately I've been wanting it to be more. If you do too, that would be amazing and we should talk about that. If not, I probably need to not see you since it's gonna mess with my head and I don't wanna go all crazy on the both of us."

No matter what your circumstances, keep it honest and watch for your own motivations and reactions. You won't always do everything perfectly, but you are far less likely to be blindsided that way.

RELATIONSHIPPING

Relationshipping is not dating. And thank Buddha, because even if you are going in with the healthiest attitude ever, dating can be really tiring.

Of course, getting boo'd up has its own set of crap to navigate. In some ways you are safer and more secure and you don't have to worry so much anymore. But on the other side, I see folx feeling too safe and secure and unworried, and then fuck things up cuz you go in all Leeerrrrroooooooy Jennnnnkiiiiiiiins style. And I don't want that for you. You've been working too hard on all this shit to biff out now.

A relationship is always ongoing work. Especially for those of us who didn't have great role models in that regard and have to be proactive in our desire to be healthier in our relationships than what we saw around us growing up. Whether you and your partner are still all new and shiny, or whether you have years under your belt, actively working on your relationship in the small ways will make the larger obstacles far easier to deal with (and may end up preventing them all together).

I realize that most of these rules aren't about sex at all . . . which makes sense because the book is called Unfuck Your Intimacy, not Unfuck Your Fuck. These are all guidelines and ideas for improving intimacy generally, which will improve physical intimacy in turn.

Love People, Not Labels

Boy or girl. Neurosurgeon or flight attendant. Labels are assignments we attach to aspects of our being. They are not the sum entirety of who we are. And they change. They change all the time. So if you become attached to the label that someone wears, you are going to be sadly disappointed when that label falls off. The only label your partner should ever get from you? "Mine."

Grow Together and Put One Another First

The strongest relationships I see are the ones that go through enormous changes together. In physical ability, career, socio-economic status, even gender.

How do you marry someone you thought was a man and be in their process of realizing they are a woman? Stay with them through all their gender confirmation treatments and surgeries even if your own sexual orientation never included women? Loving that person like a motherfucking boss, that's how.

When long-term relationships start to fall apart over longer periods of time, it's often because partners don't remain connected in their growth. People change. All the time. Life changes us, maturity changes us, and our circumstances put us in places we never thought we'd be. Losing sight of our partner as our primary person in this world happens most often when we have children. But other things can cause this to be an issue as well. Careers, other family, friends. Your partner may have interests that are wildly different from your own, or interests that you never expected.

And then, together, as a team, go tackle the world. Have you heard the term "yoke" before? It's an old-fashioned word, used to describe the crossbeam that was used to connect two farm animals together so they could effectively pull a plow. And no, I'm not calling you an ox or a cow. It became a term to later explain marriage. The idea is that two equal partners, organized to work together, can accomplish way more than two separate individuals. We work harder, stronger, and more effectively as a yoked team.

If you have kids, put each other first and then as a team put the children first. Or whatever else you are tackling. You and your partner must come first to each other. To keep from flying off in different directions and working toward different ends, stay yoked.

Spend Time Together

And I don't mean collapsed on the sofa, watching Netflix and eating ice cream in your stained sweats with boo by your side. I mean real, planned couples time. Your mate deserves to be wooed. And so do you.

This doesn't mean fancy, it just means intentional. It doesn't matter if it's a walk in the park, ice cream cones, or eating take-out and streaming the movie you missed in the theater. The point is respecting your relationship enough to make time for it in the same way you make time for everything else of importance in your life. Do you make an appointment when you go see your dentist? Plan in your schedule to run to Trader Joe's for groceries? Isn't boo (and hey, all of them if you have more than one) worth at least as much consideration?

Make a plan. To do something. Together. Once a week. It can even be at home if that is how life is rolling right now. But make that plan.

Spend Time Apart

This is stupid important if you and boo share a living space. And especially if you have kids. Once a week you should each have a chance to escape the house alone and once a week you should have a chance to have the house to yourself alone. I know how hard this is to do, but if you make an effort to make the alone time happen, you will hit the mark more often than you are hitting it now, right?

It doesn't have to be complicated. Doesn't matter if you want to go wander Target with a Starbucks in hand for an hour alone; we all need time that is just ours. Same with time alone in the house. Doesn't matter if you do laundry and watch Mozart in the Jungle with the cat. The house. Alone. No judgments on how you spend that time. It's all yours. We all need that time to reboot, recharge, and be good partners.

Establish Your Relationship "Rules"

Everyone's relationship is different, which means everyone needs a structure to support their relationships. We call this structure "rules" for lack of a better term, though most of us have enough anarchism in us to hate the idea of rules. Scaffolding of Interpersonal Respect work better? Use whatever feels right . . . but no matter what you call it? Use your fucking words to communicate your expectations. Whether we label it a want, a need, a boundary, etc., if there is an expectation you have of your partner? Y'all need to have that discussion.

Picture it. My office. Any time, because it happens at least once a week:

Partner 1: They didn't . . . .(mad, mad, hurt, upset, grump, grump, complain)

Partner 2: . . . .

Me: Did Partner 2 know you expected them to do that?

Partner 1: They should have!

Me: I see. Did you TELL them you expected that?

Partner 1: No! They should know!

Me: I flunked Mind-Reading School. I'm guessing Partner 2 did as well. Can you share with both of us what your expectations are so Partner 2 has a shot of getting out of trouble here?

Partner 2: I woulda been fine with doing what you wanted. But I'm concrete as pavement. Please tell me!

Nobody in the history of ever has run toward their lover in slow motion across a field of flowers. There isn't anything "natural" or "intuitive" about understanding someone else. Some people are good guessers, but if you really want to be understood then you better state shit up front. That's relationship rules in a nutshell.

Expect flowers on your birthday? Say it.

Expect Boo to not chat with exes on Snapchat? Say it.

Expect to meet all potential secondary partners before their first date? Say it.

Expect oral sex on Sunday afternoons? Sayyyyy the thing.

Once it's all out in the open, then you can sift through the disagreements. And bring in a therapist if you hit an impasse. But it's not rocket science. It's adulting. Which requires vulnerability and clear communication. And it isn't movie-romantic. Because we aren't living in a movie. And as uncomfortable as it is, it's better than cleaning up the damage caused by NOT having these conversations.

Everyone Has the Right to Feel Safe

We have the right to physical safety and emotional safety. Physical safety doesn't just mean free from interpersonal violence, it means feeling in control of your personal body at all times. I've worked with people who have never laid a hand on their partner, but they have a way of dominating with their physical presence that feels threatening and intimidating. That can be an intentional way of controlling the other person, and it is not safe or acceptable.

Emotional safety can be equally hard to define. I ask people to describe the sensations in their body when they feel a sense of safety. Not just their thoughts and feelings, but how they settle into themselves. Like how we feel when we crawl into a comfortable bed with soft sheets at the end of a long day. The people in our lives should support that feeling inside us, and we should do the same for them whenever we can.

Don't Fucking Lie

Don't half-truth. Don't omit. Don't answer on a technicality, Captain Semantics. Own your shit. Be honest and be authentic. Own it as yours but say it. If you are angry, say you are angry, take responsibility and say why, ask for something different and hope you will get it. But don't say you are okay when you are not. And FFS, don't play a semantics game in your mind. Don't be sneaky. Don't be sketch. Don't rationalize. If your partner would be legitimately hurt or upset by anything they saw in your phone or on your computer, don't fucking do it.

Don't Kick the Puppy

Don't allow yourself bad behavior, even if your partner does. If you kick a puppy, it may come back and lick your hand over and over again. But that is not an excuse to keep kicking. If you know your actions are hurting your partner at some level, you have to stop. Even if they say it's okay. Even if they are not brave or strong enough to ask you to stop. Have some self-accountability. Stop the behavior or get out of the relationship.

This seems to happen in relationships where one partner is not chocolate cake. If one partner has all the power in the relationship because their mate is slavishly devotional in keeping them happy and keeping them there, a lot of metaphorical puppy kicking takes place. Taking advantage of their desperation, blowing them off at the last minute, accepting gifts and favors, messing around when they didn't agree to polyamory, generally being rude and disrespectful. Just because someone lets you treat them like that does not mean it's ok. You've heard of the golden rule right? Even better? The platinum rule. Treat others the way they want to be treated. If you can't do that for your partner, or you don't want to, you need to move on.

Love Is a Behavior, Not a Feeling

Love is not a nebulous idea. It's not a vague notion of warm and fuzzies. It's the real, daily interactions of sharing our lives with someone, caring for them, and having them care for us in return. Love is what we do, day in, day out. Not what we profess in our status updates.

Love is stopping what you are doing to sit with your mate and talk about their bad day. It's making sure they have avocados in the fridge for their favorite snack. Love is making time for date night even when you've been together for years and decades. Love is sending a text saying "I was just thinking about you, how's your day? Love you." It's living our lives with this person at our side at all times, even if they aren't physically present.

Being a More Excellent You

Do you know what rocks? You not expecting a mate to fix everything wrong in your life and doing that shit yourself. Because when you are a jacked-up mess, your bat signal attracts the same. Actively working on your shit is excellent advice whether you are single or already partnered.

No one says you have to be perfect. Mr. Dr. Harper loves me for my flabby belly and scrawny butt. Not because he finds them empirically sexy (but to each their own if that's your thang), but because they are attached to someone who has worked hard to build a life we are excited about. We are both people with goals we go after with full force. We take responsibility for our fuck-ups and help each other be better people. This may mean never trusting him to take the trash out in the morning no matter how much he swears he won't forget. But hey, healthy doesn't mean flawless.

I have had clients come see me after being so fucking tired of ruining relationship after relationship because they hadn't worked on their own shit. And it's so cool to see them do that work and then, at some point, tell me with enormous surprise that they met someone amazing and are building a great relationship. "I told them about my history and they stuck around." Of course they did. Because your history stopped defining you. And they know they are dating a human being who is working on their own shit.

You deserve someone great. And they deserve someone as great as you. Yes you have baggage. Your job is to carry your own rather than expect someone else to show up with a trolley.

Fuck All the Rules

All the ideas. All the guidelines. All of them. Even these ones if they don't fit. I mean, I can't see why . . . I think they're excellent. But you know what? You and your partner need to make your own map. Hell, maybe even partner isn't the right word. Maybe you are polyamorous and "partners" is the better word. You do you.

If you and your partner are delighted with the course you have charted, keep staying true. Keep the dialogue open, make corrections as needed, and love each other silly.

UNFUCK YOUR COMMUNICATION

Man. Relationships are kind of a dick move when you think about it. Our partners see the absolute worst side of us when they are the people we love best and who love us best. We are nicer to the bratty toddler running through the aisles at Target than we are to boo, who has seen us upchuck at 3 a.m., smelled our morning breath, and cleaned our pee off the toilet seat.

It's human nature to be toughest on the people we are closest to. This is why we tend to pick fights with our mate more than with anyone else.

When someone is your partner you have to constantly negotiate and navigate boundaries. And it's an ongoing process. Relationships are fluid entities that are always morphing and reshaping themselves as we live in them. But what really needs to be navigated? And when can you just let boo be boo?

If our boundaries are the essential building blocks of our relationships, then how we communicate these boundaries is critical. So many of our relationship fights could have been headed off at the pass if we had communicated proactively to begin with. I know I've been guilty of nurturing a world of butthurt that would have been easily prevented if I had just used my words. Unless you are a total specimen of perfection, you've probably done the same at some point. Changing how we engage can make all the difference in the world. And if the fight happens anyway? We got skills for that, too.

Communication Styles

Understanding how we communicate is the first step in actually communicating. Generally speaking, we aren't taught how to do so, so we have to figure that part out first.

There are three main styles:

Aggressive communication styles tend to be excessively harsh. Aggressive communicators tend to interrupt others, disregard others' opinions, and continually reinforce their own worldview and "rightness." Have you ever met anyone like this? Seen a politician on TV act like this? You know the type. You say you like pineapple on pizza and they roll their eyes and tell you that's gross, you're wrong, and you need to stop. The meta-message of aggressive communicators is "I'm cool and you're a dumbass."

Assertive communication style is our sweet spot in most cases (unless your literal safety is on the line and being situationally aggressive makes sense). Assertive communicators are firm in their belief systems and speak in a way that is congruent with their actions. But they do so in a way that still respects differing viewpoints. If you say you want pineapple on your pizza, they may respond with "Glad to see you out there living your best life. I've heard y'all pineapple pizza folx exist. Pineapple on your half of the pie it is. Get pineapple juice on my half, though, and I may hafta cut you." The meta-message of assertive communicators is "I'm cool and you're totally cool, too. Even if we don't agree."

Passive communication style tends to be ineffective in helping people protect themselves and hold their center. Passive communicators often don't make their wants and needs known, and say that things are fine when they are really, totally, deeply not fine. Passive communicators tend to defer to others, praising them while dumping on themselves. This isn't the same thing as letting someone you know and trust help guide you to better decision-making in a crisis. This is about never feeling like you can authentically advocate for what is right for you. Passive communicators, back to the pizza example I apparently cannot let go of, might say "Oh, pineapple. That would definitely be the better choice. Let's do pineapple. I can use hydrocortisone for the rash it gives me. Yeah, I'm allergic. But not really bad. It's totally okay." The meta-message of passive communicators is "I'm a hot mess, but you're totally cool, so you make the decisions for both of us."

Some questions to reflect on:

- What is your general communication style most of the time? Is that different in different circumstances or with different people?
- What messages have you internalized about your right to healthy communication and ownership of your values and beliefs?
- If you communicate differently in certain situations, or with certain people, what about those relationships causes you to change?
- How close is your current communication style to what your ideal balance would be?
- What is the first place you can start to shift your communication style, moving closer to your ideal? How will you go about doing that?

If you don't communicate as well as you would like to, owning that is really important.

As in, "Hey partner-person! I realized recently that I don't communicate things that are important to me nearly as well as I should. Then I end up butthurt because you didn't understand what I was trying to say and you end up confused AF, which is understandable. I'm working on that. So what I've been trying to say, albeit, not well, is . . . "

If you have this conversation, I'm totally awarding you a gold star for badass adulting.

The biggest thing to remember here is that it is a process. You may need to ask each other questions and keep figuring things out. You may have to clarify what you mean until it comes out right. Your partner may resist the entire conversation (which means you have an entirely different issue). This ain't easy shit.

Communicating Like a Grown Person

Learning to communicate more assertively and effectively doesn't require a weekend Tony Robbins retreat. It just means considering effective communication as a skill, learning that skill, and practicing until it becomes second nature.

Do you remember the Pythagorean theorem? You totally just recited "a squared plus b squared equals c squared" in your head, didn't you? Did you ever use that outside of school? Yeah, me neither. You know what would have been way more helpful to learn? How to communicate with "I statements."

Try this with your partner when you are all kinds of hacked off (or all kinds of thrilled, for that matter):

I feel ______ when you ______. What I want is ______.

You know what this is? Being a grown-ass person who takes responsibility for their own feelings and actions and clearly communicates their needs, rather than blaming boo ("You made me mad!") or doing the freeze-out-no-talking thing ("If you really loved me you would read my mind!").

It's gonna feel all kinds of weird and awkward at first. I've had lots of people tell me that they burst out laughing the first few times they try it. It's just so unnatural, isn't it? Because we don't encourage people to talk like this, taking accountability and responsibility for their feelings.

But we should.

Our feelings are completely our own, and we shouldn't blame others for them. We can, however, ask them for different behaviors that better respect our boundaries. This skill works in regular communication and stays in place even if your convo has leveled up to conflict level. Staying with ownership of your own feelings completely shifts away from the blame game.

You can even take an extra step in acknowledging that they didn't intend the distress you felt, for instance by adding:

I felt uncomfortable when you made that joke just now. I know you just meant it to be funny and thought I would laugh rather than be upset. But I struggle with jokes about that topic. I would really appreciate it if you didn't tell jokes like that around me.

That's awesome shit right there. And bonus points on this, because boo can't tell you how to feel if you are taking ownership of it. It's not right or wrong, it's just what you feel. Adulting FTW.

Troubleshooting Your Communication

We are all trying to communicate mo' better. Communicating with the "I statements" model is a great strategy for being more mindful of that process. But figuring out where the breakdowns come from the most often is also hugely beneficial. I first heard this model in an online course I was streaming on Neuro-Linguistic Programming. I can't find a reference to it anywhere, so I don't know the origin story (and if you do, please drop me a line). Discussing an idea without the appropriate citation and attribution upsets my little academic heart, but it's too brilliant to not share.

The basic idea is that each exchange of verbal dialogue has four levels:

1) What we mean to say. You know, the actual idea you are trying to express.
2) What we actually say. If you are really good at only saying exactly what you mean at all times, I hope you write a book on your technique. For us regular humans, what we have in our minds and what comes out of our mouths is not always a solid match.
3) What the other person hears. Just because you said it doesn't mean they heard it without any filter.
4) What the other person thinks you mean. Even if you said "anything for dinner is fine" and you meant anything for dinner is fine, your partner may think there is a hidden agenda, or other things going on beyond the words that actually came out of your mouth.

Every couple I have worked with who is struggling with a communication breakdown has a problem in at least one of these areas. Generally, we are high achievers and are activating more than one if not all of them. Figuring out where the breakdown is informs the strategies to repair it.

Let's go back to the often-contentious decision about what to have for dinner:

1) What you mean to say. Maybe growing up, you weren't allowed to voice much opinion. Maybe you tend to think your answers are wrong. Maybe you get up in your head about what you want and get paralyzed when trying to communicate. If you don't express yourself well (or aren't great at figuring out what you want), being more measured and considered before responding can make a huge difference. Dinner example? It's okay to say, "Good question, let me think a minute," then actually check in on yourself. Maybe you genuinely don't care. Or maybe you really do want pizza and should say that.

2) What you actually say. Here is where you gotta use your words. Instead of "[mumble, mumble] like, pizza? Or maybe tacos if that's what you want. Chinese food? Um, there's soup left in the fridge . . . " say the truth. Like, "I've been jonesing for deep dish all day" or "I had tacos at lunch so anything other than Mexican food sounds good." Clear communication means that partner-person doesn't have to figure out which answer is the correct one.

3) What the other person hears. We all have our own interpretations, filters, and distractions. For this example, let's say partner-person hears the "I had tacos for lunch" part of your answer but not the "anything other than Mexican food sounds good" part and suggests fajitas for dinner. Do a gentle correction. If it's a continued problem and you are discussing bigger issues than dinner plans, it might help to ask your partner to repeat back in their words what you just told them. As in "I heard you say . . . "

4) What your partner thinks you mean. So many people have had past relationships where all responses were a death trap, they were supposed to mind read and interpret everything that was told to them, and there was hell to pay if they didn't. If you have a partner who over-interprets what you say, they may benefit from a reminder that you are responsible for your responses, and they don't have to mind-read. If you say "anything for dinner is fine" and you really mean "pizza" you better fucking say pizza, or not bitch when you get tacos for two meals in a row, right?

Resolving Conflict

Even the world's best communicators still have conflict. If the goal was never to have conflict, that would be easy. You would just have to be a total doormat and give people whatever they want all the time. If you don't want to be a doormat, the goal isn't conflict avoidance, but conflict management.

When things go sideways in your relationship, consider the following questions and strategies:

Is It Intentional?

Is your partner intentionally fucking with you? Like deliberately disrespecting your time, resources, needs, and desires? Like, "I know we had dinner plans but I went out drinking instead because fuck you"?

You have every right to be mad. But also? What the actual, literal hell are you doing with this person? If they have no fucks to give about what's important to you, get out. Believe what they are showing you about who they are. Call your bestie to request sofa surfing privileges, pack up your pooch, polish your tiara, and move on.

Fighting is worthless here. Because you are being treated like you are worthless here. Don't fight with someone who has made it clear that they don't care.

Who You Really Mad at, Cupcake?

Remember learning about Freud's defense mechanisms in Psych 101? He may have snorted too much coke, but he was right on about that shit. Displacement is a defense mechanism where we attack the safe target rather than the real cause of distress. Of course you can't tell your boss that his mother was a hamster and his father smelt of elderberries. So you get home already riled up and ready to rumble. Boo tells you they forgot to pick up your dry cleaning and you find yourself spewing venom like a champ.

If you know you are ripe for a fight, like after a hard day, do what you need to do to decompress that doesn't involve sniping at partner-person. And warn them that you are wound tight. It's totally okay to say a discussion needs to be put in the parking lot for the rest of the day, just tell your partner that's on you. Something to the end of "I'm so upset I'm afraid I'll be hurtful or mean in ways that I don't really feel. And I know I won't communicate well right now. I'm gonna go soak in the tub and figure out why I'm so upset, because I don't think this is all about you. Can we talk about this later?" The big thing is actually setting a date for later—don't use that as a sidestep technique to never have difficult conversations.

Humor Rather Than Snipe

My husband is often frustrated that I suck at hanging towels up to dry. I tend to leave them sitting in the sink. I'm trying to be better at that but I had years of living alone and not sharing that bathroom with anyone. And it doesn't bother me. I'm probably gonna use that towel to mop up the floor before I throw it in the laundry, anyway. (Which also grosses him out, but that's another story.)

If I forget to hang up the towel, he will tease me into remembering rather than yell. "Who hates to hang up towels?" And I'll wave my hand in the air and say "Me! Meeee!" It's obnoxiously cute, but it is way preferable to a stupid fight over a stupid thing, right? I remember to go hang up the towel and neither one of us feels irritated in the process.

Now, someone else having this same conversation might mean it in a mean, snarky, or demeaning way. He's being silly about it, and I take it in kind. The important point is that you find a way to communicate without the sniping, and finding avenues that rely on your shared sense of humor can really help. I've been working with a couple on communicating better with "I" statements. I made a joke about how "I feel you're an asshole" is not an I statement. That cracked them up so much that, "Well, I feel that you're being an asshole" has become their in-joke that defuses tense conversations.

Beware the Horsemen

Relationship researcher John Gottman is famous for saying he can predict divorce with 90% accuracy. All his research led him to develop what he terms "The Four Horsemen of the Apocalypse." Of his four horsemen, he has found one to be more destructive than all the others. Along with criticism, defensiveness, and stonewalling, the biggest relationship destroyer is the horseman of contempt. Contemptuous language—communication that demonstrates you don't respect your partner—not only becomes a pattern of negative dialogue between the two of you, it reinforces you in thinking about and seeing the negative in your partner.

Gottman also says that the 90% accuracy rate is predicated on people not changing. If you notice that what you are feeling is not just frustration with your partner's choices, but an actual disgust with them as a human being, ask yourself if this is something that you can change with a shift in perspective. If not, you have a pretty good idea about the path you are on.

Ask for What You Need and Negotiate on Things That Are Straight Up Preferences

Communicate your needs (the areas around which you have rigid boundaries) and ask your partner about theirs. If you can't honor these needs in each other and don't think that you would ever be able to, time to abort mission. If someone's need for safety outweighs your capacity to give, that is neither your fault nor theirs. Maybe they have a trauma history that needs more work before they can regain equilibrium. It just is what it is. And like everything else about the human experience, our needs may change over time. Admit when yours change and ask for a renegotiation. Be vulnerable enough to ask for support.

And then there are wants. We all have our preferences and idiosyncrasies. Most of them aren't worth fighting about. Being our own weird, individual selves doesn't mean we are intentionally fucking with our mate, it just means we have years of behavior patterns that are really hard to change. Ever try to give up tacos for Lent? You feel me, right?

Mr. Dr. Faith and I are pains-in-the-asses in a million different ways, but battle stations are only activated when there is a cost involved beyond irritation. I have a toilet paper roll holder that hangs over the side of the toilet tank. Mr. Dr. Faith hates the thing because he has to twist around to reach the roll. He prefers to have the roll sitting on the counter next to the toilet (what kind of monster does that???). I don't like that because it gets damp there. Guess what? We have two rolls of toilet paper in the bathroom. One sitting on the counter and one hanging on the holder. Boom.

What tend to be your relational sticking points? For a lot of people, it's how money is spent. That may mean having an agreement on "allowances"—coming up with an amount that each can spend without checking in with the other based on what you can afford and your financial goals as a couple. Sex troubles? Try out some of the sensate focus exercises in this book to rebuild physical connection. Parenting teenagers? Ugh, good luck with that one.

No matter how big or small, look at the actual cost of the issue before you decide how to proceed. It's amazing how much can be let go when you do that.

Is it Netflix and chill night and you want pizza but boo wants Chinese? Just get both.

Honestly? My goal in life is to have my house be a peaceful abode. I want it to be my favorite place in the world. My spouse feels the same, so we work hard at setting up our relationship so we maintain that peace. It's a good goal for all of us.

CHEATING

People cheat. What do I mean by cheating? Anything that doesn't pass the relationship phone test. This test is simple as fuck, and I use it with clients on the regular. If your partner were to pick up your phone and open any of your apps, would they see pictures, posts, or conversations that are in violation of what your relationship rules look like? If so, it's time to do some soul searching.

The relationship phone test is also a great way of checking in on whether or not you are headed into dangerous territory, even if you have convinced yourself that it's not cheating because nothing physical has happened. Remember that each relationship is its own entity and what's okay in one relationship may be a total no-fly in another. Yes, you can be polyamorous and still cheat, if you break relationship rules when engaging with others.

Rates of infidelity vary widely, and research does demonstrate that men cheat more than women. About 40% of men and 25% of women report having violated an agreement of monogamy with a partner overall . . . and that difference is more pronounced in same-gender relationships, where only 28% of women but 82% of men report having cheated.

As irritating as it is for a feminist to admit, there are differences on a global scale between men's and women's levels of sexual desire. It's related to testosterone production. Men think about sex more, want sex more, use porn more, and masturbate more. While I haven't yet seen any research, many trans male and transmasc people have told me anecdotally that starting T revved up their sex drive substantially. If the desire for something is higher, so is the likelihood of engaging in that desire. That doesn't let us women off the hook, though. When we cheat it is more likely to be an affair with a lot of emotional depth, which is far more difficult to recover from.

You may have picked up this book specifically for this chapter. A lot of the people I see in my practice end up there because of infidelity in their relationship. And they are now trying to figure out if the relationship should and/or can be repaired.

I work with infidelity as a form of interpersonal trauma to the partner who was cheated on. (All good therapists steal from other therapists and my approach to working with infidelity was influenced by the trauma-informed work of Barry McCarthy who was in turn influenced by Snyder, Baucom, and Gordon. References in the back of the book if you're interested.) I am first and foremost a trauma informed coach, so this approach makes intuitive sense to me. But I also take a step further, and presume the event was also traumatic to the partner who cheated.

I know I may have lost some of y'all there. Yes, I realize some people are just shitty human beings who have no regard for the feelings of others and no remorse for their behavior. They are just mad as fuck for getting busted and aren't going to do any relationship repair work. If that's the case in your relationship, the hard truth is that you don't really have a relationship based on respect for your needs and values. You've been handed an ultimatum and you need to decide whether or not it's one you can live with.

For everyone else? Yes, the person who was cheated on is clearly, unequivocally injured by what happened. But so was the person who cheated. They did something that was out of alignment to commitments they made and their personal ethical code. It's a form of moral injury that also requires attention and work. When working one-on-one with individuals in affair recovery, I have more clients who cheated than who were cheated on. This includes people who were no longer with the partner they cheated on, because they wanted to figure out what had happened and they didn't want to ever do that again. If they couldn't repair that partnership, they were determined to never hurt anyone else in the same way. I can't even begin to say how impressed I am with the level of emotional maturity that takes.

The good news? Research demonstrates that most relationships do recover from an affair. The original school of therapeutic thought was that cheating doomed everything and it was time to just go into Divorce Doula mode with the unhappy couple. Nothing is further from the truth. People fuck up, but if both parties are willing to do the work, the relationship isn't necessarily irreparable. But there are definitely certain things that will greatly increase your chances of surviving, repairing, and being stronger going forward.

Deal With the Emotional Upheaval

When everything first comes out about cheating, shit is intensely volatile. It's helpful to not try to make big decisions during this time period. It's okay to grieve and focus on self-care until you both feel you can commit to communicating with each other more effectively (with or without a therapist present). This may mean taking a break from each other. It definitely means no screaming ragequits and text message fighting. I promise you I have never seen anything accomplished by anyone engaged in those types of communication. Going back to your own self-compassion work can be of great benefit for feeling what you are feeling without becoming overwhelmed in the process.

Don't Open Wounds Unnecessarily

You need to focus on what caused the affair to happen and what will prevent it from happening in the future. I have seen lots of people become very wrapped up in needing to know all kinds of details about the affair. And I get the impulse. I really, really do. The person who was cheated on wants to feel back in control of the situation and knowing all the details seems to give a sense of that and feels like it will help them decide if they want to repair the relationship or split up.

I'm not the decider, so I'm not going to stop you. But just like with getting stuck in a volatile emotional state, I've never seen anyone benefit from going through all the minutiae of the affair. It generally only serves to re-wound them over and over again. Remember that you can't unhear information that you ask for. So you need to decide if this information is truly part of your decision making process.

If you are the person who had the affair, withholding the details that are being demanded won't work out well for you in the end. The presumption will be that there are more things you are not telling them, and suspicions will increase. I would try having a conversation about why all the details are important (this is a good time to seek professional help, BTW). Should you end up sharing all the details, be prepared to discuss the emotions that are activated.

Get the Information You Need

What kind of information about the affair might be integral to your decision-making process? Some questions that bear consideration for both the cheater and the cheated-on include:

- Is there some evidence that the affair was an escape hatch activity? That is, is there any indication that the cheating partner was looking for the relationship eject button and decided this would do the trick?
- Was the affair with someone of a different gender than that of the partner who was cheated on? That is, is there a question about the cheating partner's sexual orientation that needs to be explored?
- Has the affair ended? Is there any contact with the person with whom the cheating partner had the affair? If so, how is that being managed?
- Were drugs, alcohol, or anything else that induces an altered state of consciousness involved?
- Were barrier protection methods used to minimize the risk for sexually transmitted infections?

- Was the affair an ongoing relationship or a more limited interaction?
- Was the affair sought out in a considered way or did it happen based on opportunity?
- Did the affair contain (or even solely consist of) emotional content? That is, was it just sex or was it also a relationship? Yes, emotional affairs exist. Would the relationship with the other person fail the phone test?

That isn't to say that specific answers equate with "break up" or "stay." I wish it were that easy, but it's definitely not. And I don't need to tell you how something that seems like it should be a clear cut decision is actually one of the hardest decisions you will ever make, no matter what you decide in the end. The point of these questions is to give everyone involved an idea of what you are working with, without getting stuck in the quicksand of the minutiae.

If you and your partner decide to move forward, unpacking the impetus of the affair will be instrumental in reducing the risk of affair relapse. I have found over and over that something was going on either with the person having the affair or within the relationship itself which led them to look for something to make them feel better. Usually what they want is not even sex, but attention, someone to listen to them, or someone to make them feel special and important. But when you start heading down that road, the risk is that you end up slipping and falling into a puddle of sex. And it happens over and over again. Repair is best based on strengthening the original relationship and learning to communicate through disconnection.

Genuinely Own the Cause of the Affair

This means the partner who had the affair needs to take responsibility for their actions, understand what drove these behaviors, request forgiveness genuinely from the partner they cheated on, and commit to doing the work to re-secure their bond and prevent further episodes of cheating.

And this also means the partner who was cheated on has to believe them. The apology has to be accepted and trusted as sincere, and the partner who was cheated on has to be equally committed to strengthening the relationship and reconnecting to the person who hurt them. The affair has to stop being defined as the central element of the relationship but seen as a consequence of disconnection. This means working on the relationship in the present and planning for the future. It means bringing back basics like date nights. And it means doing things to rebuild emotional and physical intimacy, which may feel awkward and difficult after everything that happened.

Without this commitment by both parties, the chances of authentic relationship repair are pretty fucking slim. I mean, you might stay together while you continue to harbor deep rage, shame, guilt, fear, and pain. But that's not relationship repair. Bravery and vulnerability require commitment and strength from everyone involved.

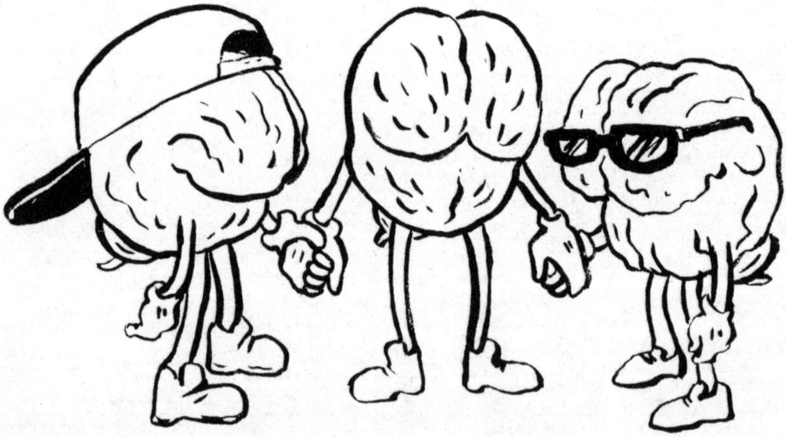

OPEN RELATIONSHIPS

Open relationships are greatly misunderstood by most people and nearly all media. There are some great books out there regarding polyamory (check out the recommended resources section for some of them). My intent here is not to reinvent the wheel, but to provide some solid science-y info about open relationships and to point out that not every book about building sexual intimacy is presuming monogamy. Which is why, you will notice, all my advice throughout this book has been polyam inclusive, too.

It's also important to present polyamory within the context of the other things we are talking about. The importance of consent and boundaries. What is and what isn't considered infidelity. Or just the simple fact that being polyam is another valid identity and way of being in the world. So if you are interested in the idea of polyamory, or just want to understand it better, here is some solid info to get you started.

Monogamy: The practice or habit of having one romantic and/or sexual relationship at a time.

Polyamory: The practice or state of being engaged in or open to the idea of having more than one romantic and/or sexual relationship at a time.

Yes, these are very general terms. That's intentional. Many people use the term polyamory to specifically mean relationships, and don't include individuals who are partnered but engage in non-relationship-based sexual exploits like orgies or swinging. However, like Dossie Easton and Janet Hardy (authors of The Ethical Slut), I use the term polyamory as an umbrella term for any relationships that are not monogamous, no matter what form they take.

Monogamy is actually pretty rare throughout the animal kingdom, especially among primates. Only 30% of primates are down for monogamy, and only 3% of mammals. Humans are a unique species in that we are wired for both monogamy and polyamory. It's a pretty much straight up 50/50 split. Half of all people prefer monogamy. So you math nerds are already with me on this: the other half dig multiple partners. This holds true of all genders. So the idea that men wanna play and women wanna stay home and raise babies with one mate doesn't hold water.

Our cultural system supports monogamy, as do most secular and spiritual moral codes. But our wiring predates all of these things. So while monogamy is what often makes our social system work, only about half of us are wired for it. And while it seems that everyone is in a monogamous relationship, research shows that only 80 to 85% of us actually are.

Hmmmm, right?

A lot of people wired for monogamy are happily monogamous. And yaaay, if you are one of them. Then there are a lot of people who are polyamorous and have slipped through the social norms and created the relationships that work for them. And things are bopping along just fine. (Lots and lots of bopping if you are doing things right!) And there are plenty of people in the middle that just aren't sure. The research does show that while 50% of us are wired for polyamory, only about 15-20% of us are practicing some form of it in our current relationship. So there are plenty of people who are maybe interested in polyamory but aren't sure they can make it work . . . and yeah, it can be difficult.

We have a lot of stigma attached to polyamorous relationships. None of the many polyamorous relationships out there have ended up ruining the fabric of society, but the idea still makes many people super uncomfortable. Different usually does. I am always surprised by the number of people who are huge advocates of marriage equality and LGBT rights but are dead set against polyamory as a viable relationship configuration. Other people's relationships are not a threat to yours or to the social structure, no matter how much it may weird you out. I promise.

If your sweetie wants to swing because he found out your neighbors do? Your sweetie was always interested in swinging. The polyam couple down the block didn't turn your sweetie any more than your gay neighbors suddenly made all the straight guys on the street drop their BBQ tongs and weed whackers, trade their Dockers for assless chaps, and develop a hankering to go to disco night at Wild Zebra.

All that being said, what if polyamory is your problem? Or interest? Or hmmmmmm moment? Or you found a pair of assless chaps in the back of your sweetie's closet? How is all that supposed to work?

CCR, Baby: Consent, Communication, and Respect

These are things that should happen in every relationship but are absolutely the keys to the successful polyamorous relationships that I have seen. And some of the healthiest relationships I have seen are polyamorous in some form or another. Yes, seriously.

What does this mean in practical terms if you are considering this? Awesome question!

Dr. Faith's Rules for Navigating Polyamory

1. Polyamory doesn't exist only in one partner's mind. It is negotiated adultery, for lack of a better term. I shouldn't have to say this part but I have had to say it and apparently continue to need to say it: If your partner doesn't know about your side activities, you are not polyamorous, you're cheating. Don't be a dick.

2. If you have a relationship fraught with all kinds of problems, and polyamory is your last-ditch effort to stay together? You won't. You will only prolong your breakup, make it messier, and create more heartache. Just break up.

3. Be open but don't be pushed. This means if you have a partner who is asking you to consider polyamory, be willing to actually consider it. But you don't have to be pushed or pressured or do anything that you absolutely don't want to do. If this is something you and your partner are exploring, look at all the different ways your relationship can be opened up and see if any are in your comfort zone. Also consider different ways you can spice up your relationship while remaining monogamous. Sometimes we need something different and we don't know what different is. Look at options before trying anything. There are plenty of meet and greet groups where you can explore without being action-oriented. Check out Meetup or FetLife scheduled events, or just do a google search for polyamory + [area you live in] to find your local folx.

4. Do what's right for you, your partner, and the relationship. The rules vary widely depending on what works for people, from "I want to meet anyone before you sleep with them" to "Don't tell me anything about them, I just know Wednesday nights are your date nights." Some people use polyamory for certain activities that their primary partner isn't into, while others prefer a fully shared third partner joining their family. What do you want it to look like? Something you do together? Something completely separate? Only people you know and trust? Only people you don't know at all? Only people who are clearly not nearly as hot as you are? (I kinda like the idea of this one, just sayin'!)

5. Negotiate the hell out of your relationship rules (scaffolding, whatever word works) and renegotiate as much as you need to. If you thought something was going to be fine and then you went bat shit crazy jealous? Own that and work through it. Don't seethe quietly in the corner while your partner is

thinking everything is okay until you go kaboom one random Sunday afternoon when your partner leaves the toilet seat up. (And yes, I know, in your defense, they do that all the fucking time and you are over it!) The authors of The Ethical Slut suggest having a plan for when jealousy hits. If you plan how to handle such feelings in a way that reconnects and strengthens the relationship, it's far less likely to reach a breaking point.

6. Depending on the level of involvement of the secondary partner(s), include them in the negotiations. I have worked with primary and secondary partners in therapy, figuring out their issues regarding an individual with whom they both had a relationship. How great is it that they brought everything to the table and worked together? Sometimes it only took one session of honest convo to get everything back on track.

7. Consider how these choices can affect other areas of your life and how you want to handle this. Whose business is it? Do you tell people? How do you discuss it if they find out? What about if you have kiddos? Have a plan for these inevitabilities so you can act rather than react.

8. Find health care providers who don't shame you for your choices. Make sure your docs know that you engage in activities that mean you need regular STI testing, for example (and, it should also go without saying, but practice safer sex, FFS!), and don't let them give you any shit about your relationships. Its generally easier to find a polyam-friendly therapist than it is a polyam-friendly MD. Those of us who specialize in intimacy will announce straight out on our Psychology Today profiles and our websites if we are polyam friendly and kink aware. Another place to look is on the site listings for Kink Aware Professionals (KAP), or you can ask around the local polyam and kink communities.

9. Don't demand that everyone have the same level of involvement and commitment. I've seen couples have healthy polyam relationships where one partner was a hardwired polyamorist and the other wasn't. They were truly okay with it, didn't have a jealous streak, had amazing communication, and wanted their partner to be happy. Some people are generally down for polyam play as a couple but not as invested in dating the way their polyam partner is. This has happened enough times that I ended up developing a new polyam label in session several years ago: sushi-polyam. It comes from the fact that one of my husband's favorite meals is sushi. He seriously digs sushi. I like sushi just fine. But it's not a hardcore favorite and so it's not on my mental rolodex of menus. If you ask me what I want for

dinner I will probably say "tacos" but if you say "sushi sound okay?" I'm likely to say "Sure!" I have zero problem saying no to things I don't want. Sushi is delicious. I just don't crave it. So if you have a sushi-polyam partner, that's OK. They don't have to be as excited about it to be perfectly content with the dynamic. And if they aren't content? They are responsible for themselves and what they agree to. If they are secretly unhappy, it's up to them to divulge that.

10. Because I am a sucker for a list of ten rules, I'm going to throw in one more: Don't let other people determine your self-worth. There are only a handful of people in this world whose opinion of me actually matters to me. The rest of the eleventy billion people on the planet don't get a vote, no matter how much they think they should. Your doctor, your therapist, and anyone else in your life do not get a vote on how you handle your intimate relationships. Only you and the individuals you are in these relationships with do. If something isn't right for you or your relationship, then don't do it. But not because Aunt Susie says so. You are allowed to seek the types of relationships that are supportive, invigorating, and fun for you, whether they be monogamous or polyamorous. Consider this a note from your doctor.

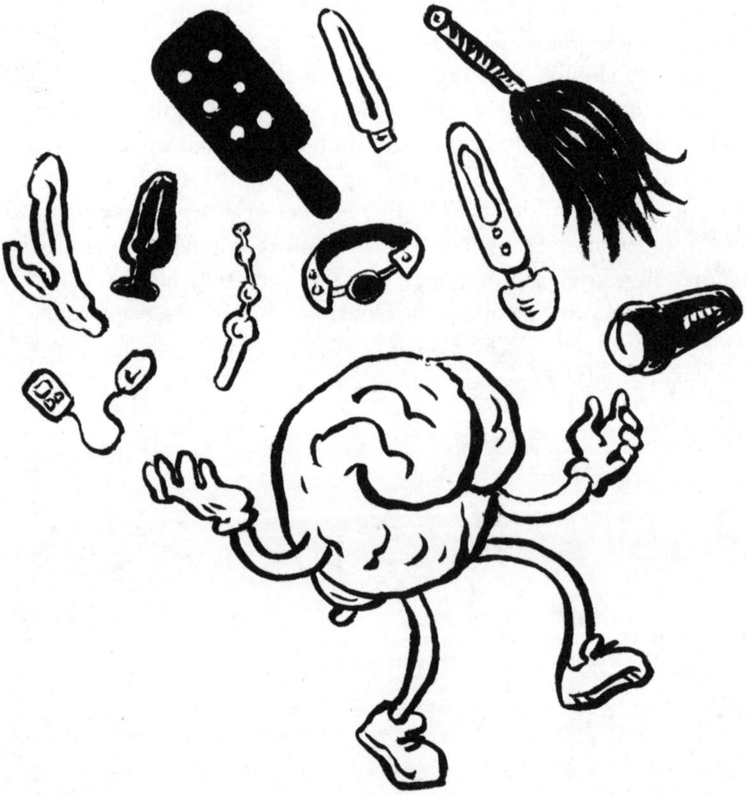

KINKS, FETS, AND BDSM (OH MYYYYYYYYY)

Maybe you want to be blindfolded or maybe you fantasize about being suspended upside down. Maybe you are intrigued by furries. Or love the idea of sex in a wading pool full of Jello. Whatever you are chatting to yourself about doesn't make you weird. There's a lot of brain science-y stuff about what makes us interested in less vanilla sexcapades. And if you fall in this category, it's all really good news. And hey, even if you don't? It's all super fascinating . . . and you may end up with a partner or a buddy that's a kinkster and you want to understand their experience better. It's more common than you'd think!

Fetishes

First, some terminology because there is always overlap and general vagueness in sexual health topics that annoys the shit out of me:

Kink is merely the overarching term used to describe sexual behaviors that are considered unconventional. Of course, unconventional is based on individual and cultural criteria of what "normal" is, so good luck defining it any further than that, right?

A fetish is something that becomes psychologically necessary for sexual gratification, either by needing to be present or imagined during sexual activity. If something exists, someone out there has a fetish for it. It could be body parts (women's feet for example), objects, or a specific behavior (like watching others have sex). Interestingly, other than the fets associated with BDSM, fetish behavior is almost exclusively something that men engage in. Which means that there is something about object fetish for stimulation that is somehow linked to testosterone. This is kinda important, because it reinforces that we have biological preferences. Meaning, because I can't say this enough in response to societal messages that state otherwise, that having a fetish doesn't mean that what you are into is a perversion, weirdness, or abuse-driven behavior.

Some fets end up getting people in serious trouble, like voyeurism. In this case, the fet itself isn't the problem, it's lack of consent. If you are watching porn about your fetish or at a venue where it's an agreed-upon activity (there are people out there who like being watched just like there are people who like to watch, after all) then it's all good. Problems happen when people try to fill their fet need but have so much shame around their interest that they end up acting out in public spaces or otherwise around people who are not consenting to the behavior they're engaging in.

Chances are, if you're into kink and fetish stuff, it's because you are a naturally hypersexual person. Research demonstrates that people of all genders who are hypersexual are the ones that are most likely to be into non-vanilla sex. Hypersexual is a bit of a loaded word, and that is such bullshit. It tends to be used to label someone as sexually dysfunctional, but unlike how it is used in the DSM (which I wrote about extensively in my book Unfuck Your Kink) really just means they have more sex than 95% of the population. And no matter what sex shamers say, liking and having lots of sex is not dysfunctional. Let's be honest "too much sex" is usually defined by people as "more sex than I have" as if that's a standard unit of measure. If you're into it? Treat. Yo. Self.

The correlation between being hypersexual and having more varied interests makes sense, right? If you are into sex and generally have a lot of sex, you are looking for ways to make it fun, interesting, and stimulating. If you only ate meals a few times a month, getting a hamburger and fries each time wouldn't be a big deal. But if you eat every day, or several times a day, you probably want some variety in your meals, right? I throw this little tidbit in here not just because I'm a research geek, but because I've had sooooo many clients find it helpful to know that their interests are a natural expansion of their sex drive.

And hopefully it's pretty obvious that it doesn't mean that the non-hypersexual people with kink and fet interests are weird and aberrant. No stats in this regard, but my clinical experience tells me that we are all wired to like what we like. And people who have kinks and fets often had interests in these things even as very young children, way before puberty. Meaning they found something intriguing and when they became sexually active adolescents and adults, sex became a natural place to express that interest.

Entire books about specific kinks and fetishes are out there, so going into great detail about all or any of them is quite impossible. But because BDSM is the most prevalent form of kink/fet sexual intimacy, and because mainstream media often portrays it so very badly, it does bear some extra consideration here.

BDSM

BDSM (also sometimes referred to as S&M) stands for Bondage / Domination / Sadism / Masochism. Depending on who you talk to, the D may stand for discipline instead of domination and the S may stand for submission instead of sadism. Either way, it's a catchall term for erotic control play, and it is nothing like the way the Fifty Shades books and movies presented it to be.

Let's go a little bit beyond the literal definition.

BDSM has what we call the "Three Cs": Consent, Control, and Communication.

Consent: BDSM is always based on consent for all parties involved. Consent fluctuates and can change and adapt over time. Consent is negotiated ahead of time and negotiated through the interaction.

Control: BDSM is about control in many different forms, not just the control of one human being by another. The dom also has to be in complete control of themself at all times in order to respect the boundaries and ensure the safety of their sub.

Communication: BDSM is seriously, seriously, seriously about communication. You have to talk about everything going on before, during, and after the experience. You may consent to something and realize later you hit a boundary you didn't know existed. Your interests may change and fluctuate over encounters or periods of time. What makes BDSM healthy is the fact that involved parties are constantly having conversations about what is going on.

There are a ton of studies out there. 10-25% of people in most studies report being turned on by aspects of BDSM, about 2-25% have actually tried BDSM in the past year (depends on how well the study defines BDSM!). The vast majority of people have said they have definitely fantasized about it. So there you go, you aren't nearly alone.

Another seriously important (and pretty cool) research point? People who are involved in BDSM tend to be more emotionally healthy than the rest of us. When studying different personality traits, BDSM practitioners reported higher levels of well-being, were more open to new experiences in general and were more extraverted, less rejection-sensitive, more conscientious, and less neurotic than the general population.

Research shows the one less desirable personality trait BDSM practitioners possess is that they are less agreeable. Which cracks me up because I take this to mean that BDSM practitioners are better at standing up for themselves and not doing things they aren't comfortable with. Yeah, not so much a negative.

BDSM is usually about sex, but not always. Sometimes BDSM is about the mindfuck rather than the act of sex. It's a turn-on, but no erogenous stimulation is taking place. You may have noticed in the initial definition of BDSM that it's about arousal and growth more than physical release.

Pain may not be involved at all, either. It's about power and control. There are many levels to this. It may be a matter of the dominant partner directing all the actions of the submissive one. It may include being tied up with scarves and tickled with a feather. It may mean spankings. It may mean hardcore needle play. YMMV. And it's your choice.

BDSM exists on a continuum. Kinda like going to the gym. Some people go every day and have serious rock hard abs. Some go a couple times a week and do a little cardio. Some people only get exercise when reaching for the box of cookies. You can do super-pervy with extra kinky sauce or a little vanilla with sprinkles.

Of course the more you play, the more careful you have to be because the more risk (emotional and physical) is involved. You stay safe by minimizing the risks and learning what you are doing before you start. And you always have an escape hatch, like a safe word. Reading and talking to others in the community is extremely beneficial for safety if you plan to go beyond anything very basic.

For example, if your interest is tying up, you don't want to knot the rope (or scarves, or whatever you are using), since a knot can easily cut off circulation and be difficult to untie in a hurry. There are resources to help you learn tying techniques that protect your sub partner. While tied up, you need to be able to maintain constant communication about your ability to maintain circulation. If you struggle to notice circulation issues in yourself (for example, you are diabetic and have neuropathy), your dom partner may ask you to push up against their hand to show that you aren't numb, and they need to have an implement available to immediately cut you free if needed.

Being a submissive in a BDSM relationship does not mean you are giving up all control. In fact, it is the polar opposite. The sub in a BDSM relationship is the one with all the power. The dom has to be in complete control of themselves in order to ensure that boundaries are not crossed, that their sub is always safe, and that they can immediately stop if the safe word is utilized. That is a lot of power and the sub has most of it. This can be a powerfully healing experience for some people with trauma backgrounds. If you are an abuse survivor, the main question to ask yourself about your BDSM relationship is: Do you feel secure and in control of the experience or not? If the answer is no or not sure, seeing a trauma-trained therapist to help you figure some of that out might make a lot of sense.

No matter what your background, each BDSM interaction should include "straight time" at the end to discuss the experience. Some people even set up contracts for their playtime, which can provide legal safety and make everyone involved feel more secure, especially if this is a new thing for you.

Don't freak out though—BDSM can be experimental and light fun. Not everything has to involve a drama llama of a contract. BDSM is like an onion. Lots of layers. Hopefully, none of them make you cry, though. Unless, of course, that's your thing.

Fantasy and Role-Play

A fantasy is a mental image, not necessarily something you act on. Role-play, on the other hand, means acting or performing a role or character that is somewhat different from your day to day life.

While BDSM can definitely have a fantasy and role-play component (and yes, you could argue that all BDSM is a form of role-play), you can also engage in fantasy and role-play without having the power differential component of BDSM.

To be honest, I hadn't really thought about role-play being its own separate entity until a number of my gender non-conforming clients talked about their use of it in sexual intimacy. If people trust me enough to talk about that stuff, I totally need to listen. And I found that, as with BDSM, the experience can be profoundly healing when approached in the right way. So let's address a few points.

Fantasy Doesn't Mean Reality

The checklist I use with clients about sexual activities has four options: yes, no, I don't know, and fantasy only. Being intrigued by an idea or turned on by it isn't the same thing as being interested in trying it out in real life.

About 75% of our sexual fantasies are about sexual activities that we have engaged in or intend to engage in. Whatever our definition of "normal" sex may be. Which means the other 25% are about things that have some level of intrigue for us but aren't something we necessarily want to try out.

When studying both heterosexual and homosexual men, Masters and Johnson Institute researchers found that both groups fantasized about having sex with a person not of their traditional orientation. That was as high on the list as BDSM fantasies, group sex fantasies, and all of the other common fantasies that people experience.

A 2015 study found that up to 62% of women in the study had experienced rape fantasies. Do 62% of women secretly harbor a desire to be raped? Maybe some losers on 4chan think so, but I seriously doubt it. The researcher looked at how often the fantasy occurred, and it wasn't often. Once a week, maybe once a month. And it wasn't tied to the idea of not having to take responsibility for a sexual encounter but was actually tied to younger generations (millennials and Zers) being experientially open and fantasy allowing them to express that without actual violation.

So much of what we fantasize about does not reflect our true interests. I've had clients tell me with great horror how they told their partners about a fantasy they had. But when their partners went to the trouble of trying to fulfill it for them, my clients were embarrassed to find that they actually had no real interest.

You may have seen articles that decry the porn industry as depicting too much violence, specifically violence towards women. Interestingly, the studies that set out to quantify violence in porn range substantially (the studies that looked to quantify the percentage of porn that contains violence show ranges of 2% to 88% percent . . . HUGE difference!). Mostly because we all define violence differently. For instance, is consensual BDSM considered violence? I wouldn't say so, but others may (she says while rolling her eyes).

Finding yourself drawn to some level of physical force doesn't make you a violent person, nor does it mean you are going to go out and act violently toward others. Brain science time: Sex and violence responses are essentially one and the same. Both activities involve stimulation of a specific part of the brain (the ventromedial hypothalamus). The only difference is in the level of the neuron activity: there is more activity during episodes of violence than during sex. So if you are an otherwise chill person who uses porn or has fantasies that involve a show of physical force, that may just be your brain amping up your neuron activity in that region for purposes of sexual excitement. You aren't automatically qualified as having a problem, okay?

Fantasy allows us to explore other ways of being in the world, expressing ourselves, and "trying things on for size." Our brains are wired for storytelling, and fantasy is just storytelling. It's how we process our perceptions and experience possibilities. If your fantasies distress you or you find yourself wanting to act on certain things that are harmful, hurtful, or illegal, that's the time to seek help. Fantasies alone are a normal human experience.

Role-Play

In my practice, I've seen a huge jump in clients who are into sexual role-play. As a Gen Xer, I definitely knew about furry parties and the like, but the internet has made it so much easier to find people with similar interests and engage in sex with them, setting up elaborate stories and settings in which we can enact certain roles that would be otherwise impossible or inappropriate. The obvious example is the dude who wants to relive his high school glory days by having his partner wear a cheerleading uniform. That's not the same as them trying to hook up with a 14-year-old cheerleader, right? Or maybe you are into firefighters but you are in a monogamous relationship with someone who isn't a firefighter. Maybe they are willing to put on the suit and come put out your metaphorical fire for you.

Role-play (within BDSM or otherwise) can also be a safe place to explore your rougher fantasies (the stuff that falls under the heading of "violent" for lack of a better term). If that's the kind of thing that gets you going, role-play can allow you to have that experience within the boundaries of safety and limits intended to protect you from unwanted harm.

I've also seen role-play be beneficial and healing for my clients who are trans or otherwise gender non-conforming. If you feel uncomfortable with your physical body presentation, role-playing as someone else allows you a new level of freedom. Many younger clients told me that non-sexual role-playing games brought their first self-awareness of their gender identity and that starting in puberty they found themselves picking characters of their authentic gender instead of birth assignment.

And it should be noted that a lot of people are just big fans of certain characters and really enjoy cosplay. Bringing that cosplay into their sexual relationships simply enhances the experience. You don't need to hate your body in order to enjoy being someone else now and then!

Things to Watch Out For

While I am totally the queen of *"you do you and let your freak flag fly,"* sexual fantasy and role-play can end up being problematic. Just like anything else fun, right? Here are some warning signs:

1) Just like with sex and porn misusage, if the fantasy and role-play take the place of real engagement with other human beings there might be a problem

2) If your fantasies do move into perseveration territory, meaning they occupy your thoughts and you feel impulses to act on things you know are wrong or find disturbing, that's another red flag

3) If your partners are violating your boundaries under the guise of the role-play, including online, it isn't real sex. It's important to set and keep boundaries (in character or out) that protect you from being hurt. (Tip from a gamer friend: Announce that you are having connection issues and log out if you don't want to have a conversation about why you're leaving.)

If you are noticing patterns of problem behavior in yourself, find a sex-positive, kink-aware professional (therapist, body worker) to work with on developing better usage strategies and coping skills.

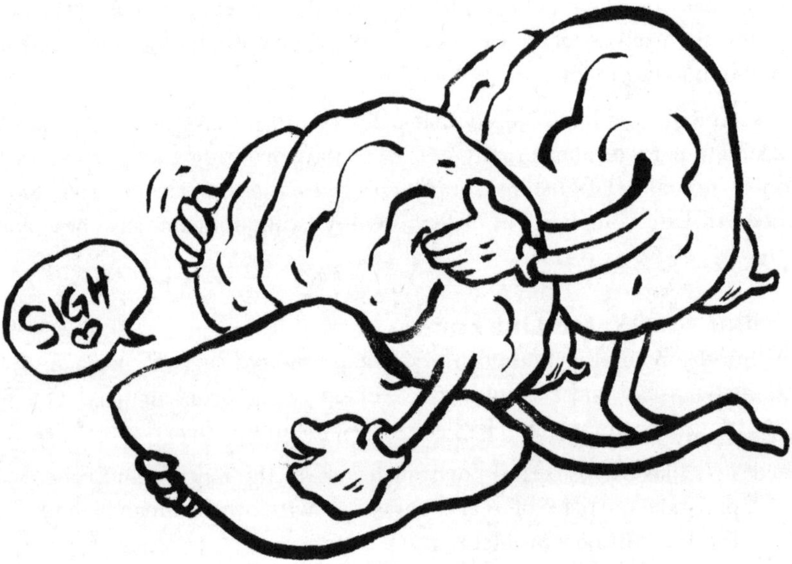
SIGH

DIFFERENTIAL DESIRES

Sometimes your partner wants something different, sexually, than you do. There doesn't seem to be any rhyme or reason to whether or not this person lets you know right away or after decades of being together. Sometimes, and usually with ungreat timing, boo drops a bombshell on you.

It could be anything from the kink, fet, and BDSM menu. It could be something utterly different like maybe they are ace, or poly, or any of the many other ways people can be in the world. Since I've been dropping some science throughout this book about all of these topics, you're with me on the fact that these are all very normal ways of being in the world.

So what do you do with that? You can part ways, totally. Consciously uncouple Gwyneth Paltrow style, sure. Or maybe there is some room for negotiation? Here are some ideas.

Negotiate Your Boundaries

Maybe your partner is the one who wants to role-play their fantasy, and you now realize that doesn't mean they have a fucked-up, psychopathic dark side but it's still something you are not OK with? Do not do a damn thing you don't want to do. This is not Fifty Shades of Grey, where someone is going to push you past your comfort zone without permission. Because even pushing you out of your comfort zone requires consent. No consent, no play.

But if it doesn't freak you out, and does lovely things for them? That's what partnership is all about, right? Boo is into diaper play? Maybe the rule will be, "Fine, I'm good with the diaper, but if you crap the thing you are on your own." Boo wants to gag you? Ok, bandana is fine, but if a ball gag shows up in the bedroom, boo gets a nut-punch. I dated a guy who was into feet. Really into feet. Feet don't do anything for me but it made him happy and I got a free pedicure out of the deal. Negotiation.

Most importantly, boundaries are not written in stone. They can be renegotiated all the time. If you both don't feel safe in having those conversations, then it really won't work. There can't be any, "Well, last week you said . . . " Consent, consent, consent. And that is as fluid as sexuality.

Consider a Pinch Hitter

Many polyamorous relationships are based on fulfilling differential desires. The thing about polyamory is, again, consent. Everyone is on the same page, everyone knows what the rules are, and everyone knows what the limits are.

Differential desires don't mean you have to dump the baby out with the bathwater. Say boo is into needle play. You are in no way into needle play. So the deal is, you go to a local club and boo gets to engage in needle play. You can go and watch. Or you can stay home and play Cards Against Humanity with your friends. Whatever. Boo is allowed to play with predetermined limits and you are needle-free. Or maybe boo is polyam and you aren't, so you go to the swingers club together to watch the action without participating. Maybe you involve porn or fantasy-talk about their polyam interests in your sex life to get them revved up without opening the relationship. Maybe Boo likes prostate stimulation and you are uncomfortable with being the stimulator so they use a toy for that while y'all are doing other sexitimes stuff together. I'm just sayin' . . . we got options here.

Figure out what you think you will be comfortable with, make a plan, and make another plan to manage any issues that may arise. The upshot is that differential desires don't have to be a deal-breaker. All relationships are a dance. Fred Astaire did just fine with a coat rack, but most of us prefer an actual partner in that dance. And if you have an excellent boo who always does the dishes when you do the cooking, there is no harm in trying to work it out.

SENSATE TOUCH

Sensate touch exercises (also called sensate focus exercises) were developed by Masters and Johnson to help couples work through intimacy issues. They are included in this book as the final chapter because they are very helpful in rebuilding partner intimacy regardless of what caused the problem to begin with. I consider sensate focus exercises another relationship skill, just like date night, effective communication, and all the other shit I yammer on about.

In Section One I talked about the levels of touch: healing, affectionate, sensual, erotic, and sexual. All forms of touch are important in our romantic partnerships and all help foster a sense of intimacy, and these exercises were designed to build on all four of these levels. One of the most important ways of doing that is not only improving our communication about touch, but also finding true enjoyment in both giving and receiving touch from our partners.

One of the biggest barriers to fostering intimate touch, both sexual and non-sexual, is the expectation of return demonstration. Instead, the giver should focus on the pleasure experienced in touching their partner, rather than focusing on what they get when it is "their turn." All relationships have a give and take, but except for the first pre-touch exercise here, time should always be set aside for the receiver to enjoy the experience without being expected to return the favor. Giving pleasure for its own sake to your partner can be its own intensely rewarding experience that fosters intimacy in and of itself.

There are many variations of these exercises out there. I designed my version to be both trauma-mindful and trauma-informed. But these exercises can be modified for any reason you need, okay?

Goals of the Exercises

- To learn how we like to be touched.
- To learn how our partners like to be touched.
- To find new ways to explore our needs and desires.
- To find new ways of receiving and giving pleasure without focusing on immediate sexual release.
- To demonstrate to ourselves and our partners a commitment to our relationships.
- To help build connection and deepen our relationships with our partners.

- To become more comfortable with our physical selves as our bodies evolve and change through childbirth, aging, and/or disability.

Establish Ground Rules

Before you begin, it's a good idea to discuss what you hope to accomplish and establish some boundaries up front:

- Determine if there are any areas that you do not want to have touched, and how you will communicate if that changes during the exercises. Consider a safe word or gesture if you are concerned that you may struggle with communicating your needs.
- Decide ahead of time if you desire to be clothed, partially clothed, or naked during the earlier stage sensate touch exercises.
- Consider how you will handle any unexpected outcomes. For example, one partner or both may become sexually aroused and want to engage in more than sensate touch. There is no rule, of course, that you cannot engage in activities other than sensate touch during your touch sessions, however neither partner should feel pressured to do so. Having a plan on how to handle those issues ahead of time will help prevent hurt feelings or unfulfilled expectations.

Afterwards, talk about your experiences and whether or not you think the goals you set at the beginning are being achieved. Discuss the positives and negatives of each encounter. Use "I" statements to demonstrate your own accountability for your thoughts and feelings.

How to Do the Exercises

Once you've talked over your goals and boundaries, pick a time and place where you will feel comfortable and won't be interrupted by other people or by the telephone, TV, or other intrusions. For the sensate focus exercises, consider doing them in the morning if a male partner is the receiver, as testosterone levels are highest in the morning. Use lighting that feels comfortable to you and music if you find that soothing. If you aren't using your bed for the initial exercises (which makes sense if that's become a source of pressure), you can still use plenty of pillows and blankets to feel comfortable wherever you are.

Use lotions, oils, or a powder for the massage exercises (make sure to use one that is face friendly for the face caress, like a moisturizing cream). Some people find lotions and oils to be slimy and prefer talc or cornstarch (which doesn't clump, is cheap AF, and is probably already in your pantry). For the exercises that include genital stimulation, you may want to use a lubricant. This can be especially helpful if a female partner has issues producing enough lubrication due to menopause or other medical conditions or if a male partner struggles to maintain a full erection. If you have not used lubricant before, read all the labels and test it out on a small area on your skin to make sure you do not have an allergic reaction. Remember not to use oil-based lubrication when using condoms or silicone-based lubricants when using silicone-based toys.

Alternate being the giver and the receiver. You can take turns during the same occasion or set separate times so the receiver can fully enjoy the experience, without having to return the favor after they are relaxed.

The person receiving the touch should state what feels good and what does not. Communicate this using "I" statements. "I like it when . . . " and "I don't like . . . " rather than "You shouldn't . . . " or "Stop that!" Positive redirection such as "I prefer . . . " always feels best to the giving partner. Positive feedback in general is always preferred, especially noises of appreciation when your partner does something you especially enjoy!

The giver should ask for feedback about areas of touch, pressure, and technique. One way to learn what the receiver likes is letting them guide your hand, especially at first. Consider using your non-dominant hand for times when a lighter touch is preferred. As you notice your partner's response to receiving certain types of stimulation, take time to focus on the sensations you feel as the giver. What does your partner's skin feel like? What does the part of your body touching them feel like as you move over their skin?

There is no time limit or limit to the number of sessions you spend on any exercise or stage. You can spend as much time as you want on each exercise before moving to the next one in order to establish comfort and trust. It is important that partners do not pressure each other to move forward until both are ready to do so. It can be very helpful to spend several weeks on a particular stage and exercise, incorporating a bit more of the body or areas of the body each time you practice.

Remember, the aim of these exercises is enjoyment, relaxation, connectedness, and pleasure. Focus on the journey rather than the end result.

Pre-Touch Shared Breathing Exercise

Sit facing each other. Maintaining eye contact, slow your breathing and focus on breathing in unison. If you don't have medical issues that disrupt your breathing patterns, try to breathe in to the count of three, hold for the count of three, and release your breath for a count of three.

Focus your thoughts on loving intent toward your partner, such as "I choose you" or "I care for you."

Continue this pattern for two minutes. Two minutes will seem like a very long time the first time you try this! You can continue these exercises over time, extending the amount of time you spend in shared breathing.

Discuss the experience with your partner. What did you notice? Did anything make you uncomfortable? Was there anything you particularly enjoyed?

The Hand Caress

Sit in a comfortable position, facing each other. Using a lotion, oil, or powder gently rub your partner's hand. Spend 5-10 minutes on each hand (10-20 minutes total). Explore each finger, the pads of their fingers, the lines of their palms. Check in with your partner about the amount of pressure you are using. Focus your thoughts on loving intent toward your partner such as "I choose you" or "I care for you."

Discuss the experience with your partner. What did you notice? Did anything make you uncomfortable? Was there anything you particularly enjoyed?

The Face Caress

Pick a position that is most comfortable for you. Many people find it works best if the giver is sitting and the receiver is lying flat on their back with their head resting on the giver's thighs. The giver should first rub a facial-friendly lubricant, like a moisturizing lotion, or powder like cornstarch on their hands. Begin with the chin, then stroke the cheeks, temples, and forehead. Check in with your partner about the amount of pressure that you are using. Explore your partner's earlobes, and the indentation just behind the earlobes on the neck. Return to massaging the temples. This exercise should take about 10-20 minutes. Focus your thoughts on loving intent toward your partner such as "I choose you" or "I care for you."

Discuss the experience with your partner. What did you notice? Did anything make you uncomfortable? Was there anything you particularly enjoyed?

Sensate Body Work

You may have noticed that the first exercises were more in the healing and possibly sensual domain. This is where we start to move into erotic and sexual!

Stage One

Limit touching and stroking to areas of the body that are not sexually stimulating. Start with areas that feel safe for your partner and incorporate more areas on future turns. Oftentimes, individuals have the first session lying on their back, being touched only on the front of their body, where they can see everything their partner is doing. If that feels comfortable, start a later session with the receiver laying on their stomach and having you work on their neck, shoulders, back, and backs of arms and legs.

You can continue to include the hands and face, but also include feet, legs, and arms. Be careful for areas that are ticklish. Continue to focus your thoughts on loving intent toward your partner such as "I choose you" or "I care for you."

Discuss the experience with your partner. What did you notice? Did anything make you uncomfortable? Was there anything you particularly enjoyed?

Stage Two

Start with the touch you used in the first stage before moving on. During the second stage, you can include genital areas in the places you touch and stroke, but the intent at this point is not sexual arousal but sensual response.

Often during stage two, individuals find it works best to start by incorporating touch of the breasts and nipples, then touching areas around the genitals. Oral touching as well as manual touching can be introduced here (or in later stages) if both partners are comfortable with it, such as light kissing, licking, or sucking.

Continue to focus your thoughts on loving intent toward your partner such as "I choose you" or "I care for you."

Discuss the experience with your partner. What did you notice? Did anything make you uncomfortable? Was there anything you particularly enjoyed?

Stage Three

Start with the touch you used in the first two stages before moving to the third. During the third stage, include touch of the genitals with intention to arouse. On a woman, stroke the clitoris and/or gently probe the vaginal opening with a finger. On men, stroke the shaft of the penis, and the head of the penis (including the frenulum, which is the spot where the head and the shaft of the penis join). On either partner, this can include stroking the anus if the receiving partner has expressed a desire for you to do so.

Continue to focus your thoughts on loving intent toward your partner such as "I choose you" or "I care for you."

Discuss the experience with your partner. What did you notice? Did anything make you uncomfortable? Was there anything you particularly enjoyed?

Stage Four

Start with the touch you used in the first three stages before moving to the fourth. And, as with the other stages, not doing this one at all is completely fine. If penetrative intercourse, however, is something you want to include in your sex life, stage four is designed to get you there.

During the fourth stage, you can attempt vaginal or anal penetration either with a finger, penis or sexual aid. The extent of penetration and what you use for penetration and where you experience penetration is entirely up to you and your partner. For example, individuals with vaginas who experience vaginismus (an involuntary contraction of the muscles around the opening of the vagina) may need to start with a q-tip or a small vaginal dilator before even a finger is a tenable option.

Continue to focus your thoughts on loving intent toward your partner such as "I choose you" or "I care for you."

Discuss the experience with your partner. What did you notice? Did anything make you uncomfortable? Was there anything you particularly enjoyed?

These are exercises you can continue using or go back to regularly as you find them helpful.

CONCLUSION

Ok, wow. That was a lot. Did you read all the way through? Are you totally exhausted? Hey, I don't blame you.

This book was intended to be full of bite-sized pieces of all the sexual and relational intimacy work I have learned and utilized over the years. It comes from the questions I've asked, and the stuck places I've seen with clients in my practice. It's not all-encompassing and it doesn't replace intensive individual or couples therapy. But hopefully, there were places where you read just the right question to help facilitate an "aha!" moment about your own life. Or you hit upon an interesting resource you had never seen before and you have a new plan of attack about something that has felt pretty overwhelming in the past.

We all deserve a healthy and fulfilling sex life. And we all get to determine what that looks like for us. Fighting for a meaningful and fulfilling life is something we do in other places, right? We vote, we floss, and we even eat broccoli instead of donuts on occasion. And this is no more frivolous work.

My hope is that this book leads to more open discussions about sexual intimacy in general. We don't have these nearly enough. If we did, I might just be out of a job and this book would fall out of print because it had become absolutely unnecessary. And I'd totally be down with that.

The topic of sexual intimacy invokes a lot of overwhelm for most people. All the blame and shame and stigma around our identities as sexual beings is hugely overwhelming. But that doesn't mean we're stuck in that place. It's not easy or intuitive work. Unfucking our intimacy issues requires practical, pragmatic strategies. If you wanted to cook a flan and didn't grow up in a flan-cooking culture you'd have to learn that shit, right? Same with a healthy sex life. That's why this book is full of practical strategies instead of romantic ideals. Because that's what unfuckening requires, right?

Let's get busy.*

*I mean, if you're consenting. And you're into that kinda thing. Of course.

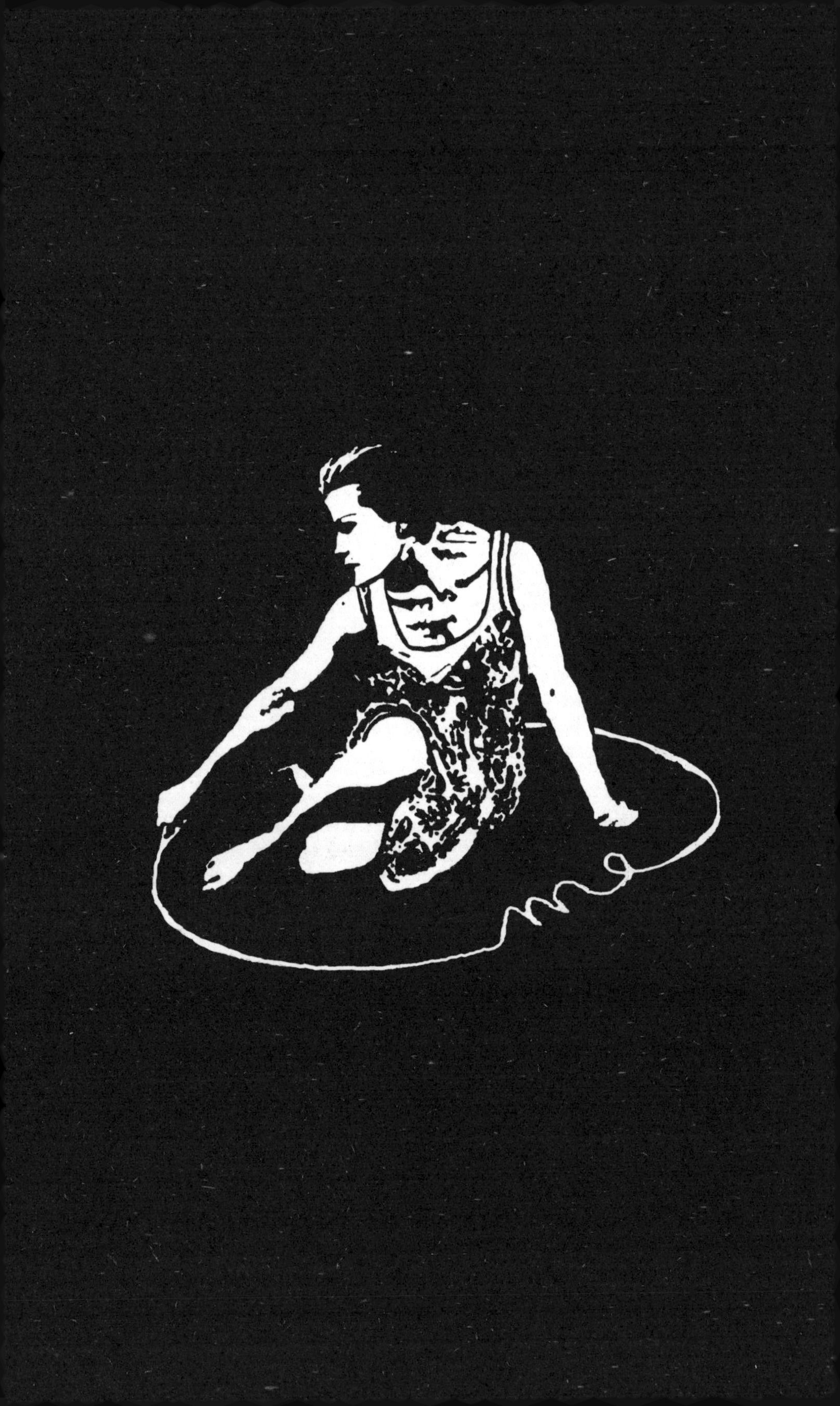
me

Unfuck Your Boundaries: Build Better Relationships through Consent, Communication, and Expressing Your Needs

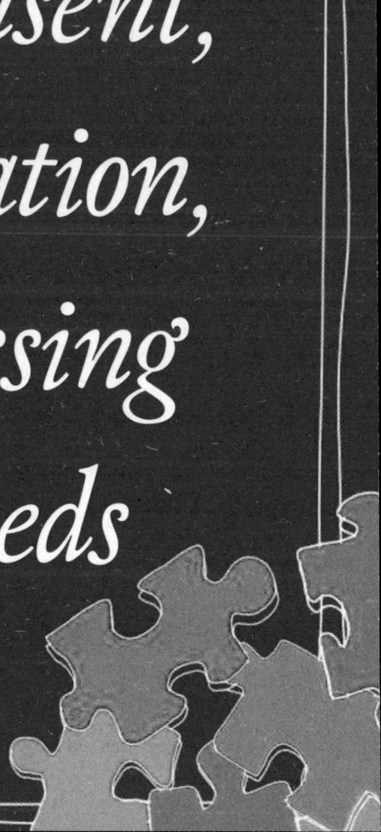

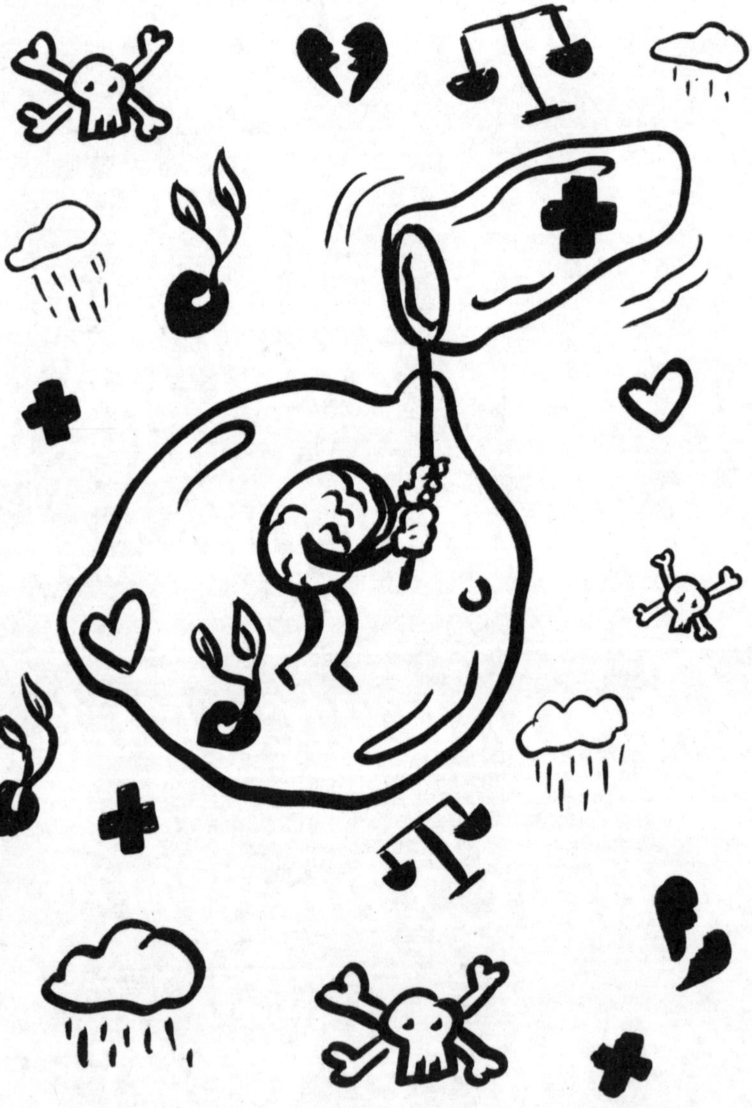

INTRODUCTION

Our boundaries are the essential building blocks of our relationships. They are how we operate in the world. They are our rules of engagement. Our everyday expressions of consent. The space in which we navigate relationships and community. Really, that's it in a nutshell.

Boundaries are the literal structure of how we live in the world. Which means that understanding them is fundamental, needful information for being a human. It should be a class in kindergarten and every grade after.

So why are conversations about boundaries devalued and diminished? Why are they made fun of? Why is the idea of standing up for our space in the world met with derision?

Healthy boundaries are as much about social justice as interpersonal effectiveness. If we don't have boundaries, we are as malleable as play-doh. And if we are malleable, we are controllable. Boundary violations may not even be overtly awful things that are happening to us. It could be the day to day chipping away at our personhood with things that are "okay."

(I mean, how many times have you said, "It's okay," but it actually wasn't good, or healthy, or wanted, and piece after piece of you disappeared?)

But what if we took it all back? What if we said, serious as a heart attack, that discussions around boundaries aren't whiny bullshit but instead are the blueprint to saving ourselves and our relationships, for moving from "okay" to healthy, good, and strong?

I wanna do that. Do you wanna do that with me? Because, fair warning, this isn't an avo toast level of book. If you have read my other stuff, you know I talk about boundaries almost as much as I talk about trauma. But I am hearing, over and over, that people want to take a deeper dive into their work around boundaries. So that's where this book came from.

This is the serious heavy lifting of conversations around topics like #metoo and #timesup. Around coercive control as a far more insidious and harmful form of abuse in relationships than violence. Around dysfunctional family systems. And people pleasing. And cultural norms that tell you to be polite.

Boundaries help us feel safer and more secure in a world that is usually anything but. They are our foundational supports for existence. Having healthy boundaries means understanding where we need space and where we need scaffolding. It means communicating those needs to the people around us.

Instead, in modern culture, boundaries are more often defined by a lack of words or actions. Not talking about things sends the message that these things aren't worth talking about. That they don't matter. That what we want, need, and desire doesn't matter. That who we are in relation to others doesn't matter. And that seeps into all our other interactions.

And it also needs to be said (I mean not to you because you get it . . . but for some of the folks in the back) that boundaries aren't a tool of manipulation. They aren't a mechanism for controlling other people and having them bow to your will. Boundaries are about claiming your own space, not claiming other people's space.

If boundaries are a relational foundation, and you realize that your foundation needs some work, putting in some support beams now may help prevent a catastrophe later. So many people are afraid that expressing their boundaries will push others away or force others to act against their own will. Generally, the opposite is true. When we do not set and maintain boundaries, we end up resentful and withdrawn from relationships and that is what leads to their eventual breakdown.

So where do we start setting positive, healthy boundaries? Boundaries are inherently unique to each person and there is no one-size-fits-all way to manage them. But we can create a framework for discussion. We can look at ourselves and start conversations that we haven't had before. And this has the power to create huge shifts not just in our lives, but within the rest of the world.

This isn't just self-changing work, it's world-changing work.

Let's get to it.

What You'll Find in This Book

Ever seen two tiny people end up having a really big kid? This book started with two small parents . . . the original boundaries zine which was really popular; and a couple of the chapters from my book Unfuck Your Intimacy, which focused on boundaries and communication in romantic relationships. So many people have asked for more on this topic, that I rewrote those sections and included them within a bigger framework around boundaries as its own thang. So now what you have in your hands is my big-assed boundaries baby, edited for duplicated material in this collected volume. And here is what this particular baby is all about:

Firstly, I am going to get up into my Professor Faith role and define boundaries, then talk about the different types and styles of boundaries and the different kinds of boundary violations. And also, because I just can't help myself, there is some info on the brain science of boundaries. It's a new field so there isn't a ton, but it's interesting (not to mention relevant as fuck to everything else we're talking about).

Then there's the hard part of the book. We are going to really look at how and why our boundaries get so fucked up to begin with. Societal messages, trauma, and attachment, ways of relating in the world. 0% fun but 100% important.

Then. Then. If you are still hanging in with me, we will use all that information to talk about all of the important work around boundary unfuckening. Learning to become more aware of our boundaries and how they are respected (or completely disrespected) by others. Plus a ton on communication. Communication is so much about boundary negotiation, isn't it? And holy shit, it's so hard to do well. So I'm gonna share all my favorite communication tools and tricks for far less than the cost of a coaching session with me.

Finally, because boundary violations at their extreme worst involve abuse to our personhood, there's a whole list of resources in the back of the book to help you find ways to either get out of or stay safe in violent relationships.

And because y'all are proactive badasses who are here to tackle shit head-on, I've sprinkled in some grounding, mindful-y type exercises throughout the book, because tackling shit head-on is fucking activating. Paying attention to the fact that this is really difficult, and taking care of yourself in the process is important. Because boundaries are a moot point if you are a puddle of emotional goo crying on the bathroom floor. And goo can't change the world, which is what we are all setting out to do.

And if workbooks help you live your best life (or if you are running boundaries workshops or similar awesome endeavors), check out the Unfuck Your Boundaries Workbook. It works just fine on its own or in conjunction with the book you currently have in hand.

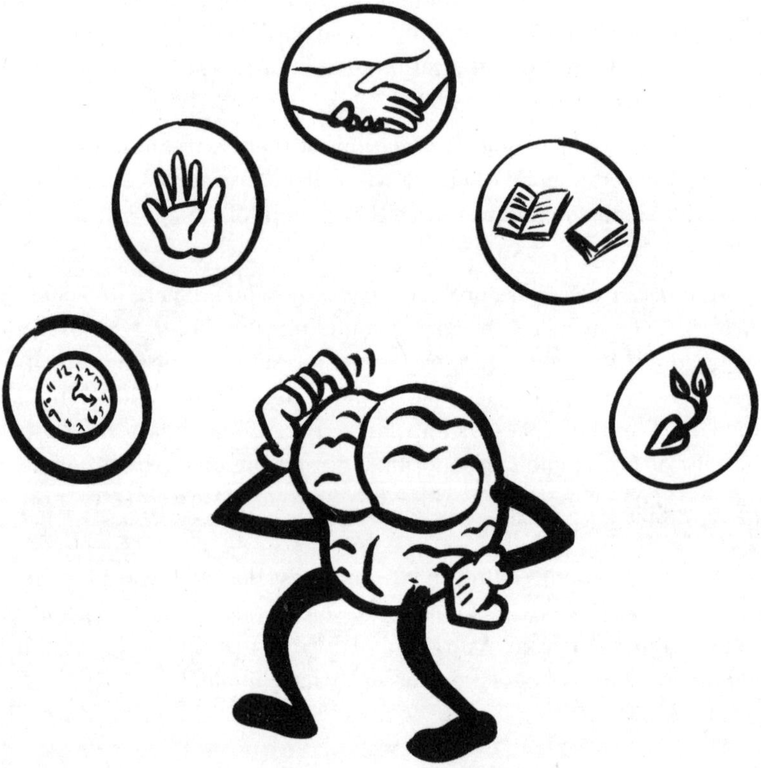

WHAT ARE BOUNDARIES?

Let's start with a pragmatic discussion about boundaries.

The term boundary really just refers to the line (literal or metaphorical) that marks the limits of a particular area. Boundaries are the edge territory of what belongs to us and what belongs to someone else.

Boundaries within any relationship, intimate or otherwise, can take many forms. They range from sexual issues ("No butt stuff, stop pressuring me!") to privacy issues ("Stay out of my journal, FFS!") to just everyday interactions ("Please don't come by my desk and chat with me today, I'm behind on that project and I'm terrible at multitasking" or "I need twenty minutes to decompress when I get home from work").

Boundaries aren't just the hard nos, they are also the maybes and the yesses-with-limits. Like, "Please knock before coming into my room," or "I'm not sure if I want to attend that event, let me see if this pain flare dissipates by Friday."

Additionally, boundaries change over time, across situations, and within different relationships. There isn't a specific trig formula you can apply in all situations that makes this easy. And any guru-type person who says otherwise is 103% full of shit. If it were all so super-simple, we wouldn't be having these conversations. I would be writing books about my cats or something. Definitely not trying to corral everything I have learned and shared about boundaries throughout my years of clinical practice into something actually usable.

Types of Boundaries

It can be helpful to think of boundaries as having seven main categories:

Physical Boundaries: These are the boundaries that deal with the pragmatics of touch (when, where, how, who, etc.)—both of others touching you and you touching others.

Property Boundaries: These are the boundaries that deal with the things we own or lay claim to. Our homes, bikes, favorite t-shirts. Of course, our primal little brains can get us into trouble in this regard, as well. People will decide that a chair in a classroom or conference room is "theirs" and no-one else should sit in it. And I have caught myself taking personal offense that someone else purchased that last ginger cookie right fucking in front of me because they totally knew I wanted it and they are trying to hurt me. Ahem. Humans definitely have territorial issues, don't we?

Sexual Boundaries: Sexual boundaries include the physical and emotional aspects of sex. They also cover information about our sexual selves: Who we like, what we like to do with the people we like, etc. They're about acceptable language, ideas, and information around sexuality. They're about terms you use surrounding sex and if jokes about sex are funny or offensive to you. Sex is such an important part of most people's lives that our boundaries around sex are way bigger than the sexual acts we engage in.

Emotional-Relational Boundaries: Emotional-relational boundaries are not just about how we want to feel and how others want to feel. They are even more about demonstrating our respect for our own personhood and the personhood of others. We respect these boundaries through how we care for others and by letting them have their own emotional experiences. But also, they are about not taking responsibility for other people's emotions (because we've all dealt with someone in a raunchy mood who tried to release that pressure valve onto us).

Intellectual Boundaries: Intellectual boundaries are about our thoughts, beliefs, and ideas and how they are respected. They are also about our access to information, ideas, and opportunities to learn. They are separate from emotional boundaries because someone can be emotionally kind (sorta) but not respect your worldview. And someone can think you are brilliant and wise, but still treat you like shit in other ways.

Spiritual Boundaries: Spiritual boundaries are about our belief systems, how we practice them, and what we choose to share around these beliefs. This is different from intellectual boundaries because spirituality is our human experience of purposeful belonging. It's a self-in-relation to something bigger than our own emotional and intellectual experiences, and that can be a point of bigger vulnerability for many people. Spiritual boundary violations could take the form of forcing someone to pray who doesn't want to, or not letting someone pray who does want to.

Time Boundaries: These are boundaries regarding one of our most precious resources: the expenditure of our minutes, hours, and days. There are plenty of things that I'm super interested in doing and that don't cross my intellectual, emotional, or other types of boundaries, but I don't have the physical time to invest in them. You totally know what I mean by that, you've been there, too, right?

There is a lot of overlap between these categories. A fairly simple boundary violation could be tied to just one category. The person who whacks your ankle with their shopping cart at the grocery store? Simple physical boundary violation. Or multiple boundaries can be pushed at once. Someone asking for your help with a project is potentially running into both your intellectual and time boundaries, right? And possibly some emotional ones, too.

And maybe that complexity of experience is what makes the whole conversation so hard. It makes figuring out our boundaries and trying to communicate about them better so complicated. Because it high-key is complicated. But hey, as the author Glennon Doyle says, "We can do hard things." And this is a worthwhile endeavor.

Questions for Consideration:

1) What are some of the boundaries that you have for each of these categories?
2) Which kinds of boundary violations do you experience the most? Which categories do those violations belong in?
3) Which kinds of boundaries do you have the most difficulty respecting for others? Which categories do those violations belong in?

How Our Boundaries are Defined

Besides having different types of boundaries, we also have the structure of the boundaries themselves to consider . . . which is more important than most people realize. Boundaries can be rigid, permeable, or flexible.

While some people have set up camp in one of these categories, most of us will operate on a continuum of these in different situations.

Rigid Boundaries are boundaries that nothing gets through, ever, and there is zero space for negotiation. Some boundaries should be rigid AF. I mean, my boundaries around not having people punch me in the face or empty my bank account are rigid because they should be. But not all boundaries need to be that hardcore. Like, you know how some people go to bed pretty early (and by some people, I mean me . . .) so they (me) don't like to be called after 9 pm? If our boundaries are super rigid in general, or super rigid around a particular issue that means we are absolutely not having any phone calls after 9 pm. Our phone is off or we don't answer it or whatever. You can't get a hold of us if it's past 8:59, which could definitely end up with some downsides for us.

Permeable Boundaries are ones that everything gets through if it wants to. These boundaries are defined for you. Attacks come from the outside, and you don't know how to hold your ground. So if I keep answering my phone when it rings late at night and having long, drawn-out conversations when I should be sleeping, my boundary around that is permeable. Meaning, I let people do whatever they want in a particular situation. Generally speaking, "permeable boundaries" is just code for "letting people walk all over you." But sometimes, some boundaries should be permeable, just like sometimes, some boundaries should be rigid. For example, in my therapy office, my life is easiest if people sit on the sofa and I sit in my comfy saucer chair. But we aren't there to make my life easier, we are there for therapy. So people can sit wherever the fuck they want (yes, including in my comfy saucer chair) and I will follow suit. I have sat on the floor with many people because that's what they needed.

Flexible Boundaries are the baby-bear middle ground that we should operate from for most of our boundary situations. Flexible boundaries are the ones that come from listening to our internal voice that wants to protect us and wants us to experience growth. That's the voice that makes continuous calibrations about our boundaries, knowing that when we are willing to compromise in certain areas it may lead to the betterment of the relationship and emotional growth for yourself. Back to the middle-aged lady who goes to bed early: I have a son who lives and works in a different time zone and is literally unable to call before 9 pm. Middle-aged lady happens to really like her son and is delighted that a busy, grown-ass man still likes to check in with his mom now and then. So if he calls and she's not conked out yet, she answers and they have a lovely chat for a few minutes. Flexible boundaries FTW.

Some boundaries should be rigid if they defend real safety and security. These are the boundaries that reflect needs rather than wants. And some rigid boundaries apply to everyone. Not attacking people with no provocation, for example.

Most are not so universal. Boundaries that are rigid for me may not be an issue at all for someone else. For instance, someone who is neurodiverse may need more alone time than other people. Someone with a trauma history may never feel comfortable with certain sexual positions. We have all had different experiences and have different needs based on them. That's part of the human condition. Our boundaries also change in different relationships, different circumstances, and different points in our lives.

I'm guessing you picked up this book because you think your boundaries are too permeable. That's the most common problem most of us face with boundaries. When message after message reinforces the notion that our boundaries have no value and are not worthy of respect, we internalize that message. And even as we mature into situations where we have more control over our surroundings, we don't know how to exercise that control. So we need to learn to firm up our boundaries, but baby bear style. Not too hard and not too soft.

Overly rigid boundaries can also be a response to past experiences, a form of overcorrection for boundaries that were too permeable in the past. For example, refusing to go on a date with anyone ever after being victimized by a romantic partner. We are the product of all our experiences, and if we had some pretty fucked up ones in the past, it entirely makes sense to overcorrect in order to protect ourselves in the present and future. Overly rigid boundaries may present us with a sense of safety in the short term because they help insulate us from situations that scare us. But that isn't the point of boundaries. Boundaries are designed to provide us safe passage through life, not as a mechanism of controlling every environment we are in and every person we interact with.

If, generally speaking, your boundaries are very strict, I'm totally not telling you to stop having boundaries. But I'm definitely saying that building ridiculous walls around yourself in the name of boundaries is going to keep you from living a full life just as much as having no boundaries at all. And honestly, being a rigid asshole is just as bad for us in the long run as letting someone stomp all over us.

With all boundaries, we need the capacity to negotiate while still maintaining our safety and not becoming a total pushover. It's that nebulous, hard-to-define difference between flexibility and permeability. For example, maybe you are starting back to school after not being in that headspace for some time. You may have to set up really rigid boundaries with others about your study time because you are feeling overwhelmed and easily distracted. But as you get into the groove of completing your coursework, you may be more open to others being in the room with you while you're studying, don't mind taking a phone call, etc. Or if you're the person who swore you'd never date again, you might be willing to go out with someone who has been vetted by a trusted friend so long as you can meet in a low-stress, easy-to-leave venue like a coffee shop.

There is a term in anthropology called liminality which refers to that uncomfortable feeling of being on the threshold between two states, like the past ways of being and how you intend the future to be different. Leaning into the discomfort of unpacking where our boundaries have been overly permeable and overly rigid allows us to cross into a different way of relating to others. Flexible boundaries mean paying attention in a proactive way instead of reacting from old patterns. And that may mean you have to make some difficult choices. Because when it comes down to it, we either let the world dictate our boundaries for us or we communicate them with what we do and say. As off-kilter as it can be at times, I would far rather experience the discomfort of difficult conversations than let the world determine what is going to happen to me.

Questions for Consideration

Here are some questions to explore your existing boundaries (whether or not you've started communicating them to others):

- What messages have you internalized about your right to healthy boundaries and the ownership of your individual needs?
- Generally speaking, are the majority of your boundaries rigid, flexible, or permeable?
- Which of your boundaries are rigid right now? Are there any that need to be challenged in that regard? Are there any that need to be more rigid?
- Which of your boundaries are permeable right now? Are there any that need to be challenged and strengthened into being flexible or even rigid? Do you have any boundaries that should remain permeable? If so, how does that permeability support, sustain, or serve you at this point in your life?
- What would your ideal boundary balance look like? How close to this ideal are you right now?
- What is something that is actively in your control that you can work on to move in the direction of your ideal?

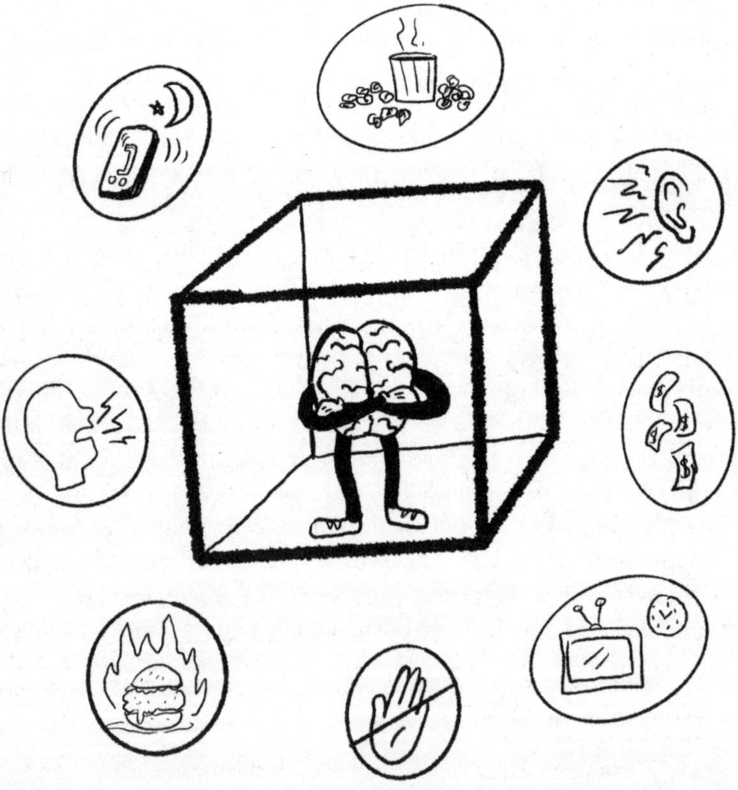

Boundary Violations (and Why Consent Is Super Important)

I've defined boundaries as the constructs that differentiate between ourselves and someone else. Boundary violations can occur when that space is not negotiated in conscious and mindful ways and our actions result in harm (regardless of our intentions).

Boundary violations are what happen when we act without consent (see Unfuck Your Intimacy for a lot more on that subject).

Pia Mellody, author of Facing Codependence, points out two main categories of boundary violations. Her categories are, simply enough, external and internal.

1) External Boundary Violations are when people do something to you in a physical way. Touching you without your permission. Taking your shit without you agreeing for them to do so. External boundary violations are tangible and measurable.

2) Internal Boundary Violations are when people violate your emotional space and try to get you to change your behavior and actions to suit their needs without requesting that change honestly. It's manipulative shit. Sometimes this takes the form of coercive control, which we get into later in the book.

What do boundary violations look like? Sara Hines Martin's book Shame on You!: Help for Adults from Alcoholic and Other Shame-Bound Families has an excellent list, which I adapted and categorized based on Pia Mellody's work. Some of these things are huge, and some are the everyday grievances we all experience, but they are all boundary violations and are important to our discussion.

I'm including a long (exhausting, depressing, and somewhat overwhelming) list of examples of boundary violations on the following pages. This list is an important part of the discussion because so many of the systemic, cultural problems that fuck up our boundaries make it so we don't often realize that boundaries are being violated right and left. That people are violating our boundaries and we are violating other people's boundaries. And yes, we stomp all over our own boundaries when we de-center our own needs in order to appease others.

I tell people on the regular "when we know better, we do better." The big cultural shifts start with recognizing these violations.

Examples of External Boundary Violations

- Sexual abuse
- Physical abuse

- Unwanted touch (including touch at times someone doesn't want to be touched, in ways they don't want to be touched, and in places the person doesn't want to be touched)
- Entering someone's living space without consent
- Cutting in front of someone in line without consent
- Not cleaning up one's own mess
- Using another person's property without consent
- Not returning or being late to return property (even if it was borrowed with consent)
- Not adhering to time agreements (being perpetually late or uncomfortably early)
- Taking control of someone else's child when their parent or guardian is present
- Moving in to live with another person without permission (IKR? But it happens)
- Smoking in front of others or in their living space without their consent

Examples of Internal Boundary Violations

- Asking personal questions outside of the depth of the relationship
- Asking others to justify their actions or viewpoints when neither impacts us
- Giving feedback about someone's behavior when it doesn't affect us
- Listening to the phone conversations of others
- Reading others' diaries, letters, emails, or private messages
- Sharing secrets or things told to us in confidence (gossiping counts here)
- Assuming the feelings of others
- Assuming the reasons for others' behavior
- Assuming others' thoughts
- Making demands instead of requests
- Expressing "advice" or "constructive criticism" when it was unsolicited and/or is offered for the sole purpose of hurting the person who is the recipient of the comments.
- Treating someone in a condescending way (talking to people as if they were a child or slow to understand)

- Judging others
- Sharing personal information about oneself without checking out if the hear-er wants to hear it
- Using abusive language
- Misgendering someone
- Using transphobic or trans-exclusionary language
- Using racist, or racially stereotyped language
- Asking for excessive or inappropriate favors
- Expecting a favor exchange (giving favors assuming favors will be given in return)
- Triangulating (trying to use a third party to control someone)

Examples of Boundary Violations That Could Be Both Internal and External

- Pushing past someone's "no" or any limits they have set
- Helping someone without first asking if they would like help
- Interrupting someone while they are talking
- Trying to force adults to live by someone else's moral and ethical standards
- Intruding at a gathering, such as joining others at a restaurant without being invited
- Continued pursuit of a relationship with someone who has indicated that they are not interested (regardless of if they had been in a relationship in the past)
- Indulging our desires at the expense or harm of another

One caution as we look at these: There's something all our brains are wired to do called the fundamental attribution error. When we mess up and violate someone else's boundaries, we attribute our actions to the situation at hand (whether this is a reasonable justification or not). When other people mess up and violate our boundaries, we attribute it to them being a fundamentally terrible person.

This is the brain's default way of thinking and until we develop an awareness of it and learn how to think through it, we end up being pretty awful to other people and expecting the worst from them. Adding a level of consideration and awareness allows us to pay attention to the details of each situation we encounter and make better decisions about whether someone is a true threat to our safety (and we will be talking more about red flags in that regard later in this book) or just a blundering human that will do better in the future if we bring our issues to their attention.

Questions for Consideration

1) Were there any boundary violations listed that you hadn't really thought of as being boundaries before?

2) Were they internal, external, or both?

3) Are there certain types of boundary violations that you have experienced more often than others historically?

4) What about in the present?

5) Are there certain types of boundary violations that you have been guilty of (even unintentionally) in the past?

6) What about in the present?

7) Are there any other boundary violations that I didn't list here that you have noticed/thought of?

Grounding Statement

I'm including grounding exercises in this book because unpacking some of our issues around boundaries can be really fucking activating. And hey, if someone recommended this book to you and you realize you are not ready, I get that. Put it aside until you are. Zero judgment . . . you know you better than anyone else does.

But if you feel that you are ready to do the work, but you know that getting through it is going to be uncomfortable and even painful, grounding exercises are designed to help with that. Grounding only means keeping yourself in the present, when facing up to the past.

Part of how the brain thinks it is keeping us safe is to tell us a story about the past, layering it onto the present so we perceive ourselves as reliving a traumatic situation. It's a great safety mechanism in actual dangerous situations . . . but it does nothing to help us deal with past issues so we can heal and move forward.

This is a simple exercise for when our brain does this. I encourage everyone to create a grounding statement that reminds them that they are in the present and doing important work. Stuff like:

1) This is only a memory. Memories suck, but they can't hurt me.

2) In the past, I was a victim. Now I am a survivor.

Come up with one that works for you, make a note of it somewhere and use the shit out of it as needed. I also suggest iced coffee as a backup option. Take care of you.

THIS IS YOUR BRAIN ON BOUNDARIES

The study of boundaries on the brain science level is part of a brand new field of science called neuroethics. *Neuroethics* refers to the overlap between social norms, philosophy, anthropology, and empirical brain science.

Imaging technology is allowing us to see that the boundaries between ourselves, others, and the environment are something that exists in the brain, not just an idea that millennials came up with to piss off boomers.

And, not at all surprising for those of you who have read my book Unfuck Your Brain, the part of the brain where these boundaries exist is the amygdala, the area of the brain that processes our emotions and regulates our fear response.

Before I get into the exact science of this, let's review what the amygdala does when it perceives a threat. To do that, we need to revisit the fight/flight/freeze response, which is our threat response system. I've talked about this in most of my previous books, but here's a refresher:

- Fight is beat their ass before your ass gets beat.
- Flight is get the fuck up out of here this isn't safe.
- Freeze is if you play possum and don't respond at all maybe all this will go away.

When this process gets out of hand and the amygdala is on a hair-trigger and freaks out all the time about things that aren't actually a threat, that's a trauma response. *Unfuck Your Brain* goes into a lot more detail about this process and how to calm it down so it just responds to actual threats again. For now, let's talk more about how our amygdala regulates our boundaries.

About ten years ago, some scientists were working with a woman with a genetic disease known as Urbach-Wiethe, which fucks up the amygdala hardcore. This patient had a serious problem with understanding personal space. So they conducted a study, comparing her comfort level with personal space (a physical boundary) against that of people who did not have this disease. People without the disease needed twice the distance between themselves and other people as the Urbach-Wiethe lady did. Her brain didn't have that switch that recognized a physical boundary and signaled, "Whoa, back the fuck up please."

The scientists said "Whoa, weird shit, here" and did more fMRI scans of the individuals in the study that did not have Urbach-Wiethe and found that the amygdala would light up when the scientists orbited into their personal space zone even if the individuals couldn't see, hear, or feel them.

Still with me? This means that the amygdala regulates distance from others even when conscious sensory cues aren't present. It's a survival instinct. So when the brain flags a boundary violation, it invokes a protective, survival-based response, tripping the switch to the sympathetic nervous system. And the sympathetic nervous system? That's the mechanism that triggers the fight/flight/freeze response.

It's not just something in a Phillip K. Dick novel anymore—we can read people's biological and mental boundaries as a physical entity, not just a philosophical idea. And this research will be hugely beneficial, not just in understanding people with weird and rare diseases, but also in understanding why boundaries are more difficult for a number of people to understand (for example, all y'all neurodivergent rock stars). Which means we can have different, and more pragmatic conversations about them while honoring that they are a very real part of our survival response.

And maybe now you are thinking, okay then, chica . . . but I'm not walking around with a portable fMRI, so how do I recognize when a boundary violation has lit up my amygdala? Especially if my past experiences in this regard have been pretty fucked up (and yes, so much more on that later in this book)? Hey, you're learning to trust yourself again and you gotta start somewhere. Let's look at some ways of doing that, ok?

Listening to Your Body

I have heard soooo many people tell me that they only realized a situation was pretty fucked up a while after it happened. I've totally done the same thing, where I responded to something in the moment based on social expectations rather than what my gut was telling me, and realized later that it wasn't okay.

Mr. Dr. Faith is a certified recovery coach working in community mental health. He's also a former private investigator who used to do the most ridiculous and dangerous jobs on the regular. So let's just say his bullshit meter is finely tuned. I asked him recently about his reads on people and how he knows someone is safe or not. He shrugged and said:

"Because the little man who lives in my stomach says so."

If you are wondering what the fuck that story has to do with boundaries the answer is "all the things." Because tuning into our bodies

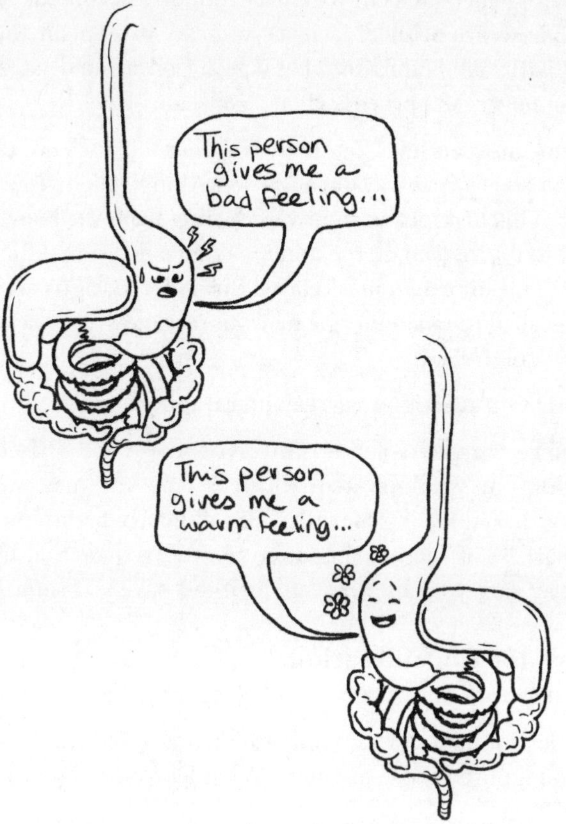

in our day to day interactions is as close as we are going to get to a 24/7 fMRI machine telling us a boundary is being violated.

Here's the thing: our subconscious is attending to far more incoming information than our conscious mind is. The study of information refers to this idea as compression theory. In a nutshell, we are taking in 11 million bits of data any given second, but can only consciously attend to about 50 of those bits in the same given second. Data compression (also called compaction) is the process of reducing the amount of information available. If we are compressing a bunch of computer files into a ZIP drive, that's lossless . . . meaning all the original data is still there. In the human brain, it is lossy (yes that's the real word), meaning that some information gets lost in the translation process.

The difference between zip drives and human brains is pretty important, right?

Physiologists were also the people to discover that we have a way of compensating for our human data compression process which lies in the body (which is why I got into hypnotherapy to begin with, it connects the entirety of the body with the working subconscious mind). It's our reflex system, which kicks in within 1/10th of a second of confronting stimulus. These are a lot of science-y terms to explain that we have a reaction with our bodies to what's going on around us, even if the information never gets processed on a conscious level.

At a subconscious level, our body is saying "oh, fuck no" to boundary violations in a very real way, through something called visceral afferent messaging. This just means an inward feeling from the body, telling the mind what to do, instead of the mind making a decision telling the body what to do. This information is relayed through the vagus nerve through something called monoaminergic neurons (and now you are super ready for bar trivia night!!).

TL;DR? Gut reactions are real, literal things.

And since the vagus nerve is involved, these body-based messages are signaling our whole system which is why you may notice things like a racing heart, feeling tearful, chills, difficulty breathing, and other physical markers of fear. Paying attention to the dude that lives in your stomach may save your life and can definitely save you some heartache.

Questions for Consideration:

1) How does your body warn you of danger? What do you notice?

2) Consider a situation where your gut instincts told you something and you ignored those instincts. What led you to ignore them?

3) Do you have experiences that may have caused faulty wiring regarding your gut instincts? An overactive danger response because of a trauma history? Or were you socially conditioned to not listen to your gut growing up? If this is the case, who are your trusted people that you can check-in with to verify if your gut instincts are on point or off-kilter?

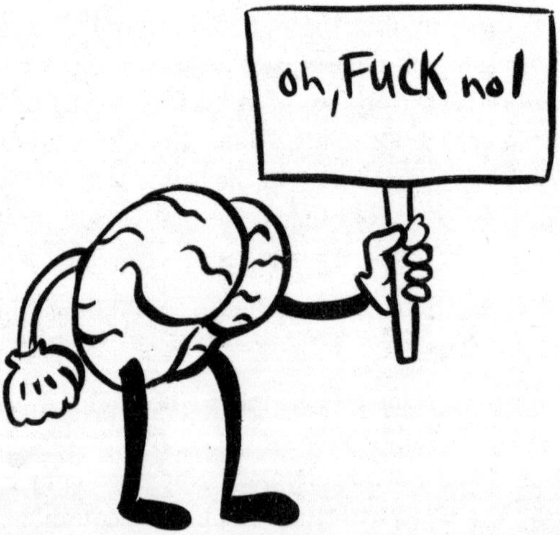

HOW OUR BOUNDARIES GET FUCKED UP

If boundaries, consent, and healthy communication were super easy, there would be zero need for this book, right? Like, if we had a culture that supported these skills and we centered teaching them from an early age I quite likely wouldn't have the job that I have.

But instead, this is really difficult, paddling-against-the-flow work. And it's desperately needed. Not just for our day-to-day interactions but for the world overall. And it would be disingenuous to discuss how to unfuck our interactions with others without first discussing how they got fucked to begin with.

There are probably eleventy-billion different reasons that boundaries get smashed to smithereens on the regular. But for the sake of not wanting to write the Encyclopedia of Boundary Fuckery, I'm sticking to four of the biggies: overall social hierarchy problems, screwed up attachment styles, high conflict personalities, and the perpetuation of coercive control. I'm focusing on these four because they are the ones that I see people struggling with day in and day out. Besides being really common, these are the issues that require examining a lot about how we live as individuals and within a society.

It's not easy. I know how hard this was to write, and I do this work on the regular. So I have a pretty good inkling about how hard it may be for a lot of people to read. And while research shows that trigger warnings are not effective at preventing individuals from experiencing trauma reactions, the least I can do is not sucker punch you with some serious shit. Because coming out the other end of this is how we change the world. And that's the real goal here.

How Society Fucks Up Our Boundaries

Originally this section focused specifically on sexual violence. The #metoo movement has opened new discussions about gender-based violence and how it has infused all aspects of our culture. And that's important as hell, but centering how cultural issues impact boundary violations solely around sexual violence does a disservice to the bigger issues at play.

(And if you are thinking "I'd kinda like to see what you wrote about sexual violence and #metoo"? All that ended up in my Unf*ck Your

Consent zine, which is more focused on navigating sexual boundaries, specifically.)

The bigger issue, according to the work of social structures scientist Riane Eisler, is that our societies are patterned around what she terms a dominator model. In cultures that are structurally maintained in this model, human hierarchies are backed up by the threat of force or actual force.

Another way to think of it is as a power-over structure (as opposed to a power-with structure). Some humans have power over others, creating a sense of ownership that is continuously reinforced. The dominator model is not just responsible for rape culture, it's responsible for slavery, mass incarceration, lack of access to healthcare by the poor, the horrific mistreatment of political refugees, and all the different ways we deny personhood to whole classes of individuals on a historical and ongoing basis.

And that's an overwhelming realization. Because the next thought is: Does that mean that all human beings are complete garbage by evolutionary design and we're all just fucked?

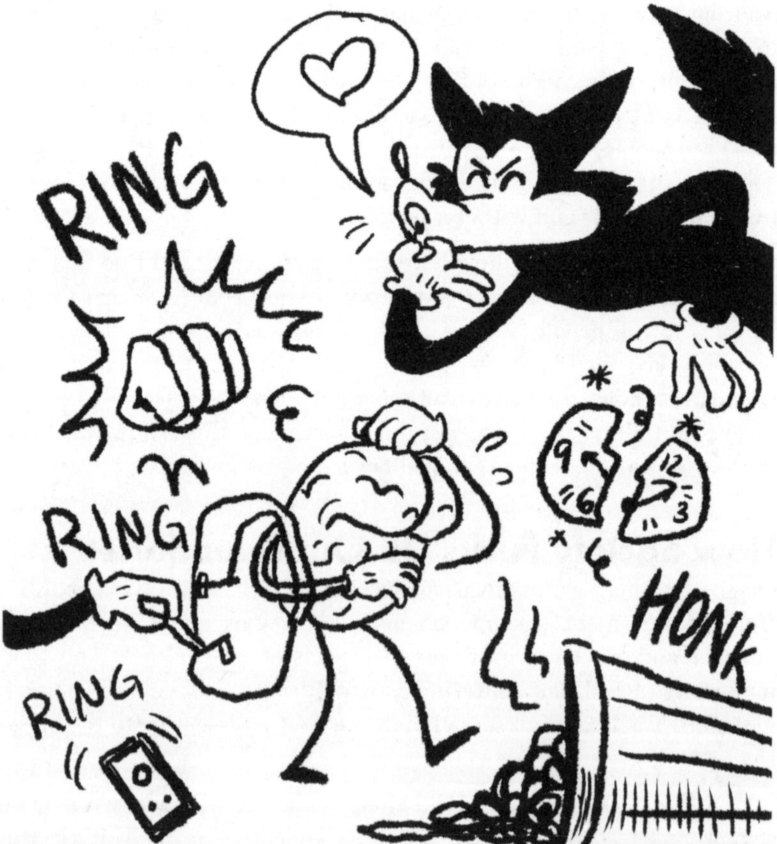

Thank the baby Buddha, no (and I don't think I could ethically do what I do every day if I thought that was true). Humans aren't total shit. Not only do we have the capacity to create more egalitarian social structures, they've always existed. Dr. Eisler calls them partnership models and points historically to the !Kung and BaMbuti, and more recently to Scandinavian nations, as evidence of our ability to develop the kind of social guidance system that redirects resources to the greater good of all people in society.

Humans have always played an active role in our own social evolution. And this evolution tends to bop along in stasis for long periods of time until we say "fuck this noise" and shake things up (Dr. Eisler would say "yeah, you mean bifurcation points but whatever"). Our history is replete with huge systemic changes in this regard. Look at how the book The Jungle by Upton Sinclair changed the rights of laborers in the meatpacking district. Or how Representative John Lewis impacted civil rights across the past decades.

You've heard the term consent culture, right? Consent culture is the normalization of asking for consent for interaction with others. For being disappointed but not butthurt when someone says no. Consent culture at its highest level-up is when we don't feel weird or embarrassed for establishing and respecting boundaries. Our current subcultural shift to consent culture means we are actively and intentionally changing our culture. And as we steer our own evolution, our laws and norms are starting to reflect these ideals.

But overall, we live in a rape culture, not a consent culture. Rape culture is a term that refers to the normalization of sexual violence. Meaning the general social attitudes and practices tolerate, excuse, condone, and even glamorize sexual violence. We have seen case after case of young men being given light sentences for sexual assault because they had "bright futures" that the judge didn't want to "ruin" (People v. Turner is one that most people remember as a particularly egregious example). Tolerating, excusing, and condoning right there.

Rape culture is the literal opposite of consent culture. If consent is how we convey boundaries then it's no wonder that rape culture has kneecapped any dialogue or standards of personal boundaries.

In consent culture, only yes means yes. Accepting this means that many people have to revisit past behaviors, to consider that maybe some past actions were actually violations, not "gray areas." Rape culture is essentially a justification culture, whereas consent culture means we, all of us, are entirely responsible for our behavior at all times. Power-with instead of power-over, right?

Violence, overall, is gendered—men are far more likely to perpetrate violence (against not just women but also other men, nonbinary individuals, and children) than any other demographic group. And sexual assault is the best-studied form of gendered violence, which is why talking about rape culture and consent culture is so powerful. But there are so many other ways that fucked up cultural power dynamics lead to a culture that tolerates systemic boundary violations.

And, yeah, I know. You didn't buy this book for a lesson in political activism and cultural paradigm shifts. You bought it for boundary help. But as Cristien Storm affirms on the very first page in her wonderful book Empowered Boundaries, "the very act of boundary setting is political whether we like it or not."

Politics is overwhelming. It's fucking awful and confusing and unending. I understand the desire to disconnect from the political nature of society, and you might be wondering why I am dragging politics into a mental health topic.

In this case, the personal is political. I mean, it always is to a certain extent, but it's hella true here. Respecting boundaries means respecting personhood. And the minute we start saying "I, too, have a personhood to be respected," we are establishing and communicating our boundaries. And by doing that, we are changing our relationships and our expectations of interactions within our surrounding community. We are evolving our concept of consent for the betterment of all humans.

All equal rights movements started with the statement of a boundary. Abolition, voting rights, desegregation, freedom to marry who you love.

When you are recognizing a boundary violation being perpetrated, the first question should be:

Do everyone's boundaries get regularly stomped on like this, or is it just certain people?

Is this a boundary that only women have to fight about? People of color? People who use wheelchairs? People who are not US citizens?

No matter how apolitical you may be in other domains, the minute you start fighting for the establishment and recognition of your boundaries and the boundaries of others, you have become a political revolutionary. Welcome to the team.

Questions for Consideration:

1) What community/social structures do you operate within that have impacted your ability to articulate your individual boundaries with the expectation of having them respected?
2) Has that changed any as you have gotten older? How so?
3) What kind of response do you anticipate when you challenge these structures?

4)How can you prepare for these anticipated challenges?

5)What's the potential payoff for doing this work?

Attachment Styles

Ok, it wouldn't be a Dr. Faith book if I didn't start talking about trauma some-damn-where, right?

Even those of us with reasonably privileged upbringings and who have a decent measure of personhood respected in the eyes of the law can really struggle with boundary setting, active consent, and clear communication. We are the product of all of our experiences, right? Not just social norms but what happened to us when we were younger and what continues to happen to us as we settle ourselves into adulthood.

Even really nice and loving parents can still struggle to teach and model healthy communication and boundary setting. And modern educational settings which operate on the need for student compliance aren't going to encourage these kinds of skills either. Many of us with otherwise happy childhoods grew up conflict avoidant or just sheerly ill-equipped to recognize, define, and articulate boundaries in our interactions with others. A lot of that has to do with our larger culture, like I talked about in the last section.

Then there are those of us who are abuse survivors, who often struggle mightily with boundaries in one extreme or another, either not holding them at all or having boundaries so rigid we become completely disconnected from those around us.

Interestingly enough, there are plenty of people who fall in a sort of weird middle space of childhood experiences that weren't totally Leave It to Beaver but also not a complete shitshow. Maybe they had parents who loved them but were wrestling with their own demons, and it affected their ability to be good parents.

Whether abusive or just kinda chaotic, these early experiences affect what therapist types call attachment styles, which basically just means the dynamics of how we navigate our interpersonal relationships. For many people, their early childhood attachment styles affect their later relationships and how they recognize and establish boundaries with friends, family, and partners.

So let's start with the three attachment styles in a nutshell:

Secure Attachment: Research shows that about 60% of us had secure attachments. (I kinda wonder about this number . . . like is it really that high? But I specialize in working with trauma so my perspective is skewed, I grant you.) Secure attachment people generally feel comfortable with others. They feel safe depending on someone and having that person depend on them. They don't freak out constantly that they are going to be abandoned or that someone is going to get too close. You know, like generally pretty healthy. Fucking weirdos. Secure attachment people tend to have healthy and flexible boundaries because they have generally found life to not be a scary place to be. They can express what they need with the expectation that that need will be honored, but also don't mind being challenged a little because they expect others to have their best interest and personal growth at heart.

Avoidant Attachment: About 20% of us have an attachment style that is termed avoidant. These are the people who have a hard time trusting or depending on others and are generally uncomfortable with the level of closeness that others want from them. Avoidant attachment people are the ones who are most likely to have pretty rigid boundaries. Their life experiences make their brains scream things like fuck all these fuckers, they aren't to be trusted.

Anxious Attachment: The final 20% of us (which you already figured out because you can math) have anxious attachment styles. They often worry that people won't love them or want to be with them or that they are going to scare their partner away. They often crave a closeness with others that they never quite get. Anxious attachment people tend to have more permeable boundaries, as they try to please others by letting themselves be walked all over on the regular.

These were the basic categories identified by researchers in the late 70s and early 80s. The attachment styles were first noticed in children and their relationships with their caregivers and were carried forth to adults to see if these attachment styles held true in adult relationships.

These categories make a lot of sense but don't really account for all the different ways these attachment styles actually show up in our day to day lives. Further research in the '90s showed that avoidant and anxious attachments are not necessarily an either/or scenario. To complete the fuckery, some people experience both. So our attachment responses can look like any of the following:

Which also explains why our boundary type may veer around all crazy sometimes between overly rigid and overly permeable depending on which of our attachment issues are being activated in any particular scenario.

Research does show that there is a moderate correlation between our childhood attachment style and our attachment style as adults. How we start out can play a big role in how we end up. We react based on our past experiences until we learn different skills. Additionally, the kinds of relationships we have as adults can either reinforce or rewire these attachment styles.

(I mean, derp, right.)

So if these attachment styles are carrying over into our adulting, they are informing how we set, enforce, and respect boundaries. If you are responding from an avoidant attachment style, you're far more likely to entrench yourself into some rigid boundaries, but if your attachment style gets into anxious territory, you may find yourself stomping all over someone else's boundaries (and/or letting them stomp all over yours) in an effort to feel closer and more connected.

Which isn't to say you're fucked forever. Notice that I said a moderate correlation? This means that being mindful of your past and recognizing how it is informing the present can help you change your responses and rewire those reaction patterns. And we are gonna do just that later in the book.

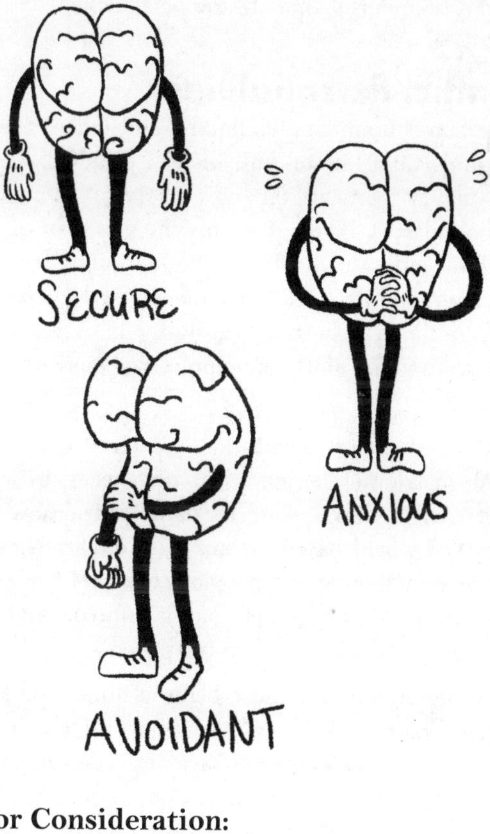

Questions for Consideration:

- How were your parents and other caretakers withdrawn or distant from you? What did they not know or understand about you? In what ways did they not support you or show up for you?
- How did that affect your view of them and the world?
- What rules about people did you develop based on these patterns?

- How were your parents and other caretakers entangled with you? How did they use you to meet their needs? What values, beliefs, and preferences did they have that they expected you to share?
- How did that affect your view of them and the world?
- What rules about people did you develop based on these patterns?
- How have these worldviews and rules affected your current relationships?
- Do you notice any correlation between your attachment patterns and having boundaries that are too rigid?
- What about boundaries that are too permeable?

High Conflict Personalities

When talking about boundary violations and where they go wonky, I would be feeding you a line of bullshit if I didn't discuss how certain types of personality traits are far more likely to lead to problems with relationship boundaries. Before I get to the worst of it, it's important to talk first about individuals who are high conflict. An individual with a high conflict personality (HCP) is someone with patterns of behavior that increase conflict rather than resolving it or reducing it in their life. It's not intentionally shitty, manipulative behavior . . . it's reactive, adaptive behavior.

I use HCP instead of terms that are clinical or diagnostic (like narcissistic or histrionic) because I'm not necessarily talking about mental illness and I don't want to pathologize how we are wired to respond to the world based on our past experiences. Getting into high-conflict mode is how many people try to feel back in control of a situation when they are feeling super out of control. And they often bust through other people's boundaries in the process.

And it's super common because being a human being isn't an easy task, is it? According to Billy Eddy, a therapist and lawyer who coined the term, about 15% of people in the US have high conflict personalities. For comparison, less than one percent of the population has been diagnosed with narcissistic personality disorder and less than two percent has histrionic personality disorder. I'd venture to guess most everyone, at some point in their life, has engaged in high conflict behavior. And some people (15% or so?) live in this space on the regular.

Oftentimes, people with more permeable boundaries have a bat-signal for high-conflict individuals because they will absorb enough crap from them that the HCP person doesn't have to examine their own shit or be held accountable for it.

The obvious question is who the fuck would want to fight with other people on the regular? Are HCPs just angry, shitty people? Not in the least, but their worldview sets them up to see conflict as a viable option for dispute resolution. If your past experiences have shown you that having your needs met is always a fight, then you are always primed to fight.

Let's look at some of the characteristics of a person with a high conflict personality, according to Eddy's High Conflict Institute:

Limited Emotional Self-Control: HCPs feel emotions very strongly and are almost entirely dominated by their negative emotions. Their responses often appear out of proportion to the event at hand. We are all hardwired to pay more attention to negative emotions because doing so is a survival instinct. We all have histories that inform our emotional responses to the world. Every one of us has had a response that seemed irrational to those around us but was absolutely our truth at the time. HCPs do so on the regular. It's not that they are wrong—they are just feeling what they are feeling, and not handling it well.

Limited Behavioral Self-Control: We are wired to react from our emotions, so if your emotions are coming in strong, your behavior is soon to follow if you don't have an awareness of what's going on. If you have limited behavioral self-control, your behaviors are very reactive and generally designed to control others so you can feel more in control.

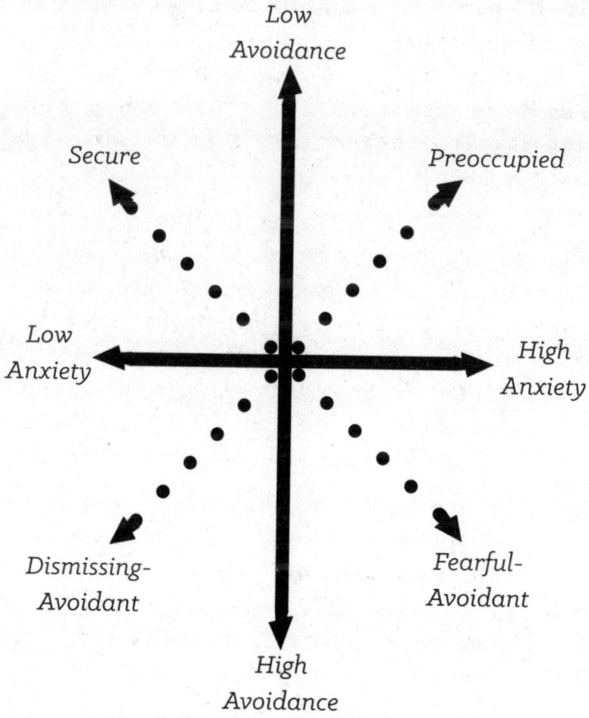

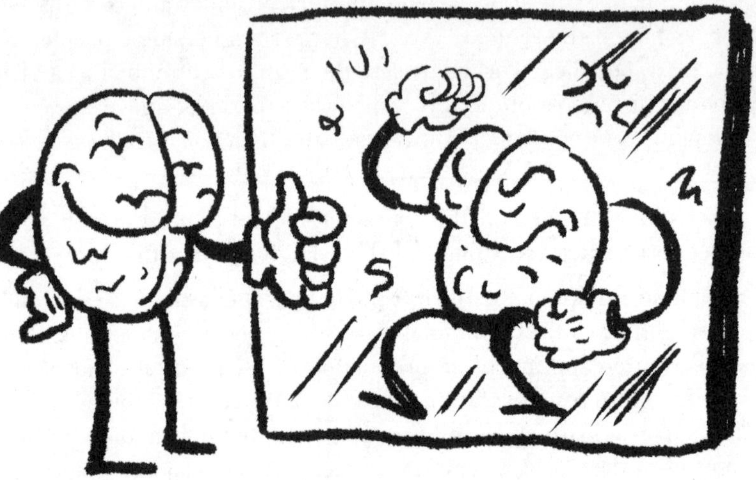

Black and White Thinking: This typical thinking error refers to the brain's default setting of labeling things as good-or-bad, right-or-wrong, yes-or-no. And if something is perceived as bad or wrong, an HCP seeks to correct that. There may be a trillion other shades of gray options that are obvious to you, but they don't see the world in that way, so are blind to them.

Externalizing: HCPs see problems as external to them. They see that they are the ones who are being hurt, and not when they are the people doing the hurting. They do not take responsibility for their part in the interaction and blame others for their problems. It's an extreme reaction to the same fundamental attribution error that's wired into all of our brains. But remember that they are black and white thinkers, so if they see problems as coming from the outside, that means whoever they perceive as the problem is the person wholly responsible for its inception and resolution.

The point of this info isn't for you to go up to people in your life and say "According to Dr. Faith, you are obviously an HCP and you should stop your shit." The point is to help you better see the worldview of someone who appears to be operating from a place of continued combativeness. And to recognize that you may fall into this mindset, as well . . . at least in certain situations. The minute we start paying attention to our own bullshit is the minute it starts to change.

A lot of the communication tricks in the next section of this book are designed specifically for containing high conflict situations. Meaning, protecting your boundaries without setting off someone in a high-conflict mindset. And TBH, these skills work well in managing all kinds of different conversations in a boss way, even if dealing with someone who doesn't constantly have their fight-face on.

The first question is: Do you even need to respond?

When someone comes at you in a high-conflict way through text, email, or social media nastiness (and sometimes even when they do so in person) sometimes the best response is simply not to. Ask yourself:

1) What are the possible consequences of responding?

2) What are the possible consequences of not responding?

If I responded to every dumb, shitty thing people say, I wouldn't have any time left to write this book on how to respond to the dumb, shitty things people say. And it's amazing how quickly a lack of response can deescalate a situation. The more you practice this the more you will realize that not responding is often the better option.

However, sometimes not responding leads to other consequences, so you have to deal with that fuckitude. For example, if a colleague insists that a problem at work was your fault, you might need to respond or you could have consequences from your supervisor. If that's your current situation, it's totally cool to skip ahead (check out the BIFF communication skill in the chapter about communicating through conflict, later on in this book).

But I have one last thing I really need to cover in this section of the book because it's far more common than we realize and needs to be talked about waywayway more than it actually is.

Coercive Control

If all the other stuff we went into about how our boundaries got fucked up wasn't enough, there is one more huge area we need to address. A form of abuse that is almost always legal and involves the strategic application of boundary violations as a means of controlling another human being.

Coercive control refers to regular patterns of boundary-violating behaviors that create fear-based compliance in someone. The term was coined by Evan Stark, whose 2007 book has the same name. His work brought to light how another person's systemic, organized boundary violations create an ongoing pattern of behavior that takes away our freedom of choice and ability to define our own personhood.

Dr. Stark's research shows that coercive control is present in up to 80% of abusive relationships. Which means only 20% of abusive relationships are defined purely by physical violence. Because it isn't something that is measured effectively (when it is measured at all), it is impossible to guess the number of relationships within the general population in which one partner abuses the other through these patterns of coercion.

Coercive control behaviors are not just a more extreme version of high conflict personality behaviors. High conflict responses are often the result of people perceiving their lives as out of control and they perceive conflict as their best means of regaining control. It is a boundary-busting behavior, and those of us who are more empathic can end up feeling attacked and manipulated by high conflict, but that's not the end goal of the person engaging in conflict.

Coercive control, by contrast, is strategic, rational, and ongoing . . . not reactive in the heat of the moment. Individuals who engage in coercive control are seeking the measurable material and social benefits they can achieve by shattering the psyche of another person in order to own them.

And because mind-games, degradation, isolation, intimidation, regulation, and an ever-changing "rule book" are not illegal actions, they are even more effective at holding another human being hostage than inflicting physical pain. It's not the physical abuse, it's the mind-fuck. It's emotional terrorism. And it's the real reason it's so hard to leave an abusive partner. And the reason that so many abuse survivors suffer from PTSD.

Once physical and sexual intimate partner violence started to become socially unacceptable in the 1970s, individuals who abused had to find other ways to maintain control over their victims . . . the uptick in coercive control in the past few decades correlates strongly with an uptick in legal consequences for perpetrating physical and sexual harm on a partner.

Dr. Stark notes that coercive control is steeped in gender-based privilege (and in case you are wondering, he is a cis/het dude), therefore the focus of his work was on cisgender, heterosexual relationships in which men used coercive control techniques against their female partners. He notes that women are more vulnerable to coercive control because of our unequal political and economic status which allows cis men to systematically take advantage of us at greater levels. Which means we are again hitting how insidiously normal rape culture is.

The numbers in this regard don't lie, but in my experience, I can absolutely attest to how coercive control extends beyond this narrow definition. Coercive control exists within all manner of intimate relationships, in LGBTQ+ communities, among family members, within friendship groups, and within employer-employee relationships.

The common denominator of unequal status still applies to the dynamic of controller and controlled. Those with less power are far more susceptible to oppressive behavior by others whom they rely on for food, shelter, financial support, and/or safety.

How do these dynamics get created? It's a systematic, conscious process. Living in a society that centers power-over dynamics allows and even encourages means of owning the bodies and spirits of others.

While most of us do not engage in that level of abusive power, there are plenty of people who do. There is a predisposition component (nature) to being a CC person, but it is far more a learned behavior (nurture). When people realize that they can perpetrate this kind of harm against another without consequence, they continue to do so.

A controlling individual sets the stage by cutting off their victim's means of support from the beginning. They seek out individuals who have vulnerabilities they can exploit. This may be people who are marginalized in significant ways (being poor, undocumented, isolated, etc.) or people who have the kind of abuse histories that have created permeable boundaries that the controlling individual can subvert almost immediately.

They set themselves up to become a rescuer in some fashion and create an indebtedness in their disempowered victim. They may rescue them financially from a bad situation. Or love bomb them with showered attention and care when they are at a low point and desperate for affection. They tether the vulnerable partner by ensuring more and more attachments to them and fewer attachments to others. At this point, resistance is worn down instead of strong-armed away.

Listed below are some of the more overt signs of being under the control of a coercive person, as well as some early-stage red flags to watch for. If you recognize yourself living these patterns, do know that there is support for getting out of an abusive situation. Even if the person has never hurt you physically, domestic violence agencies can help you strategize a plan to leave safely (or stay safely, if that is your best option currently). See the back of this book for a list of resources.

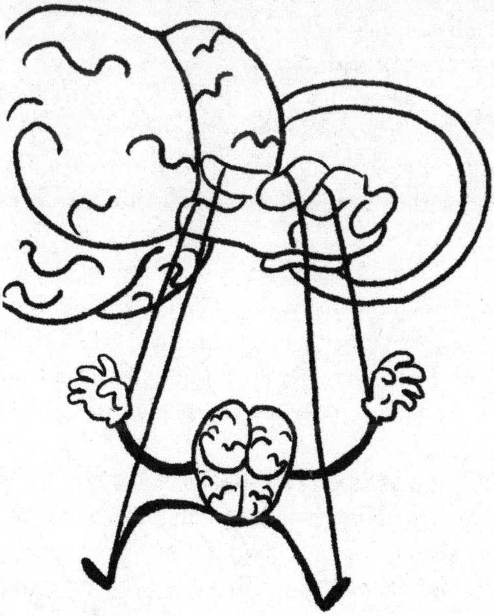

Signs of a coercively controlling person

When listed on paper, these activities seem pretty obvious, but when you are living this experience they sneak up in such a manner that we don't always see it until we step back.

The items on this list are based on the items used by researchers to measure coercive control in romantic partnerships:

- Controls/limits your contact with others (friends, family members, etc.), for instance by phone, internet, or chat
- Wants all your passwords and access to all your accounts (but you don't have access to theirs)
- Tracks your movements through your cell phone (for your "safety")
- Makes demands regarding your movements (where you go, when you go, who you go with)
- Has physically stopped you from going somewhere or leaving the house (doesn't have to be by laying hands on you—they could block your exit, hide your keys, etc.)
- Spies on you/stalks you to check in on your movements
- Checks your clothes/receipts/items in the home for signs of your activities
- Audio or video tapes you either without your consent or by threatening you into consenting
- Asks others about your activities (your children, family members, friends, neighbors)
- Makes demands about your appearance (that you look or dress a certain way for them, or maintain a certain weight)
- Controls household resources (bank accounts, vehicles, use of jointly produced income)
- Controls access to medical care
- Demands sexual intimacy in general, or specific sexual acts (either with them or with others on their demand)
- Controls use of contraceptives or STI prevention methods
- Interferes with or threatens your immigration/citizenship status
- Creates other legal trouble for you
- Threatens your housing stability (e.g., threatening to kick you out of a home they pay for, breaking rules set in a home rental to have your lease terminated and get you both evicted)
- Controls all parenting decisions and parenting tasks
- Threatens harm
- Displays physical violence towards others or property to frighten you (punching walls, hurting a family pet)
- Otherwise scares you into submission
- Threatens self-harm in retaliation for your behaviors

- Engages in self-harm in retaliation for your behaviors
- Keeps you from work/makes you late to work/disrupts your workday/gets you fired
- Destroys your property
- Destroys the property of your friends and family
- Keeps weapons and makes threats (overt or veiled) to use them against you or someone else

Red flags of a manipulative partner or early-stage coercively controlling partner

Along with the above, more overt behaviors, there are a lot of practices I see that also serve to wield power over another human being. These could be early warning sign behaviors in a new relationship that may become more intense as time goes on, or they could be occurring in longer-term relationships indicating a problem with systemic boundary violations. These behaviors are more belittling than controlling, but when done in a systematic way can invoke the process of wearing down resistance we see in coercively controlling relationships.

- Acting rude or dismissive toward your friends and family
- Does not want you doing things with friends or family without their presence
- Excuses all their behavior rather than accepting accountability
- Needs constant contact with you through the day
- Engages in behaviors outside your value system and expects you to excuse them as "no big deal" or "jokes" (such as racial comments)
- Makes "jokes" about your appearance, passions, intelligence, culture, gender, or identity
- Challenges your worldview, motives, etc. consistently (rather than asking to better understand them)
- Otherwise does not support your values and passions
- Picks fights so you feel obligated to make things up to them
- Always expects you to wait for their attention, doesn't value your time
- Never admits any fault in past relationships ending
- Expects you to be okay with their behavior when it's not okay for you to engage in same-said behavior
- Is rude to people they see as beneath them (service workers, waitstaff)
- Minimizes your feelings and dismisses how their choices and behaviors affect you in negative ways (such as accusing you of being too sensitive)
- Frames your disagreement as you not understanding or listening to them effectively
- Questions your judgment ("Oh, you're wearing that?")

- Challenges or belittles your decisions, even decisions with little consequence
- Threatens you with social embarrassment
- Disrupts the well-being of other people in your life in order to disrupt your well-being (your children, family members, loved ones)
- Makes you responsible for their happiness, stability, contentment
- Is jealous of attention you pay to others

Coercive control strategies wielded toward lesbian, gay, plurisexual, trans, and nonbinary individuals

This list of power and control tactics is created by FORGE Forward, a website with a ton of great resources for trans people. I have found that many items on the list apply to relationships in which at least one person is not heterosexual, even if they are cisgender. Their list, with my additions based on my clinical experiences and the experiences of my friends, is below:

- Disregarding, diminishing, disrespecting your identity (names, pronouns, etc.)
- Making fun of or belittling these same identity markers
- Ridiculing your appearance
- Denying your identity (that you are not a real man, woman, enby, etc.)
- Using pejorative terms to describe your identity or aspects of your identity (including terms for body parts)
- Telling you no one will love you
- Telling you you are an embarrassment to communities to which you belong (LGBT community, church community, your bowling league, etc.)
- Refusing to let you discuss issues specific to your identity
- Threatening to out you to individuals you are not yet out to
- Weaponizing others' negative feelings about you to hurt you (e.g., having a fundamentalist preacher try to "save" you)
- Weaponizing the healthcare system or judicial system against you (threatening mental health commitments, police action, etc.)
- Restricting or denying access to medical affirmative care (therapy, hormones, surgery)
- Restricting or denying access to personal affirmative items (clothing, prosthetics, etc.)
- Fetishizing your body

Is coercive control a "fixable" thing?

Most people who set out to control others don't want to change; in these cases, it's much more important to focus on the safety of the victim. But that's not the case universally. Research demonstrates that when individuals experience therapeutic support that focuses on establishing equality and appropriate boundaries in relationships, along with behavioral strategies to manage violence and systematic desire to control, they can stop treating other people this way for good.

In fact, research shows that this type of support works better than incarceration for preventing future violence. Which makes total sense: the prison system is generally designed to perpetuate power-over models and reward power-over ways of thinking. The model developed by Ellen Pence in Minnesota, the Domestic Abuse Intervention Project, has demonstrated high success rates and is now used across the country.

There are also therapists who do this work in solo practice. You can search for offender treatment providers in your area, or call your rape crisis center and ask for clinician referrals.

And yes. I have worked with individuals who saw these red flags in themselves and wanted to unpack the histories that led them to this behavior, so they could make different and better choices in the future. And I have seen them go on to have healthy relationships. We can't go back and change our pasts, but we can make a conscious decision to say this behavior stops here and now, and make significant changes.

The big indicator of success in changing abusive behavior was that the coercively controlling individual had self-awareness of what they were doing and wanted to make that change. So if you see these red flags in your own behavior and are realizing that you want to change? That level of introspection is bad-ass. If this is work that you are looking to start in your own life, the last chapter in this book, and the Unfuck Your Boundaries Workbook accountability exercises, can be a good start . . . but you will likely need support in making some serious changes in your relationships. But having healthy, fear-free relationships in the future will be well worth the effort.

The no test

Violence and abuse aren't overt in the beginning. They often start with a sense of ownership that moves into coercive control and, sometimes, external boundary violations. So even if you are in the throes of Something New (™) and things are pretty great, it's not a bad idea to see how New Person responds to boundaries.

The No Test is the brainchild of Australian domestic abuse counselor Rob Andrew, and it's amazingly simple. It is simply an evaluation of how someone responds to being told "no" for the first time.

It's far better to do this early on, and with smaller issues, before you're married and fighting over whether or not to baptize your kiddo.

Example: When Mr. Dr. Faith and I had been dating about a month, I had to attend a work holiday party. I mentioned going, and he said he would be happy to attend with me. When I responded with a "No, thank you," he understood immediately and said, "Too soon? I respect that." Well played, Woke Bae.

You are looking for signs of control in their response. Someone being disappointed at being told no is totally normal. Someone being irritated or agitated at you not going along with their plan is a sign of a controlling personality. Do they argue the point? Do they try to force a "yes" rather than negotiate around your expectations?

The No Test can be an important part of the healing process for individuals who have been victims. It's about recognizing and prioritizing your boundaries over the comfort of others. Once you truly internalize your right to say no, you are far less likely to take responsibility for someone else's response to your boundary.

Stop! Grounding time: 5 . . . 4 . . . 3 . . . 2 . . . 1

Becauuuuuse. That was more rough stuff. So here's a chance to check in with yourself, make sure you're in the present and not super-activated. This grounding skill engages the five senses, which are the ways we connect to and stay present with the world around us. Give it a whirl. Or a count. Semantics.

1. Notice and name (in your out-loud voice or inside-your-brain voice) five things you see around you.
2. Now notice and name off four things around you that you can touch. You don't have to actually touch them, but you are totally welcome to.
3. Now notice and name off three things that you hear.
4. Now notice two things you can smell. It's totally kosher to go find something like the soap in the bathroom or something.
5. Now notice one thing you can taste. You can go find something to taste if that's handy, but you can also just notice that you still taste your sandwich from lunch or your toothpaste from earlier in the morning. Whatever works.

UNFUCK YOUR BOUNDARIES

Now we are getting into the "fun" part of the book. I mean, relatively. No more discussions about the world being a dumpster fire. Just lots of information on being proactive in our day-to-day interactions. The skills in this part of the book will help us understand our own boundaries and communicate them even when it feels weird and uncomfortable to do so.

While we're at it, we'll learn how to evaluate the people around us and how we relate to them in terms of boundaries. We'll look at not just how well they respect ours, but how well we respect theirs—because we have all fucked that up at some point. And we'll talk about what to do when our boundaries are violated, and how to be accountable when we have violated the boundaries of other people.

We are creating cultural change here. Culture is everything we create, and we are engaging in the act of creation in a mindful, meaningful way. Remember when I said we are active participants in our own evolution? This is how we start.

Exploring Your Boundaries

Understanding your own boundaries is the first step.

This is where we listen to, and within, ourselves and pay attention to the answers we find. While you do this part, it's totally okay if you have stuff bubble up that surprises the shit out of you. Or if you feel completely panicked because you have zero clue as to what your answer is. That's totally okay, friend. And utterly to be expected in a culture where we don't hear "Hey, boundaries are a big thing, what's important to you?" as we grow up.

Unless you're a cat ("Touch one of my toe beans and I will end you"), you probably have had some struggles in recognizing and communicating your boundaries. We work through our boundaries issues by paying attention to our gut reactions and longer-term responses to how people interact with us.

Explore your own boundaries in a conscious and mindful way. Ask people you trust to weigh in (your awesome friends, your rock star therapist, etc.) and see how your body resonates with what they say.

You are now at the point where you have a good idea of the area you most need to work on in regards to your boundaries, whether it be stuff you are figuring out about yourself, stuff you need to work on communicating better with others (or at least certain others), etc. Here are some questions to start with. Grab a pen or paper (or your Unfuck Your Boundaries Workbook), or just give these some thought:

- What are some of your physical boundaries? Are they rigid, flexible, or permeable?
- Are there any issues you want to address regarding your physical boundaries? Anything you want to explore?
- What are some of your property boundaries? Are they rigid, flexible, or permeable?
- Are there any issues you want to address regarding your property boundaries? Anything you want to explore?
- What are some of your sexual boundaries? Are they rigid, flexible, or permeable?
- Are there any issues you want to address regarding your sexual boundaries? Anything you want to explore?
- What are some of your emotional-relational boundaries? Are they rigid, flexible, or permeable?
- Are there any issues you want to address regarding your emotional-relational boundaries? Anything you want to explore?
- What are some of your intellectual boundaries? Are they rigid, flexible, or permeable?
- Are there any issues you want to address regarding your intellectual boundaries? Anything you want to explore?
- What are some of your spiritual boundaries? Are they rigid, flexible, or permeable?
- Are there any issues you want to address regarding your spiritual boundaries? Anything you want to explore?
- What are some of your time boundaries? Are they rigid, flexible, or permeable?
- Are there any issues you want to address regarding your time boundaries? Anything you want to explore?

Now it's gut check time. Close your eyes, take a deep breath, and ask yourself the above questions again.

- When you read all those questions above, what was your emotional response? Not what you think you should have answered, not what you know the intellectual answer to be, but what your body tells you the answer actually is.
- Did anything new come up?

- Was there anything that your body reminded you about that you had initially not listed?

If you're not sure what your gut reaction is or how to interpret it, the next exercise could help . . . doesn't that work out well?

A loving-kindness boundaries meditation

Loving-kindness (also known as Metta or Maitri meditation) is about honoring our desire to be free from suffering. It's a Buddhist concept—the more secular version is self-compassion.

I've gone over both of these concepts in other books, especially Unfuck Your Brain and Unfuck Your Intimacy. But boundary work is critical to self-compassion.

Self-compassion researchers Kristen Neff and Christopher Germer suggest that in order to find a loving-kindness mantra for yourself, you ask yourself:

What do I need? What do I truly need?

This process is a wonderful tool for figuring out your boundaries and holding them mindfully. This is typically done using the phrase "May I . . ." because Buddhist teachings use "May I" as a way of pointing the heart in a positive direction. Examples may include:

May I be free from unwanted touch

May I be respected for my beliefs

May I have space to think, feel, and dream

And it's okay if you have no fucking clue what you need. It really is. Realizing that you don't know something is the first step to figuring it out. After all, you were bopping along not even realizing that there was something there you weren't attending to, right? Maybe for you, the meditation is more like:

May I learn to tune into my authentic inner voice.

May I be compassionate to myself for struggling with this process.

May I be patient with myself as I discover what is important to me.

That's a weird little trick of the mind, isn't it? The idea that noticing that doing something is hard makes actually doing it a bit easier. Getting better isn't magical and instantaneous, but if you keep at it you will see results. Pinky swear.

Dealing with backdraft

Backdraft isn't just an early '90s movie starring Kurt Russell (although he's super cute in it), it's a real term used by firefighters. It describes what happens when the oxygen a fire has been feeding on has been used up and new oxygen enters the space, causing the fire to flare up again.

Neff and Germer, the self-compassion researchers, talk about backdraft as a common part of the process of learning self-compassion. When we have shut ourselves off from our own needs for so long, paying attention to and communicating boundaries can become fresh oxygen igniting our old traumas, old attachment patterns, and old tapes about how we "should be." And then we feel like shit.

We may question our new attention to boundaries as the source of the negative feelings, rather than recognizing that the boundaries are the fresh oxygen. The old feelings are coming up so we can deal with them and release them (or, to follow the metaphor, let them die in the fire like they need to).

We may feel anxious. Or irritable. Or suddenly uncertain about things we felt pretty certain about. YMMV, so it's important to learn what backdraft feels like for you.

When discomfort arises, try the following:

1) Label it for what it is, without beating yourself up. Use the same kindness you would use if you were talking to someone you love. "Oh, ok. That's backdraft. That's really normal. In fact, that's a good sign that I'm doing difficult work."

2) Check in with yourself. Especially note your body sensations and your emotions and ask yourself "What do I need to feel safe right now so I can continue this good work instead of falling into old habits?"

3) Take any appropriate action steps toward relaying expectations about your boundary despite the discomfort you're experiencing.

4) If nothing pragmatic can be done, use a grounding skill or mindfulness skill (and what about that, I included one to try below!) to stay centered in your body until the feelings subside enough for you to feel back in control.

Measuring your breath by your footsteps

Find a place where you can walk relatively unencumbered. It doesn't have to be a straight path—walking in circles in your yard or around the parking lot of where you work is fine (and it worries people about your sanity so, bonus points, they will leave you alone).

Breathe normally. Meaning normal for you. Just however you breathe.

Cool. Walking and breathing. Got it?

Now figure out how many steps it takes for you to do an inhale and exhale cycle. There will be a rhythm to it. Everyone's a little different. Keep that shit up for a few more minutes. Walking and breathing . . . you are totally acing this whole therapeutic intervention thing like a boss. GETIT.

Okay. Now lengthen your out-breath by one extra step. Don't force it, let it ease into a longer outbreath naturally.

But you may notice a desire to lengthen your inhalation breath as well. If it feels good to do so, go ahead. Roll with this cycle for another 10 breaths.

Now lengthen the exhalation by one more footstep. Watch to see whether the inhalation also naturally lengthens by one step or not. Do the thing if your body is into it. Continue this pattern for 20 more breath cycles.

Now return to your normal breathing pattern. Are you still in the parking lot? Nobody has called for a mental health team to do a welfare check on you, have they? If you are still okay to keep walking, continue with your original (normal) breathing pattern for another 5 minutes.

If you are feeling it, move back to the lengthened breaths again, but for no more than 10 to 20 cycles before going back to your normal breathing (we don't want you getting lightheaded out there in the parking lot, after all).

Stop whenever you're ready. You're in charge of you.

How do the People in Your Life Respond to Your Boundaries?

Boundaries are fundamentally relational. And not something we can really avoid since research shows our brains are hardwired for connection. Here's a place to gain some perspective regarding your boundaries-in-relation. Because we're looking for patterns here, right?

Take another look at those lists of boundary violations in the first part of the book. Read through them again and ask these important questions:

- Which people in your life respect the boundaries that you communicate? What do these people have in common?
- Which people do not? What do these people have in common?

If, generally speaking, most people in most situations don't respect your boundaries, then it's time to look at how you are communicating them. Maybe you aren't expressing them as effectively as you thought. This part of the book will help you work on that. So yaaay . . . help is on the way!

But if you are struggling more in specific relationships or with specific people who keep blowing past your boundaries, then you might, in fact, be dealing with an asshole, or an asshole-infused situation, like a really shitty office culture. Or systemic power-over injustice at a societal level, because let's not pretend that shit doesn't happen.

Before you apply some smackdown, and especially if you're looking at a newer relationship or situation, consider a few other possibilities for why your boundaries aren't being respected:

1. This person could have other stuff going on, such as medical or emotional health issues, that make attending to what you communicate difficult for them
2. This person might be autistic, making traditional conversation cues difficult for them to suss out
3. Maybe the individual is neurodivergent in other ways (e.g., ADHD, traumatic brain injury) and has a hard time attending to relational, non-verbal signals and implicit messages
4. The person could have mental health issues that make them so internally focused that they don't have a real awareness of their impact on others
5. The person may feel so inferior to you that they don't see how their behavior impacts you
6. The person's behavioral compulsions could be so ingrained that they use violating the boundaries of others as a means of feeling more in control of the world
7. This person might be an abuse groomer digging in their heels in an attempt to get you under their emotional coercive control.

If the last scenario is the case, you know what you need to do: get out of there. Seriously, get yourself safe. If it's already escalated to violence, please get some support in making a safety plan. I'd start with the National Domestic Violence Hotline, which you can access by calling 1-800-799-7233 or logging in to chat with someone at thehotline.org.

If the other scenarios are a possibility, it's time to have a different conversation. Ask the person how they respond and learn best and try adapting your communication style.

Chances are that with scenarios 1-3, you will need to take away any need for guesswork by expressing your expectations as concretely as pavement. Ask for their attention, express yourself clearly and directly, and elicit feedback regarding their understanding. For example:

Hey, friend person, I need to chat with you about something. I recently had a "well, duh" moment when I realized that I have a boundary that I haven't communicated with you. I'm not mad at you, it's totally on me to have told you. I know you're a hugger, and you hug me whenever we hang out together. And I love that about you. But I grew up in a family where I was forced to hug everyone, whether I was comfortable with it or not. Including some people who really creeped me out. Now I feel more comfortable when people ask if they can hug me before doing so. It's a body autonomy thing that's really important to me. I know that will make sense to you and you will respect that, so I feel comfortable telling you the whole story rather than making up some bullshit story about having a cold and not wanting to hug anyone. In the future, please ask me before you hug me and understand and respect that sometimes the answer will be no, but that has to do with me, not you. Does that make sense? Do you have any questions for me?

In scenarios, 4-6 you may find that responding to them as a high conflict person is the best course of action. Check out the section below on BIFF responses, it's a great tool for high-conflict conversations.

You may be in a situation where you just have to suck it up, too. I'm well aware. You have a shitty job you can't afford to leave. Or you have a shitty family that you can't, at this time, extract yourself from. You have to weigh your options before deciding to throw down over a boundary.

This is another place where the flexibility thing comes in. You will find that tolerating others' lack of respect for your boundaries is far easier to manage when you acknowledge to yourself that you are making a choice to maintain the relationship rather than maintain the boundary. It may be the best choice for you at this moment. Remind yourself that this epic dickitude is just slightly better than the alternative, so you are choosing to accept it for right now. This perspective can really help you tolerate how upset and angry you feel. It may also propel you into creating the action plan you need to extract yourself from an increasingly shitty situation, rather than sitting in that slime pool of disrespect and disregard forever.

Questions for determining if a boundary is safely enforceable

- What kind of relationship do you have with this person (friend, family, co-worker, rando at the co-op, etc.)?
- Are y'all on the same level or does one of you have power over the other (is someone the boss, has societal privilege, a parent that pays the bills, etc.)?
- Is this relationship time-limited (are you stuck with having to deal with this mofo on the regular)?
- What would you like to tell this person if you could say everything without any consequence?
- What are the consequences if you say those things?

- Are the consequences manageable? Is there a way to make them more manageable?

Communicating Your Boundaries and Consent

Communication is how we do boundaries and consent. Changing how we engage can make all the difference in the world.

There's a linguistics theory called the Sapir-Whorf hypothesis that talks about how what we think informs how we speak (and we all get that part) and also how the way we speak starts to change how we think. Someone exposed to racist language, who starts taking on some of those linguistic tendencies, will eventually code themselves into overtly racist actions.

The brain is just a huge sponge when it comes down to it. So understanding our language patterns and making active changes in them will create better ways to negotiate the world, and better ways to recognize, uphold, and communicate boundaries.

In Unfuck Your Intimacy, there's a lot more content that's helpful for communicating about boundaries in all kinds of relationships, not just intimate ones. Head over there if you want to learn all about the different communication styles, I statements, and the four levels of communication.

Communicating what we do want instead of what we don't want

Cristien Storm's book Empowered Boundaries makes the point that while there is nothing inherently bad about a hard "no" regarding what we don't want, communicating what we do want opens up whole other avenues for dialogue and negotiation. A simple example?

Person 1: How about sushi for dinner?

Person 2, Option 1: Ugh, no.

Person 2, Option 2: I'm really in the mood for a hamburger. I'd like to go there if you are interested. Or we could grab takeout from both places and then we can both get exactly what we are feenin' for.

The second option opens up a completely different conversation and negotiation options.

But not all "what we want" communications are sushi and hamburgers. Sometimes it requires a level of vulnerability that is really hard to articulate. This means that more than just adhering to a boundary we have to authentically identify our desires and communicate them more effectively, right?

Example:

Person 1: How about I gag you and tie you up when we have sex tonight?

Person 2, Option 1: Absolutely not.

Person 2, Option 2: What I would really like to explore is prostate stimulation. How do you feel about using a toy on me designed for that?

See how the second option carries far more risk for the asker? I get into more detail regarding these kinds of interactions in my consent zine, using Betty Martin's wheel of consent, but this serves to illustrate how sometimes while a full-stop no is a perfectly acceptable answer, an expression of what you DO want can create huge shifts in understanding yourself and communicating that more effectively with the people in your life.

Question: Who would be a safe person in your life for you to experiment with on communicating your boundary about what you do want instead of what you don't want?

Communicating through conflict and disagreement

Most of the communication tools in this chapter work in power-with situations where everyone in the conversation has each other's best interests at heart. But there are tons of situations in life where there's a conflict, be it about where to get coffee or how to regulate nukes, and there isn't existing trust in the relationship or maybe you're dealing with a high conflict person, someone who is freaking out, or someone who truly doesn't care if there's a mutually beneficial resolution.

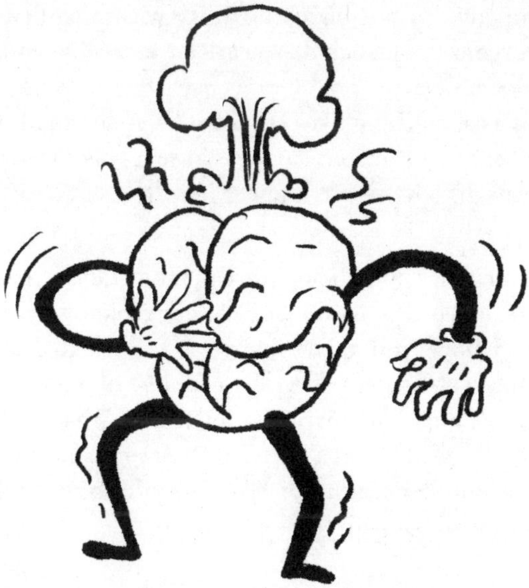

A powerful tool for these situations is the BIFF Response (Brief, Informative, Friendly, and Firm) paired with avoiding the 3 As—Advice, Admonishment, and Apologies. These are tools from Bill Eddy's High Conflict Institute and I teach them to people on the regular. They are great tools for handling conflict and also with situations that are emotionally charged in general.

If you are in the process of establishing and holding better boundaries with someone for the first time, it's going to feel emotionally charged since it's all weird and awkward and new for everyone involved. Having a bit of a recipe will help a ton. Try this one. Add extra garlic if you're feeling sassy.

Brief: Don't give any extra info. Don't over-explain. The more you write or say, the more fodder you are giving the aggrieved party for their battle, yeah? Let's say you got an angry missive from your boss, accusing you of jacking the keys to the dumpster. Instead of writing an eight-paragraph defense, try a brief, factual response: "I clocked out two hours before closing last Thursday, so I didn't carry out the garbage that day and I never used the keys."

Informative: Don't focus on their incorrect statements, focus on your accurate ones. No sarcasm, no negging, no remarks about the other person's personality, ethical choices, etc. We are looking to end the conflict, not throw down about who the real dumbass in this scenario is. In the same work example, you might add the information, "In order to refresh my memory, I double checked the calendar. I wasn't the person who closed that day, it was Xander."

Friendly: I know, it doesn't seem fair that you have to be nice when someone else is showing their ass. The best way of coming out of the conflict unscathed is to not match hostility with hostility. This doesn't mean fake nicey-nice . . . just civil. You are far more likely to get a neutral response, if not a positive one. Going back to the work example, you could phrase it as something like "Hi, Sarah! Xander and I did both work last Thursday, but I clocked out early because it was so slow and Xander closed by themself, so I don't know where the keys to the dumpster ended up."

Firm: Be firm without being threatening. Don't make comments that can invite more discussion (e.g., "Let me know if you have any questions" or "I hope you agree that . . . "). Back to Xander the key-stealer? You could close with "I wish I could be of more help, hopefully Xander will be." Think like Forrest Gump. As in "that's all I have to say about that." If you need to get a decision from someone and can't end the discussion here, another feature of "firm" is offering two choices so you don't have continued over-discussion.

If you get more communication after you have already BIFFed your response, you can either ignore it or broken-record your BIFF response with the same keywords and even less content until they give up.

Another Bill Eddy trick for BIFF communication is to avoid the three A's: Advice, Admonishments, and Apologies. So let's look at those, as well:

Advice: You don't want to give anyone advice on how to manage themselves or the situation they are ramped up about. They are already hot under the collar so you won't get anywhere. I know I don't hear much when I'm butthurt—that's a pretty universal response. Notice that rather than telling Sarah to check the timecards in my example, I said "I double checked the calendar and confirmed . . . " That avoided giving her advice on how to do her job. She will realize she should have done so herself once she calms down, so it's all good.

Admonishments: You may want to offer corrective feedback, but just like advice-giving, this isn't the time. The point of a BIFF response is to defuse an emotional conversation and end it for the time being. So avoid anything that makes it sound like you are explaining their behavior to them like they are a naughty child. Again, with Sarah the manager, imagine the continued battle if you had said, "If you had acted like an actual manager, you would have checked the schedule before having a ragefit at me"???

Apologies: Authentic apologies are a good thing. But when everyone is activated it is not the time for them. Apologizing can give the other person something to blame us for, extending the conversation. "I'm so sorry I don't know what happened to the keys" can let Sarah continue to blame you for her ridiculous insistence that you are somehow responsible. A more gentle "social apology" can be helpful to defuse the issue, if you want to add that to the mix, however. "I'm so sorry you are having to deal with such a frustrating situation with everything else on your plate!" is a show of commiseration and empathy that doesn't connect you to the blame game and doesn't give Sarah any more ammo.

Keeping your cool when communication fails

I know, I know what you are thinking. No matter how boss you are at BIFFing your communication there are some motherfuckers who aren't gonna hear shit from you. Even if you added interpretive dance to the mix, they are so wrapped up in their bullshit they are determined to hear everything you say through that world view. And in those times, absolutely nothing you do or say will lead to effective communication.

Sometimes you can't stand your ground, even politely using BIFF statements, for a multitude of reasons. Maybe they are family members on whom you are financially dependent. Maybe it's a shitty boss at a shitty job that you can't afford to quit. No matter what your circumstances, I am well aware that if "just walk away" were really that simple, everyone would do it.

And, as we've discussed, there are some situations where "just walk away" really isn't an option.

These two skills focus less on communication and more on how to protect yourself from someone else's onslaught . . . which is sometimes the only way we can set a boundary.

The pane of glass trick

Are you stuck with motherfuckers who push every last button? One of the tricks I've found that has really helped me is to imagine a clear pane of glass between me and them. I can hear and see them, but their emotional bullshit stops at the glass.

This is especially helpful for us Counselor Troi empath-type people. We can respond to the content of their words and actions without being emotionally drained by whatever forces are driving them.

And for those of us whose empathy leads us into doing more for others than we should (like rescuing, excusing, or caretaking that isn't healthy in the long run for anyone involved) it can help us remain proactive instead of reactive in a difficult relationship dynamic.

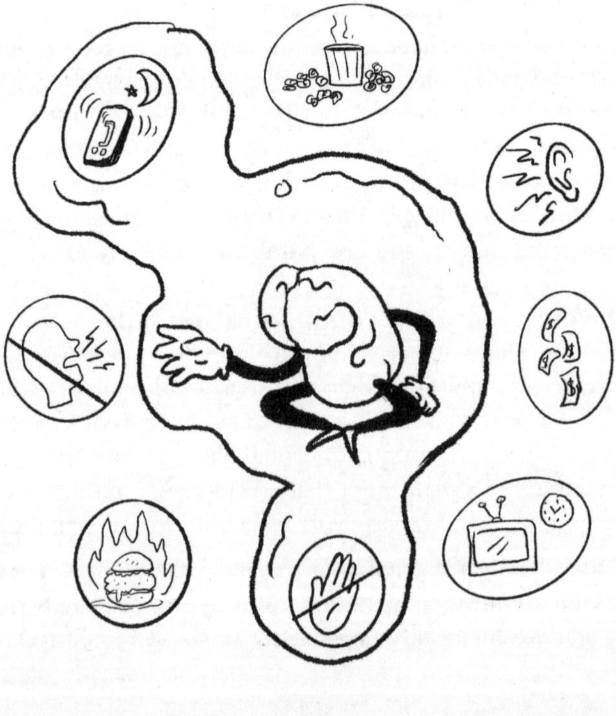

The gray rock method

Another trick for dealing with boundary-busting individuals, or just toxic, shitty situations in which someone is being harmful, is the gray rock method.

A blogger who goes by Skylar on the now-defunct 180rule.com developed what she calls the "Gray Rock Method" as a tool for convincing abusive individuals to leave you, by making yourself as boring and non-responsive as possible. You essentially become a gray rock. The more boring you are, the less fuel they have. You are essentially training them to consider you an unsatisfying conquest.

This is a tool that I had unconsciously put into practice as a teen and can testify to how well it works. I had a grandparent who commented frequently on my weight and body shape. I remember him picking up my arm when I was about 14 and declaring, "You ain't got no wrists!"

My response? "Mmmmm, ok."

The conversation ended right there, due to my complete lack of reaction.

A former intern of mine did on-call work for a local hospital that tends to be perpetually short-staffed and operating in chaos. Her supervisor was blowing up her phone, wanting her to pick up shifts outside her availability. I coached her through a BIFF response, but her supervisor continued to rant . . . trying to guilt my intern with comments like "I don't have anyone to cover! I don't know what to do! I really need help!"

My intern responded with "Yeah that's a lot" and then stopped responding. Eventually the rant ceased . . . and the haranguement was never made mention of again. If my intern had continued defending herself, her responses would have been used as proof that being short staffed was her fault, not the supervisor's.

When Do You Need to Justify Your Boundaries?

Now that we have gone on and on and on about the different types of boundaries, the range of ways we enforce them, and THEN how to communicate them (holy shit . . . I think we've all earned a graduate degree in boundary-setting at this point, what do you think?), let's talk about the complicated terrain of when and how we justify our boundaries to others (I think this means we are now getting into a PhD boundaries class, don't you?). I've found in my work that the one thing that feels worse than setting boundaries is the need to legitimize them once we set them. If your boundaries have been really permeable in the past, it's easy to fall into the trap of over-explaining as you firm them up, even in situations that are not high conflict.

In her book Empowered Boundaries, Cristien Storm explains how we sometimes get hooked into feeling a need to defend or justify our boundaries. You know, the relational labor we put into the overexplain of our boundary that is generally not nearly as necessary as we think it is.

When I read that my first thought was of Pema Chodron's definition of shenpa. The Tibetan word is usually translated as "attachment" but I prefer Chodron's translation, which means "hooked." It's that feeling of going down a well-worn path or getting caught in a record scratch that creates a continuous skip. Chodron describes it as that feeling of being trapped in a situation that doesn't feel good, causing us to tighten up and shut down.

Boundary work can trigger shenpa just like any other situation. The hook, in this case, is feeling the need to justify a boundary we are setting. Or convince someone else to understand our boundary. Advocating for ourselves can feel really uncomfortable, and a lot of people get an urge to justify their self-advocacy.

Boundary shenpa is the result. Being in our feels about setting or holding a new boundary is so uncomfortable, we go into our headspace instead. And start intellectualizing the whole process to ourselves and the person with whom we are setting the boundary. This prevents us from being authentic with ourselves and with others.

Justifying a boundary isn't always a bad thing. It depends on the situation, right? If a friend asks if I can attend her event, I can say "no" as a complete response. Or I can say "I'm sorry, I'm actually in the office that day . . . I'll be exhausted afterward and will really need to go home and rest." Some justifications are relationally relevant, which is not the same thing as boundary shenpa.

Boundary shenpa occurs when "No, I'm not comfortable with you borrowing my car" turns into an over-explanation, or even falsehoods, to justify your no. "I'd totally let you use my car, but I have errands to run/the brakes are spongy/etc, etc." Because we don't feel comfortable with our own boundary and don't want to upset the other person or have them think we're being shitty, so we get into justification mode.

What's the antidote to boundary shenpa? The Tibetan word here is shenlock. It refers to a renunciation of an old pattern. When you notice that physical response of tightening into a need to over-justify, try to recognize the habit in yourself with loving-kindness, and respond with the new boundary-setting habit we are working to become more natural. Practice how you are going to set your boundaries and how you are going to respond if someone DOES get butthurt. Some ideas:

- "No, I'm not comfortable with you borrowing my car."

- "I see that you are upset by my answer, and I respect that but I'm not going to lend you my car."
- "Be that as it may, my answer is no."

Recognizing these patterns and changing our interactions isn't one of those things where we have a huge breakthrough, make a seismic change, and then never have a problem again. It took years and years to develop our ways of communicating, and it will take a while to learn to do it differently. And all of this is like the train of dominoes, where they are laid in a row, and knocked down in a particular order. Old communication patterns that no longer serve us are some of the first dominoes we target.

How Do You Respect Other People's Boundaries?

Ok, so now that we have a better idea of your own boundaries . . . That was a fuck-ton of emotional work, wasn't it? Ugh, yeah. Let's go ahead and finish off the navel-gazing by looking at how you respond to the boundaries of others.

1. Generally speaking, do people tend to respond positively to you? Do they tell you they feel comfortable sharing with you? That you hear them without judgment?
2. Do you have people (or at least one person) in your life with whom you are able to have deep and authentic exchanges of ideas and feelings?
3. Are you able to maintain these relationships over a long period of time?
4. What kinds of situations make it hard for you to respect the boundaries of others? Is it with certain people? Or when people are making certain decisions that cause you concern?

The first three questions are a good self-examination of whether or not you are able to maintain relationships. If you struggle with the boundaries of others, it will start to eat away at all of your interpersonal relationships. Let's be honest. Do you know anyone who is bad at boundaries but somehow still maintains healthy relationships? I don't.

If you read the first three questions and had an "Oh, fuck" moment, that doesn't mean you should put down the book and immediately start emotionally self-flagellating, okay? We generally learn good or bad boundary setting from those around us. If no one modeled healthy boundaries for you in the past, how were you supposed to learn? And since no one is handed the boundaries manual at birth, a lot of us have to figure it out later. As you start being mindful of boundaries in your interactions, I bet you will see serious, positive changes in your relationships overall.

The fourth question is more universal. Because I promise we all have situations where we struggle to respect other people's boundaries. It might be with family members you care about, when you see a friend making the same dumb decision for the 97th time, or when someone engages in a behavior that you've previously seen lead to a bad end for yourself or others. Those kinds of situations can really make it hard to respect their boundaries.

And it's okay to communicate that. To say something in the vein of:

I'm having a hard time respecting your boundaries right now because I'm really worried about you. I don't want to start bossing you into doing what I want you to do. It might be better if we don't discuss this particular issue because I can't really be impartial.

It's the nicest way I can think of to avoid a "Your new bae is a piece of shit! Break up with them!" conversation that's only going to get you into trouble.

It's also okay to ask for clarification on what level of support someone is looking for. I struggle with the boundaries of my adult kiddos. Makes total sense, right? I still want to parent them. When they ask for my advice, I ask straight out: Do you want the mom answer or the supportive-adult-in-your-life answer? This gives them the opportunity to let me know how flexible their boundaries are about my interference in the situation, and has probably saved us from any number of fights over the years.

Handling no

Nobody likes to be told "no." Being told no sucks. It makes our inner toddler kick and scream, and all those toxic societal messages start to leak out in response. But the word "no" (or other words and actions that convey it) is one of the most important ways people express boundaries. What if we started paying attention to "no" messages in a conscious way, and dealt with being told no like bad-ass adults? These are some of the strategies that help:

1) Pay attention to your feelings with self-compassion. If we stuff our feelings, they are just gonna explode out later, like an overstuffed garbage bag. It's ok to think "ow, that hurt . . . I really wanted that to happen."
2) Put "no" in its proper place. No is generally the rejection of your offer, not your personhood. Quite rarely is someone saying that everything about you is wrong and unwanted and fundamentally broken. Our inner demons may tell us that when someone doesn't want to hang out with us, but it's bullshit. There are tons of good humans in the world that I don't want to work with, go to parties with, or see naked. I know you feel the same way . . . and it's important to remember that others can feel that way about you without it being symbolic of something greater.

3) Recognize the boundary you hit and learn from it. If someone tells you no, they are setting a boundary. This is good information about them and your relationship with them. This is the whole point of this book, isn't it? To recognize and communicate and respect boundaries? "No" is the space where we start seeing where the boundaries are erected.

4) Communicate this understanding. Don't wheedle or try to convince. Don't pout around slathered in butthurt. Say "I'm bummed, but I get it, no hard feelings."

Respecting people's boundaries is how we make our relationships better. People will know they can trust you with their truth and that you will respect them and understand that they aren't attacking your personhood. It makes you the embodiment of safe space. And it also serves to reinforce that if we can do that work for others then we deserve the same work done for us. Win-win.

S.T.F.U.

I have a confession to make. I get super excited about shit and tend to verbally run over people. Especially when I'm being quiet and listen-y at my clinic all day, I get way too jabbery after hours. An ex of mine called me "Mistress Interruptess" which was a nice (and funny) way of pointing out when I was on my bullshit in that regard.

Because I wasn't communicating effectively if I wasn't listening effectively. And I was definitely going to end up unintentionally hulk-smashing people's boundaries if I was being oblivious to what they were saying.

I love Sarah Mirk's book *Sex from Scratch: Making Your Own Relationship Rules.* I was skimming through my well-worn copy recently and found a hot-pink highlighted paragraph that really resonates with the ideas I am endeavoring to share here.

Sarah shares a communication strategy she learned from a tech entrepreneur named Matthew. While shutting the fuck up is something that most of us need to do at some point, his acronym is a little different and is wonderful advice for all kinds of communication. And it will improve your boundary identification game by like 33 1/2 percent. I made that stat up just now, but it WILL help. If you are listening differently, you are HEARING differently.

S.T.F.U. stands for:

Share Time: Conversation is a two-way street. Being silent and listening is just as important a role as talking. My bad-ass editrix actually saw Matthew's talk on this technique and told me that he offered a math equation to help people conceptualize how to share time in a simple way. He suggests dividing the amount of time you have for the interaction (say an hour) by the number of people in the room (say six) and make sure you don't spend more than your portion of the time talking (in this case, ten minutes).

Three Seconds: Give others a chance to continue to speak or jump into the conversation before you begin to speak. That means counting to three when there is a pause in the conversation before making your own verbal contribution.

Find Empathy: Really listen to people . . . not just the content but their backstory. Where are they coming from?

Understanding Is Not Necessary: I really love this one. Active listening is designed to help us better understand others, right? But that doesn't mean we always are successful at doing so. We've all had a what-the-literal-fuck moment in regard to someone else's worldview. It's okay to simply accept it as theirs without "getting" it. And maybe further marination on what they are saying will give you an aha moment later?

Holding Yourself Accountable for Boundary Violations

We've all had boundaries violated by others and done some boundary violating ourselves.

This can range from horrific actions like the rape and abuse we discussed earlier in this book to the more everyday crappy things we do like finishing off the last of the ice cream even though you knew your roommate was saving it for later. There are always places where we could have done so much better in terms of autonomy and respecting others.

Being an adult means examining the messages we've received our entire lives critically so we can make better and more informed choices for ourselves and the world around us. Recognizing we are the product of our experiences helps us unpack the messages we received in the past, either from family, friends, or greater culture. Part of this process includes dealing with the consequences of having violated others' boundaries. I've had a lot of people tell me that they carry deep guilt for past actions.

Guilt is not a signal that you are an irredeemable shithead, it's a signal that you have work to do. That you now know better and are committing to doing better. And that essential work happens through the process of accountability.

Accountability is the willingness or self-propelled obligation to accept responsibility for and repair the harm caused by our actions. It may mean listening to and holding space without defensiveness for another person's experience of how your actions have caused them harm (which is wayyyyyyy harder than most people think) so you can offer an apology and interact differently in the future.

It may mean doing some big soul-searching, self-examination type work about how you have walked in the world for many years. Individuals who have engaged in substance use find this to be an important part of their recovery. But they aren't the only ones. Those of us who had significant trauma histories will often continue those cycles of abuse and pain, systematically hurting others and themselves the way they have been hurt. Unpacking generations of toxic, reactive behavior takes a huge amount of work. But that work is how we heal ourselves, those around us, and future generations. You've heard the expression "hurt people hurt people and healed people heal people"? Cheesy with extra cheese, I know. But so so true. We can't change the past but we CAN say "this is where the harm stops."

Accountability work is difficult. But it's essential to having healthy relationships despite the boundary violations that we inevitably do to each other. As brain science bears out, we are a species that is hardwired for relationships. That means we need relationships to survive, but it doesn't mean we always do a good job at them. Accountability should feature prominently in our relationships, personal lives, and professional lives.

Reflect on one of the moments I know you've been thinking about where you violated someone else's boundaries. Are you still in contact with them? Do you have the sort of relationship where you could have a discussion about what happened and either request or give an apology? As in "Remember that time I ate your ice cream? I was thinking about it and I really owe you a sincere apology. You were saving it for when you had a hard day, and then your day sucked even more when it wasn't there. I can't go back in time but I can do and be better in the future." Notice that this apology didn't include any explanation about why you ate the ice cream or blame for the other person not eating it sooner. It's about healing your relationship, not excusing yourself.

Or if you're asking for accountability from someone else, you might say, "Remember last month when we went out for drinks and I said I didn't want to have more than two beers but you ordered a few rounds of shots and said 'don't worry about it, we're walking home so it's no big deal if you drink them'? I was really uncomfortable with that. I felt pressured to drink more and was frustrated that you weren't respecting my earlier request. I ended up drinking them, then was obviously mad at you about it. We can't go back in time but I can be better at expressing my boundaries so you can be clearer on respecting them."

Also? This is a personal soapbox of mine, fair warning. You need to apologize without justifying your behavior. For instance, "I'm sorry—I didn't have any money for lunch so I took yours from the fridge," is the opposite of an apology. It's a justification. It's doubling down against their hurt feelings.

Defensiveness about unintended consequences is also unhelpful. "I ran your car into the light pole but I didn't mean to" is frustratingly unhelpful, even if you add a "sorry" somewhere in the mix. Nobody assumes that intentionally running a borrowed car into a light pole was on your agenda. Instead, try, "I'm so sorry I ran your car into the light pole. It's my responsibility to have it fixed." This apology includes language of accountability, which means owning the consequences of our actions, honestly and completely.

This is a real, completely true story of a conversation I had with my late husband. He came in from the backyard and announced that my chiminea (which is a clay fire pot if you are wondering) was broken. When I asked what happened, he said "It dropped. And it broke." When I asked where it dropped from he said "Well, I was moving it. And it fell out of my hands. So it broke when it dropped from my hands."

(I know in reading this it seems like a ridiculous explanation but people explain their actions like this ALL THE TIME once you start paying attention.)

We must have gone round and round for another ten minutes of me saying "So you dropped my chiminea and broke it?" and him arguing "NO! It dropped and broke!"

When he finally said "Yes! Fine! I dropped it and broke it but I didn't MEAN to!" I replied with "Of course you didn't mean to. You're not an asshole going around breaking people's shit on purpose."

Sometimes we intended harm and there is a whole other layer of accountability work to do there, but generally, we're just dumb humans bumbling around and fucking shit up even though we're trying our best. How different would it have gone if he had said "Babe? I was trying to move your chiminea, and I broke it. I can try to fix it, but since it's clay it probably won't repair well enough to build fires in anymore. I'll replace it when I get paid on Friday."

Just apologizing isn't enough, either. If an apology is called for, do it. If you were the one stealing everyone's lunches at work, ceasing to steal those lunches isn't going to repair that trust. Think about how your actions or words impacted the other person, particularly if your actions were over a period of time. If you argue with your friend every time they tell you what they need from you, focus on listening instead. Make sure you hear and understand the nuts and bolts of their requests and commit them to memory.

Apologizing is a powerful tool for repairing relationships, but it isn't always appropriate. It may not be appropriate or safe to reach out. Or they may not be interested in what you have to say. If so, here's a new chance to respect their boundaries. This is something else that we should really consider on the regular when doing accountability work.

In twelve-step language, we make amends unless doing so would cause the other person harm. And opening up someone's healed wounds for our own sense of well-being is definitely a form of harm.

A friend of mine really biffed his relationship a year ago and tried to reach out and apologize to his ex . . . who wasn't having it. He told me "I need to respect her wanting to be left alone. It's the least I can do, right?" Friend-person realized that this was not only a boundary, but his need to apologize was really about making himself feel better and less about repairing the harm he caused the woman in question.

If you think of someone you may have hurt in the past, what do you need to do to make sure it doesn't happen again in the future? It may be as simple as realizing "I never thought about it that way. Now I know that 'convincing' someone is actually shitty and sketch and I'm over it." Or it may mean, "I really shouldn't drink that much, I'm far more likely to be a dick to other people when I do." Here's a chance to make a commitment to yourself about your future interactions.

Beyond apologizing when needed and appropriate, it's always more powerful to show change and work for change instead of telling people that you have changed. Visible allyship and peer-to-peer support are critical to the kind of evolutionary change we desperately need to survive. Many recovery programs have people who have worked the program move into sponsorship roles, helping others in the ways they have been helped. Programs like The Forgiveness Project make public the work of accountability and healing. But it doesn't take renting a billboard. It may be volunteering time to a local advocacy group. Or demonstrating your accountability around others, therefore modeling interpersonal effectiveness as a mechanism of social change (ahhhh shit, I just got all political again, didn't I? #sorrynotsorry).

Questions to consider

1) How, specifically, do you want to improve your respect for the boundaries of others? State this in positive and behaviorally focused terms, e.g., "I want to listen to the viewpoints of others without interrupting in order to understand where they are coming from" is far more doable than "I want to stop being a judgemental asshole."
2) What is your reason for wanting to make this improvement? What makes this a personal priority?
3) How will making these improvements change your life?
4) How are you hoping that these changes will improve life for people that you care about?
5) What are your best practices for moving forward? What are the actionable steps?

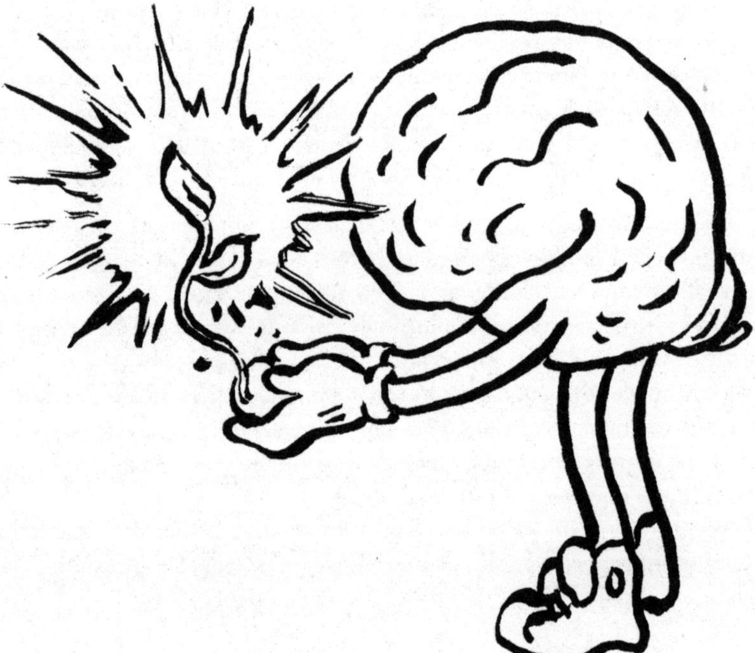

CONCLUSION

I want to tell you a little story.

My father is a person in long term recovery. He got sober through AA in the 1970s under the sponsorship of a grizzled old-timer from the Bill W. school of 12 step recovery. My father was also active duty military, so he took orders from his sponsor unblinkingly.

One day his sponsor was having him do knuckle push-ups.

Have you ever done them? Where the weight of the pushup goes into the knuckles of your hands instead of the flats of your palms? That shit HURTS, even if you are a military man in your mid-20s in fantastic shape.

My father did them, though. Complaining that they hurt. Asking if he could stop.

But every time he asked if he could stop, his sponsor told him to keep going.

Eventually, the pain got so bad, he jumped up and said "Fuck you! I don't have to do this!"

His sponsor slowly nodded his head in agreement and said "No shit."

That's it, isn't it? No matter what our past training and no matter the context of our current circumstances, we have the power to make choices that are the best for us and the world we want to live in.

What if we discussed our wants, needs, desires, and personal space as often and as matter-of-factly as we discuss football, movie star break-ups, and videogames? Our boundaries around these issues are something as real and tangible as our fingers and toes, and consent around these boundaries should be a given. What if the way we are doing it now is as useless and harmful as knuckle push-ups? If we all jumped up and said, "I don't have to do this anymore!" then the world would shift.

This book is a love letter to that idea. Because we all have so much capacity for healing. And healthy relationships. And we deserve safe passage in society.

But achieving this evolutionary shift requires such massive personal and societal change that it's hard not to feel hopeless, even as we sit here with bruised and bleeding knuckles.

This book was overwhelming to write, and now that you've read it you are probably feeling overwhelmed as well. I don't write shallow, fluffy, feel-good books where emotional wellness work is over-simplified by burying it with mantras about how the laws of attraction will create instant happiness and success (not to mention perfect boundaries).

Problems that have existed for generations don't get fixed with platitudes, they get fixed when we do the difficult work of figuring out what we truly want in life, the kinds of relationships we want and don't want, and how we best communicate these desires to those around us while holding space for them to communicate their desires to us. You thought you got a book on boundaries and instead you got a manifesto on changing the world.

Same difference, though.

You can do this.

No shit.

RECOMMENDED RESOURCES

Unfuck Your Brain

Addiction

Memoirs of An Addicted Brain: A Neuroscientist Examines His Former Life on Drugs by Marc Lewis

In The Realm of Hungry Ghosts: Close Encounters with Addiction by Gabor Mate

Eating in the Light of the Moon: How Women Can Transform Their Relationship with Food Through Myths, Metaphors, and Storytelling by Anita A. Johnston

A Woman's Addiction Workbook: Your Guide To In-Depth Healing by Lisa M. Najavits

Rational Recovery: The New Cure for Substance Addiction by Jack Trimpsey

12 Stupid Things That Mess Up Recovery: Avoiding Relapse Through Self-Awareness and Right Action by Allen Berger

Anxiety, Depression, Anger, and Other Mood Disorders

How To Not Kill Yourself: A Survival Guide for Imaginative Pessimists by Set Sytes

Bluebird: Women and The New Psychology of Happiness by Ariel Gore

Maps To The Other Side: The Adventures of A Bipolar Cartographer by Sascha Altman DuBrul

Furiously Happy: A Funny Book About Horrible Things by Jenny Lawson

Grief

Being With Dying: Cultivating Compassion and Fearlessness in the Presence of Death by Joan Halifax

A Grief Observed by C.S. Lewis

Sign Posts of Dying by Martha Jo Atkins

Good Grief by Granger E. Westberg

How Can I Help? Reaching Out To Someone Who Is Grieving by June Cerza Kolf

Self-Compassion

Self-Compassion: The Proven Power of Being Kind To Yourself by Kristen Neff

The Mindful Path to Self-Compassion: Freeing Yourself from Destructive Thoughts and Emotions by Christopher Germer

Unfuck Your Body

Polyvagal Theory

The stuff written by Stephen Porges on polyvagal theory is very dense and scientific, but interesting.

The books (and posters and flipcharts) by Deb Dana on the application of polyvagal theory to mental health are generally designed for mental health practitioners but could also def be used by anyone.

Somatic Trauma

Waking the Tiger: Healing and Trauma by Peter A. Levine

In an Unspoken Voice: How the Body Releases Trauma and Restores Goodness by Peter A. Levine

Molecules of Emotion: The Science Behind Mind-Body Medicine by Candace Pert

The Body Keeps the Score: Brain, Mind, and Body in the Healing of Trauma by Bessel van de Kolk

My Grandmother's Hands: Racialized Trauma and the Pathway to Mending Our Hearts and Bodies by Resmaa Menakem

Inflammation

The UltraMind Solution: Fix Your Broken Brain by Healing Your Body First by Dr. Mark Hyman

The Inflamed Mind: A Radical New Approach to Depression by Edward Bullmore

Stress

The Upside of Stress: Why Stress is Good for You, and how to Get Good at it by Kelly McGonigal

Burnout: The Secret to Unlocking the Stress Cycle by Amelia and Emily Nagoski

Mindfulness and Meditation

Trauma-Sensitive Mindfulness: Practices for Safe and Transformative Healing by David Treleaven

Don't Just Do Something, Sit There: A Mindfulness Retreat with Sylvia Boorstein by Sylvia Boorstein

Movement

Overcoming Trauma through Yoga: Reclaiming Your Body by David Emerson

Yoga for Depression: A Compassionate Guide to Relieve Suffering Through Yoga by Amy Weintraub

The Joy of Movement: How Exercise Helps Us Find Happiness, Hope, Connection, and Courage by Kelly McGonigal

Embracing Yoga's Roots: Courageous Ways to Deepen Your Practice by Susanna Barkataki

The Myths of the Asanas: The Stories at the Heart of the Yoga Tradition by Alanna Kaivalya and Arjuna van der Kooij

Invisible Rainbow: A Physicist's Introduction to the Science Behind Classical Chinese Medicine by Changlin Zhang

The Body Electric: Electromagnetism and the Foundation of Life by Robert O. Becker

Sleep

Why We Sleep: The New Science of Sleep and Dreams by Matthew Walker

The Sleep Revolution: Transforming Your Life, One Night at a Time by Arianna Huffington

Food

Fearing the Black Body: The Racial Origins of Fat Phobia Sabrina Strings

Body Respect: What Conventional Health Books Get Wrong, Leave Out, and Just Plain Fail to Understand about Weight by Linda Bacon and Lisa Aphramor

Stolen Harvest: The Hijacking of the Global Food Supply by Vandana Shiva

Primal Nutrition: Paleolithic and Ancestral Diets for Optimal Health by Ron Schmid

Supplements

The Emperor's New Drugs by Irving Kirsch

Drug Muggers: Which Medications Are Robbing Your Body of Essential Nutrients and Natural Ways to Restore Them by Suzy Cohen

Unfuck Your Intimacy

Abusive Relationships

If you know (or are starting to suspect) your relationship is abusive, I hope you will consider creating a safety plan for yourself. Cover what to do if you plan to stay, or for when you decide to leave. You do not have to be living with a violent partner to need or have a safety plan. Some safety planning tools I recommend include:

- The Domestic Violence Safety Plan by Kellie Holly (verbalabusejournals.com) - this is the most comprehensive plan
- The National Domestic Violence Hotline Safety Planning (thehotline.org) - specifically includes help on planning to leave when you have pets
- Scarleteen Safety Plans (available on their website, scarleteen.com) - includes a separate plan to use if you don't live with your abuser
- The military has developed a safety plan specific to the needs of having a service-member partner (DD Form 2893)

Affirming, Sex-Positive Sexuality

Sex Outside the Lines: Authentic Sexuality in a Sexually Dysfunctional Culture by Chris Donaghue - Unpacks the bullshit around the stigma of sex and encourages self-discovery and self-acceptance.

Sex From Scratch: Making Your Own Relationship Rules by Sarah Mirk - A love and dating guidebook that gleans real-life knowledge from smart people in a variety of nontraditional relationships.

BDSM, Kink, and Fet

SM 101: A Realistic Introduction by Jay Wiseman - The classic. A great overview of BDSM with good general information on getting started with exploring the lifestyle.

The Ultimate Guide to Kink: BDSM, Role Play and the Erotic Edge by Tristan Taormino - A great series of essays ranging from how-tos to think pieces about exploring power, pleasure, and human desire.

When Someone You Love Is Kinky by Dossie Easton - Very helpful for non-kinky folx who are looking to better understand and communicate with their kinky partners.

Boundaries and Consent

Learning Good Consent: Building Ethical Relationships in a Complicated World by Cindy Crabb - This compilation has fantastic information about applying boundaries and maintaining consent in real-life, sticky situations.

Ask: Building Consent Culture by Kitty Stryker - A guide to creating a culture of consent, and not just in the bedroom.

Consensuality: Navigating feminism, gender, and boundaries towards loving relationships by Helen Wildfell - A guide to creating or finding a healthy, successful relationship as well as avoiding common pitfalls.

Changing Bodies & Disabilities

The Ultimate Guide to Sex and Disability: For All of Us Who Live with Disabilities, Chronic Pain, and Illness by Miriam Kaufman, Cory Silverberg, and Fran Odette - Covers the multitude of ways disability can create obstacles to a healthy sex life along with great tips for overcoming these obstacles.

Guide To Getting It On by Paul Joannides - Recent editions of the print book have been abridged, so the chapter on sex and disability is now online for free download. Woot! But, FWIW, the book itself has great info in general.

Sexual Intelligence by Marty Klein - About communication and pragmatic expectations and the emotional work it takes to make sexual intimacy good when nobody involved in the relationship is a perfect performer. Not overtly about changing bodies but it actually totally *is* about just this topic.

Fantasies

Who's Been Sleeping in Your Head: The Secret World of Sexual Fantasies by Brett Kahr

The result of one of the largest studies ever done on sexual fantasy, with over 23,000 participants. Amazing information about what our sexual fantasies say about the nature of being human.

Tell Me What You Want: The Science of Sexual Desire and How It Can Help You Improve Your Sex Life by Justin J. Lehmiller - A researcher for The Kinsey Institute (toothbrush guy!!!) has taken his research on sexual fantasies and explored why they are super normal and how to share them with a partner to make your sex life hotter.

Orientation Spectrum

How to Understand Your Gender by Meg-John Barker and Alex Iantaffi - A comprehensive and compassionate guide to all the ways we might identify and express ourselves around gender

Bi: Notes for a Bisexual Revolution by Shiri Eisner - A wonderful political treatise on the expanse of human sexuality. Really about all the ways we can be non-monosexual, not just bi.

You and Your Gender Identity: A Guide to Discovery by Dara Hoffman-Fox and Zinnia Jones - Dara is a clinician as well as being genderqueer, and this book is about exploration more than information. Parents of gender-questioning kiddos find this very helpful.

Asexuality: A Brief Introduction by Asexuality Archive - This is my go-to reference because it focuses on the voices and lived experience of ace individuals.

Stone Butch Blues by Les Feinberg - A classic novel bringing voice to and affirming the stone experience. Newly back in print and available for free public download.

Partnering Better

Hold Me Tight: Seven Conversations for a Lifetime of Love by Sue Johnson - A helpful book full of great ideas, though with some irritating self-help lingo, based in attachment theory.

How to Fight by Thich Nhat Hanh - This little book has great information about how mindfulness and kindness to ourselves allow us to let go of anger

10 Lessons To Transform Your Marriage: America's Love Lab Experts Share Their Strategies for Strengthening Your Relationship by John and Julie Gottman - The Gottmans have done decades of research on relationship configurations (I mentioned their four horsemen in this book) and have developed excellent strategies for communicating more effectively with your partner.

Polyamory

The Ethical Slut, Third Edition: A Practical Guide to Polyamory, Open Relationships, and Other Freedoms in Sex and Love by Janet W. Hardy and Dossie Easton - This is the classic book of the consensual non-monogamy movement and is still the one I recommend most. It has great information about negotiating all types of polyamory. While pro-polyam, the authors do talk about exploring hot monogamy as an option when one partner is deeply uncomfortable with polyamory.

Opening Up: A Guide to Creating and Sustaining Open Relationships by Tristan Taormino - Another great look at all the different ways polyamory can be used to increase relationship satisfaction.

Pornography and Sex "Addiction"

The Myth of Sex Addiction by David J. Ley - Unpacks all the research that shows why comparing sex and porn usage to other addictions is a false equivalence.

Ethical Porn for Dicks: A Man's Guide to Responsible Viewing Pleasure by David J. Ley - A Q&A format book created to help men find ways of viewing and using porn responsibly.

The Feminist Porn Book: The Politics of Producing Pleasure by Tristan Taormino - Features essays by feminists in the porn and sex industry along with feminist porn scholars, including a lot of positive uses of porn.

Sex and Gender Confirmation

Sex Without Roles: Transcending Gender by Eli Sachse - A zine about exploring your sexuality in a healthy way as you transition.

Trans Bodies, Trans Selves by Laura Erickson-Schroth - This comprehensive book has a whole chapter on intimate relationships.

The Trans Partner Handbook: A Guide For When Your Partner Transitions by Jo Green - Covers a ton of different topics related to partner transition, including possible changes to sex and sexuality.

Sex Toys/Sex Aids

The Big Book of Sex Toys: From Vibrators and Dildos to Swings and Slings—Playful and Kinky Bedside Accessories That Make Your Sex Life Amazing by Tristan Taormino - Tons of information for solo and partnered use plus photos to take the guesswork of how to actually make everything work!

The Many Joys of Sex Toys: The Ultimate How-to Handbook for Couples and Singles by Anne Semans - Another illustrated guide that covers toys and toy usage techniques. Think of it as a sex cookbook with the toys as the ingredients!

Oh Joy, Sex Toy by Erica Moen and Matthew Nolan - A webcomic and four (so far!) book volumes that cover all kinds of ways of having sex, solo and partnered, for all kinds of different bodies.

Unfuck Your Sex Toys: Make Your Own DIY Tools & MacGyver Your Sexytimes by Dr. Faith G. Harper

Sexual Abuse

Things That Help by Cindy Crabb - Cindy's second zine compilation is some of my favorite writing about healing after sexual trauma, written by an incredibly articulate survivor.

Dear Sister: Letters From Survivors of Sexual Violence by Lisa Factora-Borchers - The letters are affirming and honest without veering off into being tragedy porn.

The Sexual Healing Journey: A Guide For The Survivors of Sexual Abuse by Wendy Maltz - A step by step guide on managing your trauma responses during sexual intimacy in order to reclaim a healthy, fulfilling sex life.

Spirituality

Sex, God, and the Conservative Church: Erasing Shame from Sexual Intimacy by Tina Schermer Sellers - A dense book meant for clinicians. But it has a brilliant history of Western culture and the lens of conservative religion and how that has impacted human sexuality with ideas on how to heal from the negative messages without giving up your faith tradition.

UnClobber: Rethinking Our Misuse of the Bible on Homosexuality by Colby Martin - My absolute favorite book ever on unpacking the "clobber" passages from the bible that are used to proclaim homosexuality as a sin. By an evangelical preacher whose story of coming to allyship is as important as his scriptural interpretation.

Trauma

Waking The Tiger by Peter Levine - A great book on how the body holds trauma and how that impacts all domains of our lives.

Unfuck Your Boundaries

Resources for Victims and Survivors of Interpersonal Violence

The National Domestic Violence Hotline – 1-800-799-7233 (SAFE) – ndvh.org - Speak to (or message) an advocate to seek immediate help, gain resources for survivors, or to discuss your options for leaving, should you choose to do so.

National Dating Abuse Helpline – 1-866-331-9474 – loveisrespect.org - Find ways to prevent or end an abusive relationship. This hotline is tailored to young people but offers resources for concerned friends and family, as well.

National Sexual Assault Hotline – 1-800-656-4673 (HOPE) – rainn.org - Provides strategies for prevention and safety as well as healing and recovery.

National Suicide Prevention Lifeline – 988 – 988lifeline.org - Offers support to those in distress or crisis, and provides prevention resources for loved ones.

National Center for Victims of Crime – 1-855-484-2846 (VICTIM) – victimsofcrime.org - Comprehensive advocacy program that helps victims of crimes rebuild their lives.

National Human Trafficking Resource Center/Polaris Project – Call: 1-888-373-7888 – Text: HELP to BeFree (233733) – polarisproject.org - Call or text for crisis assistance, survivor support, or to report possible trafficking. This hotline can also connect you with local anti-trafficking services in your area.

National Network for Immigrant and Refugee Rights – 1-510-465-1984 – nnirr.org - An organization whose mission is to defend and expand rights for immigrants and refugees. Call for resources, and get connected to local allies.

National Coalition for the Homeless – 1-202-737-6444 – nationalhomeless.org - Network of advocacy groups working to prevent and end homelessness. Call to get emergency assistance from your local service providers.

National Resource Center on Domestic Violence – 1-800-537-2238 – nrcdv.org and vawnet.org - Call to request individualized and comprehensive technical assistance and resources on intervention and prevention strategies.

National Center on Domestic Violence, Trauma & Mental Health – 1-312-726-7020 ext. 2011 – nationalcenterdvtraumamh.org - Offers assistance, resources, and training to advocates and service providers working with survivors.

Resources Specific to Children

Childhelp USA/National Child Abuse Hotline – 1-800-422-4453 – childhelpusa.org - Call to get help in reporting child abuse or to speak to a Childhelp counselor.

Children's Defense Fund – 202-628-8787 – childrensdefense.org - A non-profit child advocacy program that lobbies for the rights of all children in America, particularly poor children, children of color and those with disabilities.

Child Welfare League of America – 202-688-4200 – cwla.org - Coalition of private and public agencies dedicated to serving vulnerable children and families

National Council on Juvenile and Family Court Judges – 775-507-4777 – ncjfcj.org - Child Protection and custody/resource center on domestic violence, which can benefit individuals who have been victims of coercive control.

Center for Judicial Excellence – 415-444-6556 – centerforjudicialexcellence.org - Nonprofit organization focused on creating judicial accountability in the family court system, their focus on policy change is a fantastic resource for individuals who have found that their experiences of coercive control were not considered crimes by the court system.

Resources Specific to Teens

Love Is Respect – Hotline: 1-866-331-9474 or Text: loveis to 22522 – loveisrespect.org - In association with the National Domestic Violence Hotline, this organization works to empower young people to prevent and end abusive relationships.

Break the Cycle – 202-849-6289 – breakthecycle.org - Organization centered around helping young people ages 12-24 build healthy and safe relationships.

Resource Specific to Deaf Women

Deaf Abused Women's Network (DAWN) – hotline@deafdawn.org – VP: 202-559-5366 – deafdawn.org - Agency that provides crisis intervention and survivor services for the Deaf, Hard of Hearing, and DeafBlind communities.

Resources Specific to Women of Color

INCITE! Women of Color Against Violence – incite.natl@gmail.com – incite-national.org - Feminists of Color united to end state and domestic violence.

Resources Specific to Latinx Individuals

Casa de Esperanza – Línea de crisis 24-horas/24-hour crisis line – 1-651-772-1611 – casadeesperanza.org - A bilingual domestic violence hotline. Their mission is to mobilize Latin@ communities to end domestic violence.

Resource Specific to Indigenous Women

National Indigenous Women's Resource Center – 855-649-7299 – niwrc.org - Organization dedicated to ending violence amongst native and indigenous populations through education and policy development.

Resources Specific to Asian and Pacific Islander Individuals

Committee Against Anti-Asian Violence (CAAAV) – 1-212-473-6485 – caaav.org - Centered around organizing Asian communities to fight for institutional change.

Manavi – 1-732-435-1414 – manavi.org - Meeting needs (both immediate and long-term) for South Asian Women affected by violence.

Resource Specific to African American Individuals

National Center on Violence Against Women in the Black Community – 1-844-778-5462 – ujimacommunity.org - Provides resources to and advocates for the Black Community in response to domestic, sexual, and community violence.

Resources Specific to Lesbian, Gay, Plurisexual, Trans, and NonBinary Individuals

The Audre Lorde Project – 1-718-596-0342 – alp.org - Organization working towards community wellness and social/economic justice for Lesbian, Gay, Bisexual, Two-Spirit, Trans and Gender Non Conforming People of Color.

LGBT National Help Center – 1-206-350-4283 - glnh.org - Provides peer support and local resources to the LGBT community.

National LGBTQ Task Force – 1-202-393-5177 - thetaskforce.org - Organization focused on advancing justice and equality for LGBTQ people.

Northwest Network of Bisexual, Trans, Lesbian & Gay Survivors of Abuse – 1-206-568-7777 – nwnetwork.org - Network offering direct resources for victims of abuse, as well as resources for advocacy organizations.

Trans Lifeline – 877-565-8860 – translifeline.org - A hotline dedicated to improving the quality of trans lives and ending the epidemic of trans suicide by offering justice-oriented community aid.

Trevor Project – 1-866-488-7386 – thetrevorproject.org - Focused on preventing suicide and crisis intervention for LGBTQ and questioning individuals. The hotline is for those in need of immediate help.

It Gets Better – info@itgetsbetter.org – itgetsbetter.org - Aiming to uplift, empower and connect LGBTQ youth around the world.

Resource Specific to Older Adults

National Clearinghouse on Abuse in Later Life – 1-608-255-0539 – ncall.us - Provides technical assistance, training, and resources in order to advocate for elderly victims of abuse.

Resource Specific to Men

1in6 – 1in6.org - Provides men affected by sexual abuse or assault with survivor's resources.

Legal Resources

Battered Women's Justice Project – 1-800-903-0111 – bwjp.org - National resource center on civil and criminal justice responses to intimate partner violence.

Legal Momentum – 1-212-925-6635 – legalmomentum.org - Provides expert legal counsel in order to ensure economic and personal security for women and girls.

WomensLaw.org – womenslaw.org - Provides relevant legal information for all genders in regards to domestic and sexual violence.

National Clearinghouse for the Defense of Battered Women – 1-800-903-0111 x 3 - ncdbw.org - Provides customized technical assistance to victims of battery who are facing criminal charges or serving prison sentences.

Legal Network for Gender Equity - (202) 588-5180 - nwlc.org/join-the-legal-network/ -

Seeks gender justice in a variety of ways; in courtrooms, through public policies and cultural changes.

Resources Specific to Violence Prevention

National Organization for Men Against Sexism (NOMAS) – 1-720-466-3882 – nomas.org

A Call to Men – 1-917-922-6738 – acalltomen.org

Men Can Stop Rape – 1-202-265-6530 – mencanstoprape.org

Media Resources (Books, Websites, Etc.)

Learning Good Consent: Building Ethical Relationships In A Complicated World - Cindy Crabb

Empowered Boundaries: Setting Boundaries and Inspiring Social Change - Cristien Storm

Invisible Chains: Overcoming Coercive Control In Your Intimate Relationship - Lisa Aronson Fontes

Conflict Is Not Abuse – Sarah Schulman

Dare To Lead – Brene Brown

The Gift of Fear – Gavin DeBecker

Betty Martin's "Wheel of Consent" and "The Three Minute Game" - *Betty Martin.org*

How to Put Together a Consent Workshop - *tinyurl.com/ConsentWorkshopZine*

REFERENCES

Unfuck Your Brain

Chapters One through Three: All the Brain and Trauma-Wiring Stuff

Barrett, Lisa Feldman. "Solving the Emotion Paradox: Categorization and the Experience of Emotion." Personality and Social Psychology Review 10, no. 1 (2006): 20–46. Accessed September 7, 2016. affective-science.org/pubs/2006/Barrett2006paradox.pdf

Beck, Aaron T. Prisoners of Hate: The Cognitive Basis of Anger, Hostility, and Violence. New York: HarperCollins Publishers, 1999.

Beck, Aaron T., John A. Rush, and Brian F. Shaw. Cognitive Therapy of Depression. 7th ed. New York: Guilford Publications, 1987.

Beck, Judith S., Aaron T Beck, Judith V. Jordan, and Aaron Carroll. Cognitive Behavior Therapy, Second Edition: Basics and Beyond. 2nd ed. New York: Guilford Publications, 2011.

Beck, Judith S and Aaron T Beck. Cognitive Therapy for Challenging Problems: What to Do When the Basics Don't Work. New York: Guilford Publications, 2011.

Bush, G. et al. "Dorsal Anterior Cingulate Cortex: A Role in Reward-Based Decision Making. - PubMed - NCBI." 2013. Accessed September 28, 2016. ncbi.nlm.nih.gov/m/pubmed/11756669/

Foa, Edna B, Terence M Keane, and Matthew J Friedman. Effective Treatments for PTSD: Practice Guidelines from the International Society for Traumatic Stress Studies. Edited by Professor Edna B Foa, PhD Terence M Keane, and Executive Matthew J Friedman. New York: Guilford Publications, 2004.

Foster, Jane A. Gut Feelings: Bacteria and the Brain. 2013 (July 1, 2013). Accessed September 2, 2016. .ncbi.nlm.nih.gov/pmc/articles/PMC3788166/.

Hendy, David. Noise: A Human History of Sound and Listening. New York, NY, United States: HarperCollins Publishers, 2013.

Herman, Judith Lewis L. Trauma and Recovery: The Aftermath of Violence - from Domestic Abuse to Political Terror. New York, NY: Basic Books, 1992.

Mehl-Madrona, Lewis. Remapping Your Mind: The Neuroscience of Self-Transformation Through Story. United States: Bear & Company, 2015.

Miller, George A. The Magical Number Seven, Plus or Minus Two Some Limits on Our Capacity for Processing Information. 101, no. 2 (1955): 343–52.

Mitchell, Jeffrey Diplomate T and American. "TROUSSE PSYCHOTRAUMATIQUE DE DIAGNOSTIC RAPIDE." 2008.

Pessoa, Luiz. "Emotion and Cognition and the Amygdala: From 'What Is It?' to 'What's to Be Done?'."

Phelps, Elizabeth. "Human Emotion and Memory: Interactions of the Amygdala and Hippocampal Complex." Current Opinion in Neurobiology 14, no. 2 (2004): 198–202. Accessed May 18, 2016.

Porges, Stephen W. The Polyvagal Theory: New Insights into Adaptive Reactions of the Autonomic Nervous System. 76, no. Suppl 2. Accessed June 7, 2016. .ncbi.nlm.nih.gov/pmc/articles/PMC3108032/.

Stevens, FL, et al. "Anterior Cingulate Cortex: Unique Role in Cognition and Emotion. - PubMed - NCBI." 2007. Accessed September 28, 2016. ncbi.nlm.nih.gov/m/pubmed/21677237/.

Tulving, Endel. Episodic and Semantic Memory (1972). Accessed May 18, 2016. alicekim.ca/EMSM72.pdf.

HJ, Markowitsch and Staniloiu A. "Amygdala in Action: Relaying Biological and Social Significance to Autobiographical Memory. - PubMed - NCBI." 1985. Accessed January 4, 2016. .ncbi.nlm.nih.gov/m/pubmed/20933525/.

Judith. "Section 1: Foundations of the Trauma Practice Model 13 6. Tri-Phasic Model (Herman, 1992)." 2005.

Junger, Sebastian. Tribe: On Homecoming and Belonging. United States: Twelve, 2016.

Lehrer, Jonah. How We Decide. Boston: Houghton Mifflin Harcourt, 2009.

Levine, Peter A. Waking the Tiger: Healing Trauma - the Innate Capacity to Transform Overwhelming Experiences. Berkeley, CA: North Atlantic Books,U.S., 1997.

Levine, Peter A. and Maggie Kline. Trauma-Proofing Your Kids: A Parents' Guide for Instilling Joy, Confidence, and Resilience. Berkeley, CA: North Atlantic Books,U.S., 2008.

Levine, Peter A and Maggie Kline. Trauma Through a Child's Eyes: Awakening the Ordinary Miracle of Healing: Infancy Through Adolescence. Berkeley, CA: North Atlantic Books,U.S., 2006.

Levine, Peter A and Gabor Maté. In an Unspoken Voice: How the Body Releases Trauma and Restores Goodness. Berkeley: North Atlantic Books,U.S., 2010.

Lipton, Bruce. The Biology of Belief. Santa Rosa, CA: Mountain of Love/Elite Books, 2005.

Marsh, Elizabeth & Roediger, Henry. "Episodic and Autobiographical Memory." 2013 Chapter. n.p., 2013.

Mussweiler, Thomas, Birte Englich, and Fritz Strack. 0 Anchoring Effect. n.p., n.d.

National Center for PTSD "How Common Is PTSD? - PTSD: National Center for PTSD." August 13, 2015.

Sapolsky, Robert M. Why Zebras Don't Get Ulcers: An Updated Guide to Stress, Stress-Related Diseases, and Coping. 3rd ed. New York: W.H. Freeman and Company, 1998.

Schiraldi, Glenn R. The Post-Traumatic Stress Disorder Sourcebook: A Guide to Healing, Recovery, and Growth. Los Angeles, CA: McGraw-Hill Professional, 2000.

Taylor, Jill Bolte and Ph. D. Taylor. My Stroke of Insight: A Brain Scientist's Personal Journey. New York: Penguin Putnam, 2008.

Trafton, Anne and MIT News Office. "Music in the Brain | MIT News." December 16, 2015. Accessed September 6, 2016. news.mit.edu/2015/neural-population-music-brain-1216.

Treatment Innovations. "All Seeking Safety Studies - Treatment Innovations." Accessed January 4, 2016. treatment-innovations.org/evid-all-studies-ss.html

Turner, Cory. "This Is Your Brain. This Is Your Brain On Music : NPR Ed : NPR." September 10, 2014. Accessed September 6, 2016. npr.org/sections/ed/2014/09/10/343681493/this-is-your-brain-this-is-your-brain-on-music.

Van Der Hart, Onno, Paul Brown, and Bessel A Van Der Kolk. "Pierre Janet's Treatment of Post-Traumatic Stress." 2006. Accessed January 4, 2016. onnovdhart.nl/articles/treatmentptsd.pdf.

Van Der Hart, Onno, Paul Brown, and Horst, Rutger. "The Dissociation Theory of Pierre Janet." 2006.

Van der Hart, Onno. & Friedman, Barbara "Trauma Information Pages, Articles: Van der Hart Et Al (1989)." January 1930. Accessed January 4, 2016. trauma-pages.com/a/vdhart-89.php.

Van Der Kolk, Bessel. The Body Keeps the Score: Brain, Mind, and Body in the Healing of Trauma. United States: Penguin Books, 2015.

Worrall, Simon. "Your Brain Is Hardwired to Snap." News (National Geographic News), February 7, 2016.

Chapter Four: The Getting Better through Self-Care Stuff

Bass, Ellen and Jude Brister. I Never Told Anyone: Writings by Women Survivors of Child Sexual Abuse. Edited by Louise Thornton. New York, NY: William Morrow Paperbacks, 1991.

Bass, Ellen and Laura Davis. The Courage to Heal: A Guide for Women Survivors of Child Sexual Abuse. 3rd ed. New York: HarperPerennial, 1994.

Bounds, Gwendolyn. How Handwriting Boosts the Brain - WSJ. (Indiana University), October 5, 2010. wsj.com/articles/SB10001424052748704631504575531932754922518.

Burdick, Debra E and Lcsw Debra Burdick. Mindfulness Skills Workbook for Clinicians and Clients: 111 Tools, Techniques, Activities & Worksheets. New York, NY, United States: Pesi Publishing and Media, 2013.

Burns, David D. When Panic Attacks: The New, Drug-Free Anxiety Therapy That Can Change Your Life. New York: Crown Publishing Group, 2006.

Culatta, Richard. "Script Theory." 2015. Accessed September 2, 2016. instructionaldesign.org/theories/script-theory.html.

Davis, Laura, Laura Davies, and Laura Hough. Allies in Healing: When the Person You Love Is a Survivor of Child Sexual Abuse. New York: William Morrow Paperbacks, 1991.

Domonell, Kristen. "Endorphins and the Truth about Runner's High." January 8, 2016. Accessed September 7, 2016. dailyburn.com/life/fitness/what-are-endorphins-runners-high/.

Fischer, Jason B. The Two Truths about Love: The Art and Wisdom of Extraordinary Relationships. Oakland, CA: New Harbinger

McMillen, Matt. "Benefits of Exercise to Help With Depression." 2005. Accessed September 7, 2016. m.webmd.com/depression/features/does-exercise-help-depression.

Greenberger, Dennis, Christine A Padesky, and Aaron T Beck. Mind over Mood: Change How You Feel by Changing the Way You Think. New York: Guilford Publications, 1995.

Seligman, Martin E. P. Learned Optimism: How to Change Your Mind and Your Life. 2nd ed. New York, NY: Pocket Books, 1998.

Seligman, Martin E. P. and Seligman Martin. Authentic Happiness: Using the New Positive Psychology to Realize Your Potential for Lasting Fulfillment. New York: Simon & Schuster Adult Publishing Group, 2004.

Stahl, Bob and Elisha Goldstein. A Mindfulness-Based Stress Reduction Workbook. Oakland, CA: New Harbinger Publications, 2010.

Williams, Mary Beth, Soili Poijula, Soili Pojula, and Lasse A. Nurmi. The PTSD Workbook: Simple, Effective Techniques for Overcoming Traumatic Stress Symptoms. Oakland, CA: New Harbinger Publications,U.S., 2002.

Chapter Five: Treatment Options and the Variety of Care Available

Davis, Joseph A. "Critical Incident Stress Debriefing from a Traumatic Event." February 12, 2013. Accessed January 4, 2016. psychologytoday.com/blog/crimes-and-misdemeanors/201302/critical-incident-stress-debriefing-traumatic-event

Gelender, Amanda "Doctors Put Me on 40 Different Meds for Bipolar and Depression. It Almost Killed Me. - Invisible Illness - Medium." May 31, 2016. Accessed June 7, 2016. medium.com/invisible-illness/doctors-put-me-on-40-different-meds-for-bipolar-and-depression-it-almost-killed-me-c5e4fbea2816#.cadpk38ga.

Korry, Elaine. "Too Many Children In Foster Care Are Getting Antipsychotic Meds : Shots - Health News : NPR." September 2, 2015. Accessed June 7, 2016. npr.org/sections/health-shots/2015/09/02/436350334/california-moves-to-stop-misuse-of-psychiatric-meds-in-foster-care.

Kubany, Edward S and Tyler C Ralston. Treating PTSD in Battered Women: A Step-by-Step Manual for Therapists and Counselors. Oakland, CA: New Harbinger Publications, 2008.

Lieberman, Jeffrey A., T. Scott Stroup, Joseph P. McEvoy, Marvin S. Swartz, Robert A. Rosenheck, Diana O. Perkins, Richard S. E. Keefe, et al. "Effectiveness of Antipsychotic Drugs in Patients with Chronic Schizophrenia - NEJM." New England Journal of Medicine 353, no. 12 (September 22, 2005): 1209–23.

Najavits, Lisa M. Seeking Safety: A Treatment Manual for PTSD and Substance Abuse. New York: Guilford Publications, 2002.

Padesky, Christine A, Dennis Greenberger, and Mark S. Schwartz. Clinician's Guide to Mind over Mood. 2nd ed. New York: Guilford Publications, 1995.

Chapters Six through Ten: Specific Symptoms, Situations, and Diagnoses

Berger, Allen. 12 Stupid Things That Mess up Recovery: Avoiding Relapse Through Self-Awareness and Right Action. United States: Hazelden Information & Educational Services, 2008.

Blair, R. J. R. Considering Anger from a Cognitive Neuroscience Perspective. 3, no. 1. Accessed October 3, 2016. ncbi.nlm.nih.gov/pmc/articles/PMC3260787/.

Carnes, Patrick J. and Ph. D. Patrick. A Gentle Path Through the Twelve Steps: The Classic Guide for All People in the Process of Recovery. United States: Hazelden Information & Educational Services, 1994.

Doyle, Robert and Joseph Nowinski. Almost Alcoholic: Is My (or My Loved One's) Drinking a Problem? New York, NY, United States: Hazelden Publishing & Educational Services, 2012.

Evans, Katie, Michael J Sullivan, and J. Michael Sullivan. Dual Diagnosis: Counselling the Mentally Ill Substance Abuser. New York: Guilford Publications, 1990.

Gulz, Agneta. Conceptions of Anger and Grief in the Japanese, Swedish, and American Cultures– the Role of Metaphor in Conceptual Processes. n.p., n.d.

Hamilton, Tim and Pat Samples. The Twelve Steps and Dual Disorders: A Framework of Recovery for Those of Us with Addiction and an Emotional or Psychiatric Illness. United States: Hazelden Information & Educational Services, 1994.

Hazelden Publishing. The Dual Disorders Recovery Book: Twelve Step Programme for Those of Us with Addiction and an Emotional or Psychiatric Illness. United States: Hazelden Information & Educational Services, 1993.

Hendrickson, Edward L. Designing, Implementing and Managing Treatment Services for Individuals with Co-Occurring Mental Health and Substance Use Disorders: Blue Prints for Action. New York: Haworth Press, 2006.

Hahn, Thich Nhat. Anger: Wisdom for Cooling the Flames. United States: Riverhead Books,U.S., n.d.

Huesmann, Rowell L. The Impact of Electronic Media Violence: Scientific Theory and Research. 41, no. 6 Suppl 1 (April 12, 2013). Accessed January 6, 2016. ncbi.nlm.nih.gov/pmc/articles/PMC2704015/.

Kubler-Ross, Elisabeth. On Death and Dying: What the Dying Have to Teach Doctors, Nursers, Clergy and Their Own Families. New York, NY: Simon & Schuster Adult Publishing Group, 1997.

Lakoff, George and Kovecses, Zoltan. "The Cognitive Model of Anger Inherent in American English" 1983. n.p., 2011. georgelakoff.files.wordpress.com/2011/04/the-cognitive-model-of-anger-inherent-in-american-english-lakoff-and-kovecses-1983.pdf

Lingford-Hughes, Ann and Nutt, David."Neurobiology of Addiction and Implications for Treatment | The British Journal of Psychiatry." EDITORIAL 182, no. 2 (February 1, 2003): 100–197. Accessed October 3, 2016. bjp.rcpsych.org/content/182/2/97.

Maté, Gabor. In the Realm of Hungry Ghosts: Close Encounters with Addiction. Berkeley, CA: North Atlantic Books, 2011.

Zwaan, Rolf A. "Experiential Framework for Language Comprehension: The Immersed Experiencer: Toward An Embodied Theory of Language Comprehension." Learning and Motivation 44 (2003)

Unfuck Your Body

Introduction

Chan, C., Gan, R., Shah, N. P., & Corke, H. (2018). Polyphenols from selected dietary spices and medicinal herbs differentially affect common food-borne pathogenic bacteria and lactic acid bacteria. Food Control, 92, 437-443.

Mccraty, R., & Zayas, M. A. (2014). Cardiac coherence, self-regulation, autonomic stability, and psychosocial well-being. Frontiers in Psychology, 5.

Breathing

Benson, H. (1976). The relaxation response. New York: William Morrow.

Bhasin MK, Dusek JA, Chang BH, Joseph MG, Denninger JW, et al. (2017) Correction: Relaxation Response Induces Temporal Transcriptome Changes in Energy Metabolism, Insulin Secretion and Inflammatory Pathways. PLOS ONE 12(2): e0172873. doi.org/10.1371/journal.pone.0172873

Bhasin, Manoj K., et al. "Relaxation Response Induces Temporal Transcriptome Changes in Energy Metabolism, Insulin Secretion and Inflammatory Pathways." PLoS ONE, vol. 8, no. 5, 2013.

Brulé, D. (2020). Just breathe: Mastering breathwork. New York: Atria/Enliven Books.

Cebolla, A. M., & Cheron, G. (2019). Understanding Neural Oscillations in the Human Brain: From Movement to Consciousness and Vice Versa. Frontiers in Psychology, 10.

Cope, S. (2001). Yoga and the quest for the true self. New York: Random House International.

Emerson, D. and Hopper , E, (2011). Overcoming trauma through yoga: reclaiming your body. California: North Atlantic Books.

Harrold, E. (2017). Life with breath: IQ + EQ = new you. Draper, UT: Go BE Great.

Herrero JL, Khuvis S, Yeagle E, Cerf M, Mehta AD. Breathing above the brain stem: volitional control and attentional modulation in humans. J Neurophysiol. 2018;119(1):145-159.

Joseph, Chacko N., et al. "Slow Breathing Improves Arterial Baroreflex Sensitivity and Decreases Blood Pressure in Essential Hypertension." Hypertension, vol. 46, no. 4, 2005, pp. 714–718.

Jovanov, E. "On Spectral Analysis of Heart Rate Variability during Very Slow Yogic Breathing," 2005 IEEE Engineering in Medicine and Biology 27th Annual Conference, Shanghai, 2005, pp. 2467-2470.

Saoji, A. A., Raghavendra, B., & Manjunath, N. (2019). Effects of yogic breath regulation: A narrative review of scientific evidence. Journal of Ayurveda and Integrative Medicine, 10(1), 50-58.

Simpkins, C. A., & Simpkins, A. M. (2014). Yoga and mindfulness therapy workbook for Clinicians & Clients. Eau Claire, WI: Pesi Publishing & Media.

Treleaven, D. (2018). Trauma-sensitive mindfulness: practices for safe and transformative healing. New York, NY: W. W. Norton and Company, Inc.

van der Kolk, B. (2014). The body keeps the score: brain, mind, and body in the healing of trauma. New York, NY: Penguin Books.

Yackle, Kevin, et al. "Breathing Control Center Neurons That Promote Arousal in Mice." Science, vol. 355, no. 6332, 2017, pp. 1411–1415.

Pain

Abdo, Hind, et al. "Specialized Cutaneous Schwann Cells Initiate Pain Sensation." Science, vol. 365, no. 6454, 2019, pp. 695–699.

Coleman, M. (2019, July/August). Working Mindfully With Physical Pain. Spirituality and Health, 20–22.

Darnall, B. D., Mackey, S. C., Lorig, K., Kao, M.-C., Mardian, A., Stieg, R., Porter, J., DeBruyne, K., Murphy, J., Perez, L., Okvat, H., Tian, L., Flood, P., McGovern, M., Colloca, L., King, H., Van Dorsten, B., Pun, T., & Cheung, M. (2020). Comparative Effectiveness of Cognitive Behavioral Therapy for Chronic Pain and Chronic Pain Self-Management within the Context of Voluntary Patient-Centered Prescription Opioid Tapering: The EMPOWER Study Protocol. Pain Medicine (Malden, Mass.), 21(8), 1523–1531. doi.org/10.1093/pm/pnz285

Davies, N. (2018, February/March). Acceptance and Commitment Therapy for Pain. Pain-Free Living.

Dinsmoor, R. S. (2018, February/March). Qi Gong. Pain-Free Living.

Dolan, L. C., Matulka, R. A., & Burdock, G. A. (2010). Naturally occurring food toxins. Toxins, 2(9), 2289–2332. doi.org/10.3390/toxins2092289

Geneen, L., Smith, B., Clarke, C., Martin, D., Colvin, L. A., & Moore, R. A. (2014). Physical activity and exercise for chronic pain in adults: An overview of Cochrane reviews. Cochrane Database of Systematic Reviews.

Gibson, E. M., Nagaraja, S., Ocampo, A., Tam, L. T., Wood, L. S., Pallegar, P. N., . . . Monje, M. (2019). Methotrexate Chemotherapy Induces Persistent Tri-glial Dysregulation that Underlies Chemotherapy-Related Cognitive Impairment. Cell, 176(1-2).

Gilam, G., Gross, J. J., Wager, T. D., Keefe, F. J., & Mackey, S. C. (2020). What Is the Relationship between Pain and Emotion? Bridging Constructs and Communities. Neuron, 107(1), 17–21. doi.org/10.1016/j.neuron.2020.05.024

Jahnke, R., Larkey, L., Rogers, C., Etnier, J., & Lin, F. (2010). A comprehensive review of health benefits of qigong and tai chi. American journal of health promotion : AJHP, 24(6), e1–e25. doi.org/10.4278/ajhp.081013-LIT-248

Klein, P. J., Baumgarden, J., & Schneider, R. (2019). Qigong and Tai Chi as Therapeutic Exercise: Survey of Systematic Reviews and Meta-Analyses Addressing Physical Health Conditions. Alternative therapies in health and medicine, 25(5), 48–53.

Lima, L. V., Abner, T., & Sluka, K. A. (2017). Does exercise increase or decrease pain? Central mechanisms underlying these two phenomena. The Journal of physiology, 595(13), 4141–4150. doi.org/10.1113/JP273355

Markus, M. A., & Morris, B. J. (2008). Resveratrol in prevention and treatment of common clinical conditions of aging. Clinical interventions in aging, 3(2), 331–339.

McManus DE. Reiki Is Better Than Placebo and Has Broad Potential as a Complementary Health Therapy. J Evid Based Complementary Altern Med. 2017;22(4):1051-1057.

Natri, H., Garcia, A. R., Buetow, K. H., Trumble, B. C., & Wilson, M. A. (2019). The Pregnancy Pickle: Evolved Immune Compensation Due to Pregnancy Underlies Sex Differences in Human Diseases. Trends in Genetics, 35(7), 478-488.

Omoigui, S. (2007). The biochemical origin of pain – Proposing a new law of pain: The origin of all pain is inflammation and the inflammatory response. Part 1 of 3 – A unifying law of pain. Medical Hypotheses, 69(1), 70-82.

Omoigui S. (2007). The biochemical origin of pain: the origin of all pain is inflammation and the inflammatory response. Part 2 of 3 - inflammatory profile of pain syndromes. Medical hypotheses, 69(6), 1169–1178. doi.org/10.1016/j.mehy.2007.06.033

Omoigui S. The Interleukin-6 inflammation pathway from cholesterol to aging—role of statins, bisphosphonates and plant polyphenols in aging and age-related diseases. Immun Ageing. 2007 Mar 20;4:1.

Shockley, S., & Siegel, B. S. (2018). The pain companion: Everyday wisdom for living with and moving beyond chronic pain. Novato, CA: New World Library.

Schweder, M. (2018, July/August). Mother Earth Living, 44-49.

Vowles, K. E., Fink, B. C., & Cohen, L. L. (2014). Acceptance and Commitment Therapy for chronic pain: A diary study of treatment process in relation to reliable change in disability. Journal of contextual behavioral science, 3(2), 74–80. doi.org/10.1016/j.jcbs.2014.04.003

Vowles, K. E., Witkiewitz, K., Levell, J., Sowden, G., & Ashworth, J. (2017). Are reductions in pain intensity and pain-related distress necessary? An analysis of within-treatment change trajectories in relation to improved functioning following interdisciplinary acceptance and commitment therapy for adults with chronic pain. Journal of consulting and clinical psychology, 85(2), 87–98. doi.org/10.1037/ccp0000159

Vowles, K. E., Witkiewitz, K., Sowden, G., & Ashworth, J. (2014). Acceptance and commitment therapy for chronic pain: evidence of mediation and clinically significant change following an abbreviated interdisciplinary program of rehabilitation. The journal of pain : official journal of the American Pain Society, 15(1), 101–113. doi.org/10.1016/j.jpain.2013.10.002

Whiteside, A. (2004). Exercise lowers pain threshold in chronic fatigue syndrome. Pain, 109(3), 497-499.

Sleep

Burkhart, K, and J R Phelps. "Amber Lenses to Block Blue Light and Improve Sleep: a Randomized Trial." Advances in Pediatrics., U.S. National Library of Medicine, Dec. 2009, ncbi.nlm.nih.gov/pubmed/20030543.

Buysse DJ. Sleep health: can we define it? Does it matter? SLEEP 2014;37(1):9-17.

"Circadian Rhythm." Psychology Today, Sussex Publishers, psychologytoday.com/us/basics/circadian-rhythm.

Czeisler, Charles A. "Perspective: Casting Light on Sleep Deficiency." Nature News, Nature Publishing Group, 22 May 2013, nature.com/articles/497S13a.

webmd.com/diet/features/natural-good-sleep-tips-on-melatonin-valerian#1.

Figueiro, M G, et al. "The Impact of Light from Computer Monitors on Melatonin Levels in College Students." Advances in Pediatrics., U.S. National Library of Medicine, ncbi.nlm.nih.gov/pubmed/21552190.

Gillette, M U, and S A Tischkau. "Suprachiasmatic Nucleus: the Brain's Circadian Clock." Advances in Pediatrics., U.S. National Library of Medicine, ncbi.nlm.nih.gov/pubmed/10548871.

Gooley, Joshua J., et al. Advances in Pediatrics., U.S. National Library of Medicine, Mar. 2011, ncbi.nlm.nih.gov/pmc/articles/PMC3047226/.

Hartmann, E. "Effects of L-Tryptophan on Sleepiness and on Sleep." Advances in Pediatrics., U.S. National Library of Medicine, ncbi.nlm.nih.gov/pubmed/6764927/.

"Kava Lactones and the Kava-Kava Controversy." Egyptian Journal of Medical Human Genetics, Elsevier, 29 Aug. 2003, sciencedirect.com/science/article/abs/pii/S0031942203003819.

Purves, Dale. "Neuroglial Cells." Advances in Pediatrics., U.S. National Library of Medicine, 1 Jan. 1970, ncbi.nlm.nih.gov/books/NBK10869/.

Shaw, K, et al. "Tryptophan and 5-Hydroxytryptophan for Depression." Advances in Pediatrics., U.S. National Library of Medicine, ncbi.nlm.nih.gov/pubmed/11869656.

Singh, D, et al. "Severity of Pain and Sleep Problems during Kratom (Mitragyna Speciosa Korth.) Cessation among Regular Kratom Users." Advances in Pediatrics., U.S. National Library of Medicine, ncbi.nlm.nih.gov/pubmed/29558272/.

"Touch for Socioemotional and Physical Well-Being: A Review." Egyptian Journal of Medical Human Genetics, Elsevier, 25 Feb. 2011, sciencedirect.com/science/article/pii/S0273229711000025.

Walker, Matthew P. Why We Sleep: Unlocking the Power of Sleep and Dreams. Scribner, 2018.

Inflammation and Toxins

Abbott NJ and Yusof SR (2010). Structure and function of the blood-brain barrier. Front. Pharmacol. Conference Abstract: Pharmacology and Toxicology of the Blood-Brain Barrier: State of the Art, Needs for Future Research and Expected Benefits for the EU.

Albert, P. R., & Benkelfat, C. (2013). The neurobiology of depression—revisiting the serotonin hypothesis. II. Genetic, epigenetic and clinical studies. Philosophical transactions of the Royal Society of London. Series B, Biological sciences, 368(1615), 20120535. doi.org/10.1098/rstb.2012.0535

Alpert, M., Friedhoff, A. J.: Receptor sensitivity modification in the treatment of tardive dyskinesia. Clin. Pharmacol. Ther. 19, 103–104 (1976)

"Ancestral Diet Gone Toxic." Los Angeles Times, Los Angeles Times, 13 Jan. 2004, latimes.com/archives/la-xpm-2004-jan-13-me-inuit13-story.html.

Augusto-Oliveira, M., Arrifano, G. P., Lopes-Araújo, A., Santos-Sacramento, L., Takeda, P. Y., Anthony, D. C., Malva, J. O., & Crespo-Lopez, M. E. (2019). What Do Microglia Really Do in a Healthy Adult Brain?. Cells, 8(10), 1293. doi.org/10.3390/cells8101293

Bone I. The increasing importance of inflammation in neurological disease. Curr Opin Neurol. 2007;20(3):331-333.

Bullmore, Edward T. The Inflamed Mind: a Radical New Approach to Depression. Short Books, 2019.

Calkins, Beverly M. "A Meta-Analysis of the Role of Smoking in Inflammatory Bowel Disease." Digestive Diseases and Sciences, vol. 34, no. 12, 1989, pp. 1841–1854.

Callaghan BL, Fields A, Gee DG, et al. Mind and gut: Associations between mood and gastrointestinal distress in children exposed to adversity. Dev Psychopathol. 2020;32(1):309-328.

Carrington, D. (2020). Microplastic particles now discoverable in human organs. Retrieved October 29, 2020, from amp.theguardian.com/environment/2020/aug/17/microplastic-particles-discovered-in-human-organs

Carrington, Damian, and Matthew Taylor. "Air Pollution Is the 'New Tobacco', Warns WHO Head." The Guardian, Guardian News and Media, 27 Oct. 2018, theguardian.com/environment/2018/oct/27/air-pollution-is-the-new-tobacco-warns-who-head

Cowen, P. J., & Browning, M. (2015). What has serotonin to do with depression?. World psychiatry : official journal of the World Psychiatric Association (WPA), 14(2), 158–160. doi.org/10.1002/wps.20229

Davies N, Thwaites G. Infections of the nervous system. Pract Neurol. 2011;11(2):121-131.

Duman, R. S., & Li, N. (2012). A neurotrophic hypothesis of depression: role of synaptogenesis in the actions of NMDA receptor antagonists. Philosophical Transactions of the Royal Society B: Biological Sciences, 367(1601), 2475–2484.

"Endocrine-Disrupting Chemicals EDCs." Hormone Health Network, hormone.org/your-health-and-hormones/endocrine-disrupting-chemicals-edcs.

Feighner, J. P., Boyer, W. F., Merideth, C. H., & Hendrickson, G. G. (1989). A double-blind comparison of fluoxetine, imipramine and placebo in outpatients with major depression. International Clinical Psychopharmacology, 4(2), 127–134. ncbi.nlm.nih.gov/pubmed/2663975

Fung,Thomas C., Helen E. Vuong, Cristopher D. G. Luna, Geoffrey N. Pronovost, Antoniya A. Aleksandrova, Noah G. Riley, Anastasia Vavilina, Julianne McGinn, Tomiko Rendon, Lucy R. Forrest, Elaine Y. Hsiao. Intestinal serotonin and fluoxetine exposure modulate bacterial colonization in the gut. Nature Microbiology, 2019.

Gennings, C., Ellis, R., & Ritter, J. K. (2012). Linking empirical estimates of body burden of environmental chemicals and wellness using NHANES data. *Environment international*, *39*(1), 56–65. doi.org/10.1016/j.envint.2011.09.002

"Greenland: Love in a Very Cold Climate." The Independent, 20 Oct. 2011, independent.co.uk/environment/greenland-love-in-a-very-cold-climate-525188.html.

"How Dirty Air Could Be Affecting Our Gut Health." BBC Future, BBC, bbc.com/future/article/20190128-how-dirty-air-could-be-affecting-our-gut-health.

Hemmings, S., Malan-Müller, S., van den Heuvel, L. L., Demmitt, B. A., Stanislawski, M. A., Smith, D. G., Bohr, A. D., Stamper, C. E., Hyde, E. R., Morton, J. T., Marotz, C. A., Siebler, P. H., Braspenning, M., Van Criekinge, W., Hoisington, A. J., Brenner, L. A., Postolache, T. T.,

Hillhouse, T. M., & Porter, J. H. (2015). A brief history of the development of antidepressant drugs: From monoamines to glutamate. Experimental and Clinical Psychopharmacology, 23(1), 1–21.

McQueen, M. B., Krauter, K. S., Knight, R., . . . Lowry, C. A. (2017). The Microbiome in Posttraumatic Stress Disorder and Trauma-Exposed Controls: An Exploratory Study. Psychosomatic medicine, 79(8), 936–946. doi.org/10.1097/PSY.0000000000000512

Hyman, Mark. The Ultramind Solution: Fix Your Broken Brain by Healing Your Body First. Simon & Schuster, 2010.

Kaplan GG, Tanyingoh D, Dixon E, et al. Ambient ozone concentrations and the risk of perforated and nonperforated appendicitis: a multicity case-crossover study. Environ Health Perspect. 2013;121(8):939-943.

Kim, Doe-Young, and Michael Camilleri. "Serotonin: a Mediator of the Brain-Gut Connection." The American Journal of Gastroenterology, vol. 95, no. 10, 2000, pp. 2698–2709.

Kirsh, Irving. The Emperor's New Drugs: Exploding the Antidepressant Myth. Bodley Head, 2009.

Kish, Lisa, et al. "Environmental Particulate Matter Induces Murine Intestinal Inflammatory Responses and Alters the Gut Microbiome." PLoS ONE, vol. 8, no. 4, 2013.

Li, N., Lee, B., Liu, R.-J., Banasr, M., Dwyer, J. M., Iwata, M., . . . Duman, R. S. (2010). mTOR-Dependent Synapse Formation Underlies the Rapid Antidepressant Effects of NMDA Antagonists. Science, 329(5994), 959–964.

López-Muñoz, F., Alamo, C., Juckel, G., & Assion, H.-J. (2007). Half a century of antidepressant drugs: on the clinical introduction of monoamine oxidase inhibitors, tricyclics, and tetracyclics. Part I: monoamine oxidase inhibitors. Journal of Clinical Psychopharmacology, 27(6), 555–559.

Ma Q. (2013). Role of nrf2 in oxidative stress and toxicity. Annual review of pharmacology and toxicology, 53, 401–426. doi.org/10.1146/annurev-pharmtox-011112-140320

Malan-Muller S, Valles-Colomer M, Raes J, Lowry CA, Seedat S, Hemmings SMJ. The Gut Microbiome and Mental Health: Implications for Anxiety- and Trauma-Related Disorders. OMICS. 2018;22(2):90-107.

Ming He, Hou-Hsien Chiang, Hanzhi Luo, Zhifang Zheng, Qi Qiao, Li Wang, Mingdian Tan, Rika Ohkubo, Wei-Chieh Mu, Shimin Zhao, Hao Wu, Danica Chen. An Acetylation Switch of the NLRP3 Inflammasome Regulates Aging-Associated Chronic Inflammation and Insulin Resistance. Cell Metabolism, 2020;

Mu, Q., Kirby, J., Reilly, C. M., & Luo, X. M. (2017). Leaky Gut As a Danger Signal for Autoimmune Diseases. *Frontiers in Immunology, 8.*

Nguyen, T., Nioi, P., & Pickett, C. B. (2009). The Nrf2-antioxidant response element signaling pathway and its activation by oxidative stress. The Journal of biological chemistry, 284(20), 13291–13295. doi.org/10.1074/jbc.R900010200

Pahwa R, Goyal A, Bansal P, et al. Chronic Inflammation. [Updated 2020 Nov 20]. In: StatPearls [Internet]. Treasure Island (FL): StatPearls Publishing; 2020 Jan-. Available from: ncbi.nlm.nih.gov/books/NBK493173/

Prozac. (2005). Chemical & Engineering News, 83(25). Retrieved from pubs.acs.org/cen/coverstory/83/8325/8325prozac.html

Salomon, R. M., Miller, H. L., Krystal, J. H., Heninger, G. R., & Charney, D. S. (1997). Lack of behavioral effects of monoamine depletion in healthy subjects. Biological Psychiatry, 41(1), 58–64.

Schmaal, L., Hibar, D. P., Sämann, P. G., Hall, G. B., Baune, B. T., Jahanshad, N., . . . Veltman, D. J. (2017). Cortical abnormalities in adults and adolescents with major depression based on brain scans from 20 cohorts worldwide in the ENIGMA Major Depressive Disorder Working Group. Molecular Psychiatry, 22(6), 900–909.

Schmaal, L., Veltman, D. J., van Erp, T. G. M., Sämann, P. G., Frodl, T., Jahanshad, N., Hibar, D. P. (2016). Subcortical brain alterations in major depressive disorder: findings from the ENIGMA Major Depressive Disorder working group. Molecular Psychiatry, 21(6), 806–812.

Udenfriend, S., Weissbach, H., & Bogdanski, D. F. (1957). Biochemical Findings Relating to the Action of Serotonin. Annals of the New York Academy of Sciences, 66(3), 602–608.

Wong, D. T., Perry, K. W., & Bymaster, F. P. (2005). The Discovery of Fluoxetine Hydrochloride (Prozac). Nature Reviews Drug Discovery, 4(9), 764–774.

Takahiro Masuda, Roman Sankowski, Ori Staszewski, Chotima Böttcher, Lukas Amann, Christian Scheiwe, Stefan Nessler, Patrik Kunz, Geert van Loo, Volker Arnd Coenen, Peter Christoph Reinacher, Anna Michel, Ulrich Sure, Ralf Gold, Josef Priller, Christine Stadelmann, Marco Prinz. Spatial and temporal heterogeneity of mouse and human microglia at single-cell resolution. Nature, 2019.

Tian L, Ma L, Kaarela T, Li Z. Neuroimmune crosstalk in the central nervous system and its significance for neurological diseases. J Neuroinflammation. 2012;9:155. Published 2012 Jul 2.

Trade Secrets: Chemical Body Burden. (n.d.). Retrieved August 01, 2020, from pbs.org/tradesecrets/problem/bodyburden.html

Weder N, Zhang H, Jensen K, et al. Child abuse, depression, and methylation in genes involved with stress, neural plasticity, and brain circuitry. J Am Acad Child Adolesc Psychiatry. 2014;53(4):417-24.e5.

Yano, J. M., Yu, K., Donaldson, G. P., Shastri, G. G., Ann, P., Ma, L., Nagler, C. R., Ismagilov, R. F., Mazmanian, S. K., & Hsiao, E. Y. (2015). Indigenous bacteria from the gut microbiota regulate host serotonin biosynthesis. Cell, 161(2), 264–276. doi.org/10.1016/j.cell.2015.02.047

Young S. N. (2007). How to increase serotonin in the human brain without drugs. Journal of psychiatry & neuroscience : JPN, 32(6), 394–399.

Zhang, J. M., & An, J. (2007). Cytokines, inflammation, and pain. International anesthesiology clinics, 45(2), 27–37. doi.org/10.1097/AIA.0b013e318034194e

Eating

Adams, J., White, M. Characterisation of UK diets according to degree of food processing and associations with socio-demographics and obesity: cross-sectional analysis of UK National Diet and Nutrition Survey (2008–12). Int J Behav Nutr Phys Act 12, 160 (2015). doi.org/10.1186/s12966-015-0317-y

Bacon, L., & Aphramor, L. (2014). Body respect: What conventional health books get wrong, leave out, and just plain fail to understand about weight. Dallas, TX: BenBella Books.

Bailey, L.R. (1966). "Indian Slave Trade in the Southwest". Los Angeles, CA: Westernlore Press.

Benjamin W. Bellet, Payton J. Jones, Richard J. McNally, Trigger warning: Empirical evidence ahead, Journal of Behavior Therapy and Experimental Psychiatry, Volume 61, 2018, Pages 134-141, doi.org/10.1016/j.jbtep.2018.07.002.

Campbell, P. C. T., Campbell, C. T., Campbell, T. M., Trainor, T., Robbins, J., & Lyman, H. B. (2006). The china study: The most comprehensive study of nutrition ever conducted and the startling implications for diet, weight loss and long-term health. Dallas, TX, USA: Benbella Books.

Carroccio A, D'Alcamo A, Iacono G, Soresi M, Iacobucci R, Arini A, Geraci G, Fayer F, Cavataio F, La Blasca F, Florena AM, Mansueto P. Persistence of Nonceliac Wheat Sensitivity, Based on Long-term Follow-up. Gastroenterology. 2017 Jul;153(1):56-58.e3.

Cerulli, T. (2013). The Mindful Carnivore: A vegetarian's hunt for sustenance. United States: Pegasus Books.

Cheng E, Um CY, Prizment A, Lazovich D, Bostick RM. Associations of evolutionary-concordance diet, Mediterranean diet and evolutionary-concordance lifestyle pattern scores with all-cause and cause-specific mortality. Br J Nutr. 2018 Dec 18:1-10.

Choi HR, Kim J, Lim H, Park YK. Two-Week Exclusive Supplementation of Modified Ketogenic Nutrition Drink Reserves Lean Body Mass and Improves Blood Lipid Profile in Obese Adults: A Randomized Clinical Trial. Nutrients. 2018 Dec 3;10(12):1895.

Colbin, A. (1986). Food and healing. United States: Random House Publishing Group.

Davis, W., Davis, M. d. W., & Philpott, W. H. (2013). Wheat belly: Lose the wheat, lose the weight, and find your path back to health. United States: Rodale Books.

Durant, J. (2014). Paleo manifesto: Ancient wisdom for lifelong health. United States: Harmony Books.

Eating Disorder Statistics. General & Diversity Stats: ANAD. (2020, November 16). Retrieved November 24, 2020, from anad.org/education-and-awareness/about-eating-disorders/eating-disorders-statistics/

Emery, P. (2003). PROTEIN | Digestion and Absorption of Protein and Nitrogen Balance. Encyclopedia of Food Sciences and Nutrition, 4854–4858.

Farm Bill Spending. (n.d.). Retrieved December 03, 2020, from ers.usda.gov/topics/farm-economy/farm-commodity-policy/farm-bill-spending/

Farooqi IS, O'Rahilly S. The Genetics of Obesity in Humans. [Updated 2017 Dec 23]. In: Feingold KR, Anawalt B, Boyce A, et al., editors. Endotext [Internet]. South Dartmouth (MA): MDText.com, Inc.; 2000-. Available from: ncbi.nlm.nih.gov/books/NBK279064/

Friend, Y. (2019, October 18). The Bizarre and Racist History of the BMI. Retrieved November 27, 2020, from elemental.medium.com/the-bizarre-and-racist-history-of-the-bmi-7d8dc2aa33bb

Gómez-Ambrosi, J., Silva, C., Galofré, J. C., Escalada, J., Santos, S., Gil, M. J., Valentí, V., Rotellar, F., Ramírez, B., Salvador, J., & Frühbeck, G. (2011). Body adiposity and type 2 diabetes: increased risk with a high body fat percentage even having a normal BMI. Obesity (Silver Spring, Md.), 19(7), 1439–1444. doi.org/10.1038/oby.2011.36

Finlay, B. B., & Finlay, J. M. (2019). The whole-body microbiome: How to harness microbes—inside and out—for lifelong health. Madeira Park, British Columbia: Douglas and McIntyre.

Francis, H. M., Stevenson, R. J., Chambers, J. R., Gupta, D., Newey, B., & Lim, C. K. (2019). A brief diet intervention can reduce symptoms of depression in young adults – A randomised controlled trial. Plos One, 14(10).

Fuel Your Gut With Prebiotics. (2019, Fall). Nutrition Health Review, (124), 9.

Glickman, Dan, and Dariush Mozaffarian. "Our Food Is Killing Too Many of Us." The New York Times, The New York Times, 26 Aug. 2019, nytimes.com/2019/08/26/opinion/food-nutrition-health-care.html.

Health Benefits of Fermented Foods. (2019, Fall). Nutrition Health Review, (124), 9.

Ives, G. C., Fein, L. A., Finch, L., Sluiter, E. C., Lane, M., Kuzon, W. M., & Salgado, C. J. (2019). Evaluation of BMI as a Risk Factor for Complications following Gender-affirming Penile Inversion Vaginoplasty. Plastic and reconstructive surgery. Global open, 7(3), e2097. doi.org/10.1097/GOX.0000000000002097

Jackson, A., Stanforth, P., Gagnon, J. et al. The effect of sex, age and race on estimating percentage body fat from body mass index: The Heritage Family Study. Int J Obes 26, 789–796 (2002). doi.org/10.1038/sj.ijo.0802006

Kaplan, Hillard, et al. "Coronary Atherosclerosis in Indigenous South American Tsimane: a Cross-Sectional Cohort Study." The Lancet, vol. 389, no. 10080, 2017, pp. 1730–1739.

Kolata, G. (2016, December 12). One Weight-Loss Approach Fits All? No, Not Even Close. Retrieved December 02, 2020, from nytimes.com/2016/12/12/health/weight-loss-obesity.html

Loh, W., & Tang, M. (2018). The Epidemiology of Food Allergy in the Global Context. International journal of environmental research and public health, 15(9), 2043. doi.org/10.3390/ijerph15092043

Moss, M. (2013, February 20). The Extraordinary Science of Addictive Junk Food. Retrieved October 01, 2020, from nytimes.com/2013/02/24/magazine/the-extraordinary-science-of-junk-food.html

Mozaffarian D, Mande J, Micha R. Food Is Medicine—The Promise and Challenges of Integrating Food and Nutrition Into Health Care. JAMA Intern Med. 2019;179(6):793–795.

Negative Affect, Intrusive Thoughts, and Avoidance. Clinical Psychological Science, 7(4), 778–793. doi.org/10.1177/2167702619827018

Nova groups for food processing. (n.d.). Retrieved September 30, 2020, from world.openfoodfacts.org/nova

O'connor, A. (2016, July 19). How the Government Supports Your Junk Food Habit. Retrieved December 02, 2020, from well.blogs.nytimes.com/2016/07/19/how-the-government-supports-your-junk-food-habit/

Pace, T. W., Negi, L. T., Adame, D. D., Cole, S. P., Sivilli, T. I., Brown, T. D., Issa, M. J., & Raison, C. L. (2009). Effect of compassion meditation on neuroendocrine, innate immune and behavioral responses to psychosocial stress. Psychoneuroendocrinology, 34(1), 87–98. doi.org/10.1016/j.psyneuen.2008.08.011

Processed Foods. What they are, how they affect our bodies, and how to avoid them.. (2019, Spring). Nutrition Health Review, (124), 7-9.

"Public Impact Initiative: Food Is Medicine." Public Impact Initiative: Food Is Medicine | Friedman School of Nutrition Science and Policy, nutrition.tufts.edu/about/public-impact-initiative-friedman-school/food-is-medicine.

Susan B Racette, Susan S Deusinger, Robert H Deusinger, Obesity: Overview of Prevalence, Etiology, and Treatment, Physical Therapy, Volume 83, Issue 3, 1 March 2003, Pages 276–288, doi.org/10.1093/ptj/83.3.276

Rahman, M., & Berenson, A. B. (2010). Accuracy of current body mass index obesity classification for white, black, and Hispanic reproductive-age women. Obstetrics and gynecology, 115(5), 982–988. doi.org/10.1097/AOG.0b013e3181da9423

Reducing Chronic Inflammation. (Jan-Feb, 2020). Nutrition Health Review, (126), 15-17.

Sacks, F. M., Bray, G. A., Carey, V. J., Smith, S. R., Ryan, D. H., Anton, S. D., . . . Williamson, D. A. (2009). Comparison of Weight-Loss Diets with Different Compositions of Fat, Protein, and Carbohydrates. New England Journal of Medicine, 360(9), 859-873.

Strings, S. (2019). Fearing the Black Body. New York University Press.

The Endocrine Society. (2009, June 22). Widely Used Body Fat Measurements Overestimate Fatness In African-Americans, Study Finds. ScienceDaily. Retrieved November 22, 2020 from sciencedaily.com/releases/2009/06/090611142407.htm

The Gut Microbiota-Obesity Connection. (2019, Fall). Nutrition Health Review, (127), 6-8.

The Gut Microbiota-Obesity Connection. (2019, Fall). Nutrition Health Review, (124), 9.

The Role of Nutrition in Brain Health. (2020, March-APril). Nutrition Health Review, (124), 9.

Wood, R., Pitchford, P., & Markel, P. (1999). The new whole foods encyclopedia: A comprehensive resource for healthy eating. New York, NY: Penguin/Arkana.

Why Processed Food Is Cheaper Than Healthier Options. (2013, March 01). Retrieved October 01, 2020, from npr.org/2013/03/01/173217143/why-process-food-is-cheaper-than-healthier-options

Willett WC, Koplan JP, Nugent R, et al. Prevention of Chronic Disease by Means of Diet and Lifestyle Changes. In: Jamison DT, Breman JG, Measham AR, et al., editors. Disease Control Priorities in Developing Countries. 2nd edition. Washington (DC): The International Bank for Reconstruction and Development / The World Bank; 2006. Chapter 44. Available from: ncbi.nlm.nih.gov/books/NBK11795/ Co-published by Oxford University Press, New York.

Jensen, B., & Anderson, M. (2000). Empty harvest: Understanding the link between our food, our immunity and our planet. United States: Avery Publishing Group Inc.,U.S.

Johnston, A. (2000). Eating in the light of the moon: How women can transform their relationship with food through myths, metaphors and storytelling. United States: Gurze Books.

Levin, P., & Lee, J. (2002). Perfect bones: A Six-Point plan for healthy bones. United States: Celestial Arts.

Medford, L., & C.N, E. C. (1999). Why can't I lose weight? United States: L D N Publishing.

Moss, M., & Professor of History Michael Moss (2013). Salt, sugar, fat: How the food giants hooked us. New York: Random House Publishing Group.

Möller, G. (2006). Animal drug residues in food. Retrieved from webpages.uidaho.edu/foodtox/lectures/lecture22/L22-Animal%20Drug%20Residues%20in%20Food.pdf

National Research Council (1999). The use of drugs in food animals. Retrieved July 2, 2016, from nap.edu/read/5137/chapter/7

NCBI Bookshelf (1980). Antibiotics in Animal Feeds - The Effects on Human Health of Subtherapeutic Use of Antimicrobials in Animal Feeds. Retrieved from ncbi.nlm.nih.gov/books/NBK216502/

News, F. S. (2010, April 1). How Sulfa-Loaded Beef Gets To Market | Food Safety News. Retrieved July 2, 2016, from foodsafetynews.com/2010/04/how-sulfa-loaded-beef-gets-to-market/

Paul, G. (2014). Eat yourself calm. United States: Hamlyn (UK).

Philpott, T. (2014, April 23). Monsanto GM Soy Is Scarier Than You Think | Mother Jones. Retrieved July 2, 2016, from m.motherjones.com/tom-philpott/2014/04/superweeds-arent-only-trouble-gmo-soy

Quillin, P. (2010). Wisdom and healing power of whole foods: The ultimate handbook for using whole foods and lifestyle changes to bolster your body's ability to repair and regulate itself. United States: Leader Company

Schimke, D., Grumdahl, D. M., Staff, E. L., Olson, K., Wachter, H., Terry, B., . . . Anthony, M. (2004, March). Big Fat Controversy □ Experience Life. Retrieved July 3, 2016, from experiencelife.com/article/big-fat-controversy/

Schmidt, R. (1987). Traditional foods are your best medicine. (1st ed.). New York: Ballantine.

Somer, E. (1995). Food and mood. New York: Holt.

Steinman, D., & Marcus, W. (2006). Diet for a poisoned planet: How to choose safe foods for you and your family - the Twenty-first century edition (21st ed.). United States: Running Press.

Stitt, B. R. (1997). Food & behavior. Natural Press.

The National Academies Press (1999). 5 Drug Residues and Microbial Contamination in Food | The Use of Drugs in Food Animals: Benefits and Risks. Retrieved from nap.edu/read/5137/chapter/7

Movement

Benias, P.C., Wells, R.G., Sackey-Aboagye, B. et al. Structure and Distribution of an Unrecognized Interstitium in Human Tissues. Sci Rep 8, 4947 (2018). doi.org/10.1038/s41598-018-23062-6

Borghouts, L. B., & Keizer, H. A. (2000). Exercise and Insulin Sensitivity: A Review. International Journal of Sports Medicine, 21(1), 1-12.

Muehsam, D., Lutgendorf, S., Mills, P. J., Rickhi, B., Chevalier, G., Bat, N., et al. (2017). The embodied mind: a review on functional genomic and neurological correlates of mind-body therapies. Neurosci. Biobehav. Rev. 73, 165–181.

Craig, A.D.. (2003). Interoception: The Sense of the Physiological Condition of the Body. Current opinion in neurobiology. 13. 500-5. 10.1016/S0959-4388(03)00090-4.

Healthy Ways To Deal With Stress. (2020). Nutrition Health Review, (129), 4–7.

Mond, J. M., Hay, P. J., Rodgers, B., & Owen, C. (2006). An update on the definition of "excessive exercise" in eating disorders research. International Journal of Eating Disorders, 39(2), 147-153.

Reducing Chronic Inflammation. (Jan-Feb, 2020). Nutrition Health Review, (126), 15-17.

Sullivan, Marlysa B., et al. "Yoga Therapy and Polyvagal Theory: The Convergence of Traditional Wisdom and Contemporary Neuroscience for Self-Regulation and Resilience." Frontiers in Human Neuroscience, vol. 12, 2018.

Taylor, A. G., Goehler, L. E., Galper, D. I., Innes, K. E., and Bourguignon, C. (2010). Top-down and Bottom-up mechanisms in mind-body medicine: development of an integrative framework for psychophysiological research. Explore 6, 29–41.

Trivedi, M. H., Greer, T. L., Church, T. S., Carmody, T. J., Grannemann, B. D., Galper, D. I., . . . Blair, S. N. (2011). Exercise as an Augmentation Treatment for Nonremitted Major Depressive Disorder. The Journal of Clinical Psychiatry, 72(05), 677-684.

Young SN. How to increase serotonin in the human brain without drugs. J Psychiatry Neurosci. 2007;32(6):394-399.

Stress

"Adrenaline and Noradrenaline." Encyclopedia of Life Sciences, els.net/WileyCDA/ElsArticle/refId-a0001401.html

Asbert, M. (1976). Serotonin depression: A biochemical subgroup with the affective disorders? Science,191, 478-80; Asberg, M., (1976). 5-HIAA in the cerebrospinal fluid. Archives of General Psychiatry, 33, 1193-97.

Asbert, M. (1976). Serotonin depression: A biochemical subgroup with the affective disorders? Science,191, 478-80; Asberg, M., (1976). 5-HIAA in the cerebrospinal fluid. Archives of General Psychiatry, 33, 1193-97.

Bellono NW, Bayrer JR, Leitch DB, et al. Enterochromaffin Cells Are Gut Chemosensors that Couple to Sensory Neural Pathways. Cell. 2017;170(1):185-198.e16.

Berk, M., Kapczinski, F., Andreazza, A. C., Dean, O. M., Giorlando, F., Maes, M., . . . & Magalhães, P. V. S. (2011). Pathways underlying neuroprogression in bipolar disorder: focus on inflammation, oxidative stress and neurotrophic factors. Neuroscience & biobehavioral reviews, 35(3), 804-817.

Breit, S., Kupferberg, A., Rogler, G., & Hasler, G. (2018). Vagus Nerve as Modulator of the Brain-Gut Axis in Psychiatric and Inflammatory Disorders. Frontiers in psychiatry, 9, 44. doi.org/10.3389/fpsyt.2018.00044

Bullmore, Edward T. The Inflamed Mind: a Radical New Approach to Depression. Short Books, 2019.

Butts KA, Weinberg J, Young AH, & Phillips AG (2011). Glucocorticoid receptors in the prefrontal cortex regulate stress-evoked dopamine efflux and aspects of executive function. Proceedings of the National Academy of Sciences of the United States of America, 108 (45), 18459-64 PMID: 22032926

Callaghan, B. L., Fields, A., Gee, D. G., Gabard-Durnam, L., Caldera, C., Humphreys, K. L., . . . & Tottenham, N. (2019). Mind and gut: Associations between mood and gastrointestinal distress in children exposed to adversity. Development and psychopathology, 1-20.

Chang, T. T., Yen, Y-C., (2010). Cytokines and Major Psychiatric Disorders. Taiwanese Journal of Psychiatry (Taipei) Vol. 24 No. 4, 257-268.

Charmandari E, Nicolaides NC, Chrousos GP. Adrenal insufficiency. Lancet.

2014 Jun 21;383(9935):2152-67.

Crawford LE, Knouse LE, Kent M, et al. Enriched environment exposure accelerates rodent driving skills. Behav Brain Res. 2020;378:112309.

Dietrich J, Han R, Yang Y, Mayer-Pröschel M, Noble M. CNS progenitor cells and oligodendrocytes are targets of chemotherapeutic agents in vitro and in vivo. J Biol. 2006;5(7):22.

Dobbin, J. P., Harth, M., McCain, G. A., Martin, R. A., & Cousin, K. (1991). Cytokine production and lymphocyte transformation during stress. Brain, behavior, and immunity, 5(4), 339-348.

Field, Tiffany, et al. "Cortisol Decreases and Serotonin and Dopamine Increase Following Massage Therapy." The International Journal of Neuroscience, U.S. National Library of Medicine, Oct. 2005, ncbi.nlm.nih.gov/pubmed/16162447/.

Foster, J. A., Rinaman, L., & Cryan, J. F. (2017). Stress & the gut-brain axis: regulation by the microbiome. Neurobiology of stress, 7, 124-136.

Gallup, Inc. "Gallup 2018 Global Emotions Report." Gallup.com, gallup.com/analytics/241961/gallup-global-emotions-report-2018.aspx?utm_source=link_newsv9&utm_campaign=item_242117&utm_medium=copy.

Gershon, M. D. (1999). The enteric nervous system: a second brain. Hospital Practice, 34(7), 31-52

Gibson, E. M., Nagaraja, S., Ocampo, A., Tam, L. T., Wood, L. S., Pallegar, P. N., . . . Monje, M. (2019). Methotrexate Chemotherapy Induces Persistent Tri-glial Dysregulation that Underlies Chemotherapy-Related Cognitive Impairment. Cell, 176(1-2).

Guilliams , Thomas G. The Role of Stress and the HPA Axis in Chronic Disease Management Principles and Protocols for Healthcare Professionals. Point Institute.

Haas, Robert, et al. "Lactate Regulates Metabolic and Pro-Inflammatory Circuits in Control of T Cell Migration and Effector Functions." PLOS Biology, vol. 13, no. 7, 2015.

Haroon, E., Raison, C. L., & Miller, A. H. (2012). Psychoneuroimmunology meets neuropsychopharmacology: translational implications of the impact of inflammation on behavior. Neuropsychopharmacology, 37(1), 137.

He, Ming, et al. "An Acetylation Switch of the NLRP3 Inflammasome Regulates Aging-Associated Chronic Inflammation and Insulin Resistance." Cell Metabolism, vol. 31, no. 3, 2020.

Hemmings, S. M., Malan-Muller, S., van den Heuvel, L. L., Demmitt, B. A., Stanislawski, M. A., Smith, D. G., . . . & Marotz, C. A. (2017). The microbiome in posttraumatic stress disorder and trauma-exposed controls: an exploratory study. Psychosomatic medicine, 79(8), 936.

Hong-Ji, Kim. "South Koreans Lock Themselves up to Escape Prison of Daily Life." Reuters, Thomson Reuters, widerimage.reuters.com/story/south-koreans-lock-themselves-up-to-escape-prison-of-daily-life.

Hyman, Mark. The UltraMind Solution: Fix Your Broken Brain by Healing Your Body First: the Simple Way to Defeat Depression, Overcome Anxiety, and Sharpen Your Mind. Scribner, 2010.

Keller, Abiola, et al. Current Neurology and Neuroscience Reports., U.S. National Library of Medicine, Sept. 2012, ncbi.nlm.nih.gov/pmc/articles/PMC3374921/#R21.

Kirsch, Irving. The Emperor's New Drugs: Exploding the Antidepressant Myth. Basic Books, 2011.

Koopman, F. A., Chavan, S. S., Miljko, S., Grazio, S., Sokolovic, S., Schuurman, P. R., Tak, P. P. (2016). Vagus nerve stimulation inhibits cytokine production and attenuates disease severity in rheumatoid arthritis. Proceedings of the National Academy of Sciences, 113(29), 8284-8289.

Lacasse, JR & Leo, J. (2005). Serotonin and Depression: A Disconnect between the Advertisements and the Scientific Literature. PLOS Medicine.

Larochelle, C. (2020, February 04). More than a knee injury: ACL tears cause harmful changes in our brain structure. Retrieved July 28, 2020, from news.umich.edu/more-than-a-knee-injury-acl-tears-cause-harmful-changes-in-our-brain-structure/

Martin, C. R., Osadchiy, V., Kalani, A., & Mayer, E. A. (2018). The Brain-Gut-Microbiome Axis. Cellular and Molecular Gastroenterology and Hepatology, 6(2), 133-148.

Michopoulos, V., Powers, A., Gillespie, C. F., Ressler, K. J., & Jovanovic, T. (2017). Inflammation in fear-and anxiety-based disorders: PTSD, GAD, and beyond. Neuropsychopharmacology, 42(1), 254.

Milaniak, I., & Jaffee, S. R. (2019). Childhood socioeconomic status and inflammation: A systematic review and meta-analysis. Brain, behavior, and immunity.

Monje, M. L. (2003). Inflammatory Blockade Restores Adult Hippocampal Neurogenesis. Science, 302(5651), 1760-1765.

Papierska, L., & Rabijewski, M. (2013). Delay in diagnosis of adrenal insufficiency is a frequent cause of adrenal crisis. International journal of endocrinology, 2013, 482370. doi.org/10.1155/2013/482370

Renna, M. E., O'toole, M. S., Spaeth, P. E., Lekander, M., & Mennin, D. S. (2018). The association between anxiety, traumatic stress, and obsessive–compulsive disorders and chronic inflammation: A systematic review and meta□analysis. Depression and anxiety, 35(11), 1081-1094.

Smith S. R. (1997). Immunological Evidence Supporting The Immune-Cytokine Model of Depression. Cytokines and Depression.

Smith, Sean M., and Wylie W. Vale. Current Neurology and Neuroscience Reports., U.S. National Library of Medicine, Dec. 2006, ncbi.nlm.nih.gov/pmc/articles/PMC3181830/.

Stanley, et al. "Stressed out and Not Thinking Straight? Blame Dopamine Release in Your Prefrontal Cortex." Neurotic Physiology, 14 Sept. 2017, scicurious.scientopia.org/2012/12/05/stressed-out-and-not-thinking-straight-blame-the-dopamine-in-your-prefrontal-cortex/.

Sylvia, K. E., & Demas, G. E. (2018). A gut feeling: microbiome-brain-immune interactions modulate social and affective behaviors. Hormones and behavior, 99, 41-49.

Tattersall RB. Hypoadrenia or "a bit of Addison's disease". Med Hist.

1999 Oct;43(4):450-67.

Toft, H., Bramness, J. G., Lien, L., Abebe, D. S., Wampold, B. E., Tilden, T., . . . & Neupane, S. P. (2018). PTsD patients show increasing cytokine levels during treatment despite reduced psychological distress. Neuropsychiatric disease and treatment, 14, 2367.

Werbner, M., Barsheshet, Y., Werbner, N., Zigdon, M., Averbuch, I., Ziv, O., . . . & Koren, O. (2019). Social-Stress-Responsive Microbiota Induces Stimulation of Self-Reactive Effector T Helper Cells. mSystems, 4(4), e00292-18.

Valles-Colomer, Mireia, et al. "The Neuroactive Potential of the Human Gut Microbiota in Quality of Life and Depression." Nature Microbiology, vol. 4, no. 4, 2019, pp. 623–632.

Valles-Colomer, M., Falony, G., Darzi, Y. et al. The neuroactive potential of the human gut microbiota in quality of life and depression. Nat Microbiol 4, 623–632 (2019). doi.org/10.1038/s41564-018-0337-x

Taylor, Alan. "A Weekend in a Prison Cell to Escape Modern Life." The Atlantic, Atlantic Media Company, 26 Nov. 2018, theatlantic.com/photo/2018/11/weekend-in-a-prison-cell-to-escape-modern-life/576652/.

Treadway, M. T., Cooper, J. A., & Miller, A. H. (2019). Can't or Won't? Immunometabolic Constraints on Dopaminergic Drive. Trends in Cognitive Sciences, 23(5), 435-448.

Weintraub, Karen. "'Stress Hormone' Cortisol Linked to Early Toll on Thinking Ability." Scientific American, 25 Oct. 2018, scientificamerican.com/article/ldquo-stress-hormone-rdquo-cortisol-linked-to-early-toll-on-thinking-ability/

Whitaker, R. (2010). Anatomy of an Epidemic: Magic Bullets, Psychiatric Drugs and the Astonishing Rise of Mental Illness in America. Crown Publishing.

Viena TD, Banks JB, Barbu IM, Schulman AH, Tartar JL. Differential effects of mild chronic stress on cortisol and S-IgA responses to an acute stressor. Biol Psychol. 2012;91(2):307-311.

Yano, J., Yu, K., Donaldson, G., Shastri, G., Ann, P., Ma, L., . . . Hsiao, E. (2015). Indigenous Bacteria from the Gut Microbiota Regulate Host Serotonin Biosynthesis. Cell, 161(2), 264-276.

You and Your Hormones, yourhormones.info/hormones/adrenaline/.

Zhang, Maochen, et al. "Illness Perceptions and Stress: Mediators between Disease Severity and | PPA." Journal of Pain Research, Dove Press, 23 Nov. 2016.

Supplements

Chaparro, C. M., & Dewey, K. G. (2010). Use of lipid-based nutrient supplements (LNS) to improve the nutrient adequacy of general food distribution rations for vulnerable sub-groups in emergency settings. Maternal & child nutrition, 6 Suppl 1(Suppl 1), 1–69. doi.org/10.1111/j.1740-8709.2009.00224.x

Cortese, M., Riise, T., Bjørnevik, K., Holmøy, T., Kampman, M. T., Magalhaes, S., Pugliatti, M., Wolfson, C., & Myhr, K. M. (2015). Timing of use of cod liver oil, a vitamin D source, and multiple sclerosis risk: The EnvIMS study. Multiple sclerosis (Houndmills, Basingstoke, England), 21(14), 1856–1864. doi.org/10.1177/1352458515578770

DeDea, Larissa PharmD, BCPS, PA-C When to take statins; Lovaza versus OTC fish oil supplements, Journal of the American Academy of PAs: May 2011 - Volume 24 - Issue 5 - p 23

DiNicolantonio JJ, O'Keefe JH, Wilson W. Subclinical magnesium deficiency: a principal driver of cardiovascular disease and a public health crisis. Open Heart 2018;5:e000668.

Doleyres, Y. and Lacroix, C. (2005) Technologies with free and immobilised cells for probiotic bifidobacteria production and protection. Int Dairy J 15, 973–988.

D'Souza, A.L., Rajkumar, C., Cooke, J. and Bulpitt, C.J. (2002) Probiotics in prevention of antibiotic associated diarrhoea: meta-analysis. BMJ 324, 1361–1366.

Eseceli, H. (2020). Pro-/Anti-Inflammatory Food Supplements: Probiotics and Prebiotics. In Gün□en, U., & Atan, R. M. (Eds.), Role of Nutrition in Providing Pro-/Anti-Inflammatory Balance: Emerging Research and Opportunities (pp. 142-168). IGI Global.

Fast foods make flu shot even less effective. (2019, April 7). Experimental Biology Annual Meeting.

Fuller, R. (1989) Probiotics in man and animals. J Appl Bacteriol 66, 365–378.

Gill, H.S. and Guarner, F. (2004) Probiotics and human health: a clinical perspective. Postgrad Med J 80, 516–526.

Gordon, D. (2019, May/June). 10 Concerns About Supplements. Spirituality and Health.

Gruner, T., & Arthur, R. (2012). The accuracy of the Zinc Taste Test method. Journal of alternative and complementary medicine (New York, N.Y.), 18(6), 541–550. doi.org/10.1089/acm.2011.0298

Ito M. K. (2015). A Comparative Overview of Prescription Omega-3 Fatty Acid Products. P & T : a peer-reviewed journal for formulary management, 40(12), 826–857.

Khan, A., Zaman, G., & Anderson, R. A. (2009). Bay leaves improve glucose and lipid profile of people with type 2 diabetes. Journal of clinical biochemistry and nutrition, 44(1), 52–56. doi.org/10.3164/jcbn.08-188

Karadima V, Kraniotou C, Bellos G, Tsangaris GT. Drug-micronutrient interactions: Food for thought and thought for action. EPMA J. 2016;7:10.

LaValle JB. Hidden disruptions in metabolic syndrome: drug-induced nutrient depletion as a pathway to accelerated pathophysiology of metabolic syndrome. Altern Ther Health Med. 2006;12(2):26-31.

Levine, H. (n.d.). Can Your Medications Cause Depression? Retrieved July 28, 2020, from consumerreports.org/drugs/can-medications-cause-depression/

Swardfager, W., Herrmann, N., McIntyre, R. S., Mazereeuw, G., Goldberger, K., Cha, D. S., Schwartz, Y., & Lanctôt, K. L. (2013). Potential roles of zinc in the pathophysiology and treatment of major depressive disorder. Neuroscience and biobehavioral reviews, 37(5), 911–929. doi.org/10.1016/j.neubiorev.2013.03.018

Markowitz JS, Donovan JL, DeVane CL, et al. Effect of St John's wort on drug metabolism by induction of cytochrome P450 3A4 enzyme. JAMA. 2003;290:1500-1504.

Maret W, Sandstead HH. Zinc requirements and the risks and benefits of zinc supplementation. J Trace Elem Med Biol 2006;20:3-18.

Maxfield L, Crane JS. Zinc Deficiency. [Updated 2020 Jul 2]. In: StatPearls [Internet]. Treasure Island (FL): StatPearls Publishing; 2020 Jan-. Available from: ncbi.nlm.nih.gov/books/NBK493231/

Mehta, N. M., & Duggan, C. P. (2009). Nutritional deficiencies during critical illness. Pediatric clinics of North America, 56(5), 1143–1160. doi.org/10.1016/j.pcl.2009.06.007

Mohn, E. S., Kern, H. J., Saltzman, E., Mitmesser, S. H., & McKay, D. L. (2018). Evidence of Drug-Nutrient Interactions with Chronic Use of Commonly Prescribed Medications: An Update. Pharmaceutics, 10(1), 36. doi.org/10.3390/pharmaceutics10010036

Paredes, S. D., Marchena, A. M., Bejarano, I., Espino, J., Barriga, C., Rial, R. V., Reiter, R. J., & Rodríguez, A. B. (2009). Melatonin and tryptophan affect the activity-rest rhythm, core and peripheral temperatures, and interleukin levels in the ringdove: changes with age. The journals of gerontology. Series A, Biological sciences and medical sciences, 64(3), 340–350. doi.org/10.1093/gerona/gln054

Prasad AS, Beck FW, Grabowski SM, Kaplan J, Mathog RH. Zinc deficiency: changes in cytokine production and T-cell subpopulations in patients with head and neck cancer and in noncancer subjects. Proc Assoc Am Physicians 1997;109:68-77.

Rashrash, M., Schommer, J. C., & Brown, L. M. (2017). Prevalence and Predictors of Herbal Medicine Use Among Adults in the United States. Journal of patient experience, 4(3), 108–113. doi.org/10.1177/2374373517706612

Reducing Chronic Inflammation. (Jan-Feb, 2020). Nutrition Health Review, (126), 15-17.

Richard, D. M., Dawes, M. A., Mathias, C. W., Acheson, A., Hill-Kapturczak, N., & Dougherty, D. M. (2009). L-Tryptophan: Basic Metabolic Functions, Behavioral Research and Therapeutic Indications. International journal of tryptophan research : IJTR, 2, 45–60. doi.org/10.4137/ijtr.s2129

Romani A. M. (2011). Cellular magnesium homeostasis. Archives of biochemistry and biophysics, 512(1), 1–23. doi.org/10.1016/j.abb.2011.05.010

Sandstead HH. Understanding zinc: recent observations and interpretations. J Lab Clin Med 1994;124:322-7.

Singh, V., Mohammad, S., & Singh, N. (2012). Herbs and surgery. National journal of maxillofacial surgery, 3(1), 101–106. doi.org/10.4103/0975-5950.102180

Temple University. "Novel Protein In St. John's Wort Found To Suppress HIV-1 Gene Expression." ScienceDaily. ScienceDaily, 25 October 2005. sciencedaily.com/releases/2005/10/051025074707.htm>.

The Truth About Antibiotics. (2016, December). Family Circle.

Van Zyl M. The effects of drugs on nutrition. S Afr J Clin Nutr. 2011;24(3):S38-S41.

Vitamin D and Magnesium for Managing Depression. (2012, March-April). Nutrition Health Review, (127), 6-8.

Young SN. How to increase serotonin in the human brain without drugs. J Psychiatry Neurosci. 2007;32(6):394-399.

Vagal System

Bargas, J., & Pérez-Ortega, J. (2017). Microcircuits neuroscience to understand pathophysiology. Oncotarget, 8(5), 7226–7227. doi.org/10.18632/oncotarget.14792

Bracha H. S. (2004). Freeze, flight, fight, fright, faint: adaptationist perspectives on the acute stress response spectrum. CNS spectrums, 9(9), 679–685. doi.org/10.1017/s1092852900001954

Bordoni, B., Morabito, B., Mitrano, R., Simonelli, M., & Toccafondi, A. (2018). The Anatomical Relationships of the Tongue with the Body System. Cureus, 10(12), e3695. doi.org/10.7759/cureus.3695

Breit, S., Kupferberg, A., Rogler, G., & Hasler, G. (2018). Vagus Nerve as Modulator of the Brain-Gut Axis in Psychiatric and Inflammatory Disorders. Frontiers in psychiatry, 9, 44. doi.org/10.3389/fpsyt.2018.00044

Burton, C. M., & King, L. A. (2004). The health benefits of writing about intensely positive experiences. Journal of Research in Personality, 38(2), 150-163.

Csikszentmihalyi, Mark. (2006). Readings in Han Chinese Thought. Indianapolis and Cambridge: Hackett Publishing Company, Inc. ISBN 0-87220-710-2.

Craig A. D. (2002). How do you feel? Interoception: the sense of the physiological condition of the body. Nature reviews. Neuroscience, 3(8), 655–666. doi.org/10.1038/nrn894

Critchley, Hugo D., and Neil A. Harrison. "Visceral Influences on Brain and Behavior." Neuron, vol. 77, no. 4, 2013, pp. 624–638.

Dana, D., & Porges, S. W. (2020). Polyvagal exercises for safety and connection: 50 client-centered practices. New York: W.W. Norton & Company.

Dana, D., & Porges, S. W. (2018). The polyvagal theory in therapy: Engaging the rhythm of regulation. New York: W.W. Norton & Company

Porges, S. W., & Dana, D. (2018). Clinical applications of the polyvagal theory: The emergence of polyvagal-informed therapies. New York (N.Y.): W.W. Norton & Company.

Darwin C. The Expression of Emotions in Man and Animals. D Appleton; New York, NY: 1872.

Kandel, E. R., Dudai, Y., & Mayford, M. R. (2014). The molecular and systems biology of memory. Cell, 157(1), 163–186. doi.org/10.1016/j.cell.2014.03.001

Koopman, F. A., Chavan, S. S., Miljko, S., Grazio, S., Sokolovic, S., Schuurman, P. R., . . . Tak, P. P. (2016). Vagus nerve stimulation inhibits cytokine production and attenuates disease severity in rheumatoid arthritis. Proceedings of the National Academy of Sciences, 113(29), 8284–8289.

Kok, B. E., Coffey, K. A., Cohn, M. A., Catalino, L. I., Vacharkulksemsuk, T., Algoe, S. B., . Fredrickson, B. L. (2013). How Positive Emotions Build Physical Health. Psychological Science, 24(7), 1123-1132.

Karen-Anne McVey Neufeld, John Bienenstock, Aadil Bharwani, Kevin Champagne-Jorgensen, YuKang Mao, Christine West, Yunpeng Liu, Michael G. Surette, Wolfgang Kunze & Paul Forsythe. "Oral Selective Serotonin Reuptake Inhibitors Activate Vagus Nerve Dependent Gut-Brain Signalling." Scientific Reports (First published: October 3, 2019)

Laborde, S., Mosley, E., & Thayer, J. F. (2017). Heart Rate Variability and Cardiac Vagal Tone in Psychophysiological Research - Recommendations for Experiment Planning, Data Analysis, and Data Reporting. Frontiers in psychology, 8, 213. doi.org/10.3389/fpsyg.2017.00213

Levine, P. A. (2010). In an unspoken voice: How the baby releases trauma and restores goodness. Barkeley, CA: North Atlantic Books.

Levine, P. A., & Frederick, A. (1997). Waking the tiger: Healing trauma: The innate capacity to transform overwhelming experiences. Berkeley, CA: North Atlantic Books.

Maehle A. H. (2004). "Receptive substances": John Newport Langley (1852-1925) and his path to a receptor theory of drug action. Medical history, 48(2), 153–174. doi.org/10.1017/s0025727300000090

Murray, A. R., Atkinson, L., Mahadi, M. K., Deuchars, S. A., & Deuchars, J. (2016). The strange case of the ear and the heart: The auricular vagus nerve and its influence on cardiac control. Autonomic Neuroscience, 199, 48-53.

Novella, Steven (25 January 2012). "What Is Traditional Chinese Medicine?". sciencebasedmedicine.org. Society for Science-Based Medicine. Retrieved 13 May 2015.

Porges, S. W. (2011). The polyvagal theory: Neurophysiological foundations of emotions, attachment, communication, and self-regulation. New York: Norton.

Porges S. W. (2009). The polyvagal theory: new insights into adaptive reactions of the autonomic nervous system. Cleveland Clinic journal of medicine, 76 Suppl 2(Suppl 2), S86–S90. doi.org/10.3949/ccjm.76.s2.17

Porges S. W. (2007). The polyvagal perspective. Biological psychology, 74(2), 116–143. doi.org/10.1016/j.biopsycho.2006.06.009

Porges S. W. (2001). The polyvagal theory: phylogenetic substrates of a social nervous system. International journal of psychophysiology : official journal of the International Organization of Psychophysiology, 42(2), 123–146. doi.org/10.1016/s0167-8760(01)00162-3

Price, C. J., & Hooven, C. (2018). Interoceptive Awareness Skills for Emotion Regulation: Theory and Approach of Mindful Awareness in Body-Oriented Therapy (MABT). Frontiers in psychology, 9, 798. doi.org/10.3389/fpsyg.2018.00798

Rao, M., Gershon, M. The bowel and beyond: the enteric nervous system in neurological disorders. Nat Rev Gastroenterol Hepatol 13, 517–528 (2016). doi.org/10.1038/nrgastro.2016.107

Schmidt, J. E., Carlson, C. R., Usery, A. R., & Quevedo, A. S. (2009). Effects of tongue position on mandibular muscle activity and heart rate function. Oral surgery, oral medicine, oral pathology, oral radiology, and endodontics, 108(6), 881–888. doi.org/10.1016/j.tripleo.2009.06.029

Squires, S. (1985, August 21). Molecules of Emotion. Retrieved October 27, 2020, from washingtonpost.com/archive/lifestyle/wellness/1985/08/21/molecules-of-emotion/b9357aaa-a702-425c-a832-0dd3a182b2c3/

Tanida, M., Niijima, A., Shen, J., Nakamura, T., & Nagai, K. (2005). Olfactory stimulation with scent of essential oil of grapefruit affects autonomic neurotransmission and blood pressure. Brain research, 1058(1-2), 44–55. doi.org/10.1016/j.brainres.2005.07.048

Trampe D, Quoidbach J, Taquet M (2015) Emotions in Everyday Life. PLoS ONE 10(12): e0145450. doi.org/10.1371/journal.pone.0145450

Unfuck Your Intimacy

Addington, D. (1997). *A hand in the bush.* San Francisco, CA: Greenery Press.

Addington, D. (2006). *Play piercing.* San Francisco, Calif.: Greenery.

Alman, I. (1993). *Let's talk sex.* Freedom, CA: Crossing Press.

Apps, A. (n.d.). *Intersex.*

Asexuality Archive. (2012). *Asexuality: A brief introduction.*

Barker, M. and Hancock, J. (n.d.). *Enjoy sex.*

Barker, M. and Scheele, J. (2016). *Queer.* London: Icon Books Ltd.

Barnes-Svarney, P. (2012). *Why Do Women Crave More Sex in the Summer?.* Penguin Group (USA) Incorporated.

Bass, E. and Davis, L. (1992). *The courage to heal.* New York: HarperPerennial.

Becker, G. (1997). *The gift of fear.* Boston: Little, Brown and Company.

Belge, K. and Bieschke, M. (2012). *Queer.* San Francisco, Calif.: Zest.

Berkowitz, E. (2013). *Sex and punishment.* Berkeley, Calif.: Counterpoint.

Bernstein, R. (2009). *The East, the West, and sex.* New York: Vintage Books.

Binaohan, B. (2014). *Decolonizing Trans/Gender 101.* biyuti publishing.

Blank, H. (2000). *Big big love.* Emeryville, CA: Greenery Press.

Blank, J. and Corinne, T. (2011). *Femalia.* San Francisco, CA: Last Gasp.

Blank, J. and Whidden, A. (2000). *Good vibrations.* San Francisco, Calif.: Down There Press.

Blue, V. (2006). *The adventurous couple's guide to sex toys.* San Francisco, Calif.: Cleis Press.

Blum, D. (2014). *Sex on the brain.* New York: Penguin Books.

Blume, E. (1998). *Secret survivors.* New York: Ballantine Books.

Bongiovanni, A., Jimerson, T., Crank! and Yarwood, A. (n.d.). *A quick & easy guide to they/them pronouns.*

Bornstein, K. (1220). *A queer and pleasant danger.* Boston, Mass: Beacon.

Bornstein, K. (2013). *Gender Outlaw.* Hoboken: Taylor and Francis.

Bornstein, K. and Bergman, S. (2010). *Gender outlaws.* Berkeley, CA: Seal Press.

Boyd, H. (2007). *She's not the man I married.* New York: Seal Press.

Breaking silence. (1995). New York: Xanthus Press.

Britton, P. and Lerma, H. (2003). *The complete idiot's guide to sensual massage illustrated.* Indianapolis, Ind.: Alpha.

Britton, P. (n.d.). *The art of sex coaching.*

Brody, M. (n.d.). *Stop the fight!.*

Carnes, P. (1989). *Contrary to love.* Minneapolis: CompCare.

Carnes, P. (1992). *Don't call it love.* New York: Bantam.

Carnes, P. (2001). *Facing the shadow.* Wickenburg, AZ: Gentle Path.

Carnes, P. and Carnes, P. (2001). *Out of the shadows.* Center City, MN: Hazelden Information & Edu.

Carnes, P. and Moriarity, J. (1997). *Sexual anorexia.* Center City (Minn.): Hazelden.

Carnes, P., Delmonico, D. and Griffin, E. (2008). *In the shadows of the net.* Center City, Minn.: Hazelden.

Chodorow, N. (n.d.). *Femininities, masculinities, sexualities.*

Cockrill, K., Gimeno, L. and Herold, S. (2015). *Untold stories.* North Charleston: CreateSpace Independent Publishing Platform.

Cohen Greene, C. and Garano, L. (n.d.). *An intimate life.*

Corinna, H. (2007). *S.E.X.*. New York: Da Capo.

Cottrell, S. (2014). *Mom, I'm gay.* Freedhearts.

Davis, L. (1991). *Allies in healing.* New York, N.Y.: HarperPerennial.

Davis, L. (1991). *The Courage to Heal Workbook.* New York, N.Y.: Harper & Row.

Diamond, L. (2009). *Sexual fluidity.* Cambridge, Mass.: Harvard University Press.

Diamond, M. (2011). *Trans/love.* San Francisco: Manic D Press.

Dodson, B. (1996). *Sex for one.* New York: Crown Trade Paperbacks.

Dohrenwend, A. (2012). *Coming around.* Far Hills, N.J.: New Horizon Press.

Duron, L. (2013). *Raising my rainbow.* New York: Broadway Books.

Durve, A. (2012). *The power to break free workbook.* [United States]: Power Press LLC.

Easton, D. and Hardy, J. (2004). *Radical ecstasy.* Oakland, Calif.: Greenery Press.

Easton, D. and Liszt, C. (n.d.). *The ethical slut.*

Easton, D., Hardy, J. and Easton, D. (2003). *The new topping book.* Oakland, CA: Greenery Press.

Easton, D., Liszt, C. and Beck, A. (1997). *The bottoming book, or, how to get terrible things done to you by wonderful people.* Greenery.

Ehrensaft, D. (n.d.). *The gender creative child.*

Eisner, S. (n.d.). *Bi.*

Emberley, M. and Harris, R. (2009). *It's Perfectly Normal.* Somerville: Candlewick Press.

Emerson, D. (n.d.). *Trauma-sensitive yoga in therapy.*

Emme, M. (2013). *In your hands.* Berlin: Bruno Gmander.

Erickson-Schroth, L. (n.d.). *Trans bodies, trans selves.*

Evans, P. (2003). *Verbal abuse survivors speak out.* Holbrook, Mass.: Adams Media.

Factora-Borchers, L. and Simmons, A. (n.d.). *Dear sister.*

Feinberg, L. (2005). *Transgender warriors.* Boston, Mass: Beacon Press.

Feinberg, L. (2006). *Drag king dreams.* New York: Carroll & Graf Publishers.

Feinberg, L. (2007). *Trans liberation.* Boston, Mass: Beacon Press.

Fernbach, A. (2003). *Fantasies of fetishism.* New Brunswick, NJ [u.a.]: Rutgers Univ. Press.

Fields, R. Douglas (2015) *Why we snap.* New York: Dutton.

Fincham, F., Fernandes, L. and Humphreys, K. (1993). *Communicating in relationships.* Champaign, IL: Research Press.

Finley, K. (2000). *A different kind of intimacy.* New York: Thunder's Mouth Press.

Ford, J. (1997). *Child of the universe.* [Ellsworth, Me.]: [Epigrammata Press].

Forssberg, M. and Lundin, M. (2007). *Sex for guys.* Toronto [Ont.]: Groundwood Books.

Garbacik, J. and Lewis, J. (n.d.). *Gender & sexuality for beginners.*

Germer, C. (2009). *The mindful path to self-compassion.* New York: Guilford Press.

Glasser, W. (1995). *Staying together.* New York: HarperCollins.
Glenum, L. (2010). *Gurlesque.* Philadelphia, PA: Saturnalia Books.
Goad, J. (2007). *Jim Goad's gigantic book of sex.* Los Angeles, Calif.: Feral House.
Goldberg, S. and Brushwood Rose, C. (2009). *And Baby Makes More: Known Donors, Queer Parents, and Our Unexpected Families.* Insomniac Press.
Gottman, J., Gottman, J. and DeClaire, J. (n.d.). *Ten lessons to transform your marriage.*
Haberman, H. (n.d.). *Family jewels - a guide to male genital play and torment.*
Haines, S. (1999). *The survivor's guide to sex.* San Francisco: Cleis Press.
Hardy, J. (2006). *21st century kinkycrafts.* San Francisco, Calif.: Greenery.
Hasler, N. and Capozzola, M. (n.d.). *Sex.*
Heath, H. and White, I. (2002). *The challenge of sexuality in health care.* Osney Mead, Oxford: Blackwell Science.
Helminiak, D. (n.d.). *What the Bible really says about homosexuality.*
Henderson, E. and Armstrong, N. (n.d.). *100 questions you'd never ask your parents.*
Herek, G. (1998). *Stigma and sexual orientation.* London: SAGE.
Hills, R. (n.d.). *The sex myth.*
Hitt, S. (1997). *Cooking with less salt, less sugar, less fat . . . in less time.* Windmore Writers.
Hoffman-Fox, D., Jones, Z., Finch, S. and Keig, Z. (n.d.). *You and your gender identity.*
Hogan, S. (2003). *Gender issues in art therapy.* London: Jessica Kingsley Pub.
Holly, K. (n.d.). *Domestic violence safety plan.*
Hochschild, Arlie Russell. *The Managed Heart: Commercialization of Human Feeling.* University of California Press, 2012.
Jarvis, C. (2002). *The marriage sabbatical: the journey that brings you home.* Broadway Books/Jan.
Joannides, P., Gross, D. and Johnson, T. (n.d.). *Guide to getting it on.*
Johnson, S. (n.d.). *Hold me tight.*
Judson, O. (2003). *Dr. Tatiana's sex advice to all creation.* Metropolitan Owl Book.
Kahr, B. and Kahr, B. (2009). *Who's been sleeping in your head.* New York: Basic Books.
Kaufman, M., Silverberg, C. and Odette, F. (2010). *The ultimate guide to sex and disability.* Read How You Want.
Keel, P. (2000). *All about us.* New York: Broadway Books.
Kendrick, S., Kendrick, A. and Kimbrough, L. (2008). *The love dare.* Nashville, Tenn.: B & H Publishing Group.
Kerner, I. (2008). *Passionista.* New York: William Morrow.
Kerner, I. and Rinna, L. (2014). *The big, fun, sexy sex book.* New York: Gallery Books.
Kerner, I. (n.d.). *She comes first.*
Killermann, S. (2013). *The social justice advocate's handbook.* Austin, Tx.: Impetus Books.
Komisaruk, B. (2010). *The orgasm answer guide.* Baltimore: Johns Hopkins University Press.
Kort, J. (n.d.). *Gay affirmative therapy for the straight clinician.*
Kramer, P. (1997). *Should you leave?.* New York: Scribner.
Kuklin, S. (2015). *Beyond magenta.* Somerville: Candlewick Press.
Lee, J. (n.d.). *Coming out like a porn star.*
Lee, J. (n.d.). *Torn.*
Leiblum, S. and Rosen, R. (2000). *Principles and practice of sex therapy.* New York: Guilford Press.
Leman, K. (n.d.). *Sheet music.*
Lerner, H. (1990). *The dance of intimacy.* New York, N.Y.: Harper Perennial.
Ley, D. (n.d.). *The myth of sex addiction.*
Linssen, L. and Wik, S. (2010). *Love unlimited.* Forres, Scotland: Findhorn Press.
Lotney, K. (2000). *The ultimate guide to strap-on sex.* San Francisco, Calif.: Cleis.
Love, P. and Robinson, J. (1995). *Hot monogamy.* New York: Plume.
Maltz, W. (2001). *The sexual healing journey.* New York: HarperCollins World.
Marr, L. (2007). *Sexually transmitted diseases.* Baltimore: Johns Hopkins University Press.
Martin, C. (n.d.). *Unclobber.*
Masters, P. (2001). *Look into my eyes.* San Francisco, Calif.: Greenery Press.
Masters, P. (2007). *The Control Book.* Rinella Editorial Services.
Matik, W. (2002). *Redefining our relationships.* Oakland, CA: HMPH! Press.

Maxfield, G. (1998). *The Novel approach to sexuality and disability.* Sparks, Nev.: Northern Nevada Amputee Support Group.

Mazza, J. (2001). *Exploring your sexual self.* Cincinnati, OH: Walking Stick Press.

McCarthy, B. (n.d.). *Sex made simple.*

McKay, M., Fanning, P. and Paleg, K. (1996). *Couple skills.* Oakland, Calif.: New Harbinger Publ.

Melton, G. (2016). *Love warrior.* Flatiron Books.

Merck, M. (1993). *Perversions.* London: Virago.

Mirk, S. (n.d.). *Sex from scratch.*

Moon, A. (n.d.). *Bad dyke.*

Moser, C. and Hardy, J. (2002). *Sex disasters, and how to survive them.* San Francisco, Calif.: Greenery Press.

Nagoski, E. (n.d.). *Come as you are.*

Neff, K. (2011). *Self-compassion.* New York: HarperCollins.

Northrup, C., Schwartz, P. and Witte, J. (2012). *The normal bar.* New York: Crown Archetype.

Oliver, G. and Oliver, C. (2007). *Mad about us.* Minneapolis, Minn.: Bethany House Publishers.

Our bodies, ourselves. (2008). New York: Touchstone Book/Simon & Schuster.

Parker-Pope, Tara. "More People Appear to Be Cheating on Their Spouses, Studies Find." *The New York Times, The New York Times,* 27 Oct. 2008, nytimes.com/2008/10/28/health/28well.html.

Pascoe, C. (2012). *Dude, you're a fag.* Berkeley, Calif.: University of California Press.

"Path to Safety - National Domestic Violence Hotline." The National Domestic Violence Hotline, thehotline.org/help/path-to-safety/.

Prooyen, Eva Van. "This One Thing Is the Biggest Predictor of Divorce." *The Gottman Institute,* The Gottman Institute 4 Min Read 10,856 The Meaning of Life Is to Make Other People's Lives More Meaningful. 15 Feb. 2018, gottman.com/blog/this-one-thing-is-the-biggest-predictor-of-divorce/

Queen, C. (2009). *Exhibitionism for the shy.* Gardena, Calif.: Down There Press.

Richo, D. (2005). *The five things we cannot change.* Boston, Mass.: Shambhala.

Robnoxious (n.d.). *Alive with vigor.*

Ross, C. and Dodson, B. (n.d.). *Betty Dodson bodysex basics.*

Rothblum, E.D., Krueger, E.A., Kittle, K.R. et al. Asexual and Non-Asexual Respondents from a U.S. Population-Based Study of Sexual Minorities. Arch Sex Behav 49, 757-767 (2020). doi.org/10.1007/s10508-019-01485-0

Rubel, R. (2007). *Master/slave relations.* Las Vegas, Nev.: Nazca Plains.

"Safety Planning for Domestic Violence and Abuse Victims." Abusive Relationships, Verbal Abuse in Marriage and Domestic Violence, Verbal Abuse Journals, verbalabusejournals.com/how-stop-abuse/safety-planning/.

"Safety Plan: When You Live With the Abuse." Scarleteen, 22 Apr. 2014, scarleteen.com/safety_plan_when_you_live_with_the_abuse.

Salmansohn, K. and Krauss, T. (2002). *The clitourist.* New York: Universe.

Savage, D. and Miller, T. (n.d.). *It gets better.*

Semans, A. and Winks, C. (2001). *The mother's guide to sex.* New York: Three Rivers Press.

Sewell, J. (2007). *I'd rather eat chocolate.* New York: Broadway Books.

Sex. (2014). Quiver.

Smith, R., Gingrich, C. and Taylor, G. (n.d.). *Speaking out.*

Sprinkle, A. (2005). *Dr. Sprinkle's spectacular sex.* New York: Jeremy P. Tarcher/Penguin.

Stahl, B. and Goldstein, E. (2010). *A mindfulness-based stress reduction workbook.* Oakland, Calif.: New Harbinger Publications.

Stern, D. (n.d.). *Swingland.*

Stewart, E. and Spencer, P. (2002). *The V book.* New York: Bantam Books.

Strayed, C. (n.d.). *Tiny beautiful things.*

Strict, M. (2003). *Intimate invasions.* San Francisco, Calif.: Greenery.

Stryker, S. (2008). *Transgender history.* Berkeley, Calif.: Seal Press.

Sukel, K. (2014). *This is your brain on sex.* Free Press.

Taormino, T. (1998). *The ultimate guide to anal sex for women.* San Francisco, Calif.: Cleis Press.

Taormino, T. (2007). *Opening up.* San Francisco, Calif.: Cleis.

Taormino, T. (2009). *The anal sex positions guide.* Beverly, MA: Quiver.

Taormino, T. (2010). *The big book of sex toys.* Gloucester, Mass.: Quiver.

Taormino, T. (n.d.). *New sex.*

Tempest. (2006). *The toybag guide to medical play.* San Francisco, Calif.: Greenery.`

The "go ask Alice" book of answers. (1998). New York: H. Holt.

Tilsen, J. (2013). *Therapeutic conversations with queer youth.* Lanham: Jason Aronson.

"Tinder: Swiping Self Esteem?" ScienceDaily, ScienceDaily, 4 Aug. 2016, sciencedaily.com/releases/2016/08/160804172410.htm.

Tipping, C. (1997). *Radical forgiveness.* Atlanta, GA: GOLDENeight Publishers.

Two Knotty Boys. and Utley, L. (2008). *Showing you the ropes.* San Francisco, Calif.: Green Candy.

Varrin, C. (2005). *Female dominance.* New York: Citadel.

Verdolin, J. (n.d.). *Wild connection.*

Waxman, J. (2007). *Getting off.* Emeryville, CA: Seal Press.

Westheimer, R. and Lehu, P. (2009). *Dr. Ruth's top 10 secrets for great sex.* San Francisco: Jossey-Bass.

"White Mountain Waldorf School." *White Mountain Waldorf,* whitemountainwaldorf.org/articles/touch/.

Wijsmeijer, AA. and van Assen, MA. "Psychological characteristics of BDSM participants." J Sex Med. 2013 Aug;10(8):1943-52

Winks, C. (1999). *The g-spot.* Down There.

Wiseman, J. (2000). *Jay Wiseman's erotic bondage handbook.* Emeryville, CA: Greenery Press.

Yoe, C. (n.d.). *The best of Sexology.*

Unfuck Your Boundaries

2015 U.S. Transgender Survey Report. (n.d.). Retrieved from vawnet.org/material/2015-us-transgender-survey-report

Aravind VK, Krishnaram VD, Thasneem Z. Boundary crossings and violations in clinical settings. *Indian J Psychol Med.* 2012;34(1):21–24.

Breit, S., Kupferberg, A., Rogler, G., & Hasler, G. (2018). Vagus Nerve as Modulator of the Brain-Gut Axis in Psychiatric and Inflammatory Disorders. *Frontiers in psychiatry, 9,* 44.

Boas, F. (1997). *Handbook of American Indian languages: Franz Boas.* London: Routledge/Thoemmes.

Bottalico, B. (2009). Neuroscience, accountability and individual boundaries. *Frontiers in Human Neuroscience, 3.*

Chapman, S., & Routledge, C. (2005). *Key thinkers in linguistics and the philosophy of language.* Edinburgh: Edinburgh University Press.

Chödrön, P., & Sell, E. H. (2018). *Comfortable with uncertainty: 108 teachings.* Boulder: Shambhala.

Chödrön, P. (2018, November 23). How We Get Hooked By Shenpa. Retrieved from lionsroar.com/how-we-get-hooked-shenpa-and-how-we-get-unhooked/

Crabb, C. (2017). *Learning good consent.* Microcosm Publishing.

DeBecker, G. (2000). *The gift of fear.* London: Bloomsbury.

Dutton, M. A., Goodman, L., & Schmidt, R. J. (2008). Development and Validation of a Coercive Control Measure for Intimate Partner Violence in Boston, Massachusetts and Washington, DC, 2004. *ICPSR Data Holdings.*

Edwards, S. R., Bradshaw, K. A., & Hinsz, V. B. (2014). Denying Rape but Endorsing Forceful Intercourse: Exploring Differences Among Responders. *Violence and Gender, 1*(4), 188-193.

Fontes, L. A. (2015). *Invisible chains: Overcoming coercive control in your intimate relationship.* New York, NY: Guilford Press.

Gender Differences in Heterosexual College Students' Conceptualizations and Indicators of Sexual Consent: Implications for Contemporary Sexual Assault Prevention Education. (n.d.). Retrieved from tandfonline.com/doi/full/10.1080/00224499.2013.792326

Hunter, M. (2007, June 22). How To Write A BIFF Response. Retrieved from highconflictinstitute.com/free-articles/2018/1/12/how-to-write-a-biff-response

Jenkins, A. (2001). *Invitations to responsibility: The therapeutic engagement of men who are violent and abusive.* Adelaide: Dulwich Centre Publications.

Kitzinger, C., & Frith, H. (1999). Just Say No? The Use of Conversation Analysis in Developing a Feminist Perspective on Sexual Refusal. Retrieved from journals.sagepub.com/doi/abs/10.1177/0957926599010003002

Lorde, A. (2007). *Sister outsider: Essays and speeches.* New York: Crossing Press.

Mirk, S. (2017). *Sex from scratch: Making your own relationship rules.* Portland, OR: Microcosm Publishing.

"Monoaminergic." Monoaminergic - an Overview | ScienceDirect Topics, sciencedirect.com/topics/biochemistry-genetics-and-molecular-biology/monoaminergic.

Mythcommunication: It's Not That They Don't Understand, They Just Don't Like The Answer. (2011, March 21). Retrieved from yesmeansyesblog.wordpress.com/2011/03/21/mythcommunication-its-not-that-they-dont-understand-they-just-dont-like-the-answer/

Neff, K., & Germer, C. K. (2018). *The mindful self-compassion workbook: A proven way to accept yourself, build inner strength, and thrive.* New York, NY: Guilford Press.

Ng, Wee Keong, et al. "Lossless and Lossy Data Compression." Evolutionary Algorithms in Engineering Applications, 1997, pp. 173-188.

O'Shea, T. (2011) *Green Paper Report: Consent in History, Theory and Practice.* Essex Autonomy Project: autonomy.essex.ac.uk/wp-content/uploads/2016/11/Consent-GPR-June-2012.pdf

Rockwell, I. N. (2002). *The five wisdom energies: A Buddhist way of understanding personalities, emotions, and relationships.* Boston: Shambhala.

Schulman, S. (2017). *Conflict is not abuse: Overstating harm, community responsibility and the duty of repair.* Vancouver: Arsenal Pulp Press.

Shepherd, B. (2019, January 31). How a simple tool called the 'No Test' could help identify a potentially abusive partner. Retrieved from abc.net.au/news/2019-01-31/how-the-no-test-could-help-prevent-domestic-violence/10764100

Skene, L., & Smallwood, R. (2002, January 05). Informed consent: Lessons from Australia. Retrieved from bmj.com/content/324/7328/39.long

Stark, E. (2009). Rethinking Coercive Control. Violence Against Women, 15(12), 1509–1525. doi.org/10.1177/1077801209347452

Stark, E. D. (2009). *Coercive control: The entrapment of women in personal life.* Oxford: Oxford University Press.

Storm, C. (2018). *Empowered boundaries: Speaking truth, setting boundaries, and inspiring social change.* Berkeley, CA: North Atlantic Books.

The History Behind Sexual Consent Policies. (2014, October 05). Retrieved from npr.org/2014/10/05/353922015/the-history-behind-sexual-consent-policies

Thelilynews. (2019, February 14). It's not enough to hope for the best. Millennials are writing contracts for their relationships. - The Lily. Retrieved from thelily.com/its-not-enough-to-hope-for-the-best-millennials-are-writing-contracts-for-their-relationships/

Trans-Specific Power and Control Tactics. (n.d.). Retrieved from vawnet.org/material/trans-specific-power-and-control-tactics

Violence Against Trans and Non-Binary People. (n.d.). Retrieved from vawnet.org/sc/serving-trans-and-non-binary-survivors-domestic-and-sexual-violence/violence-against-trans-and

"Visceral Influences on Brain and Behavior." Neuron, Cell Press, 20 Feb. 2013, sciencedirect.com/science/article/pii/S0896627313001402.

Vrangalova, Z. (2018, November 02). Everything You Need to Know About Consent

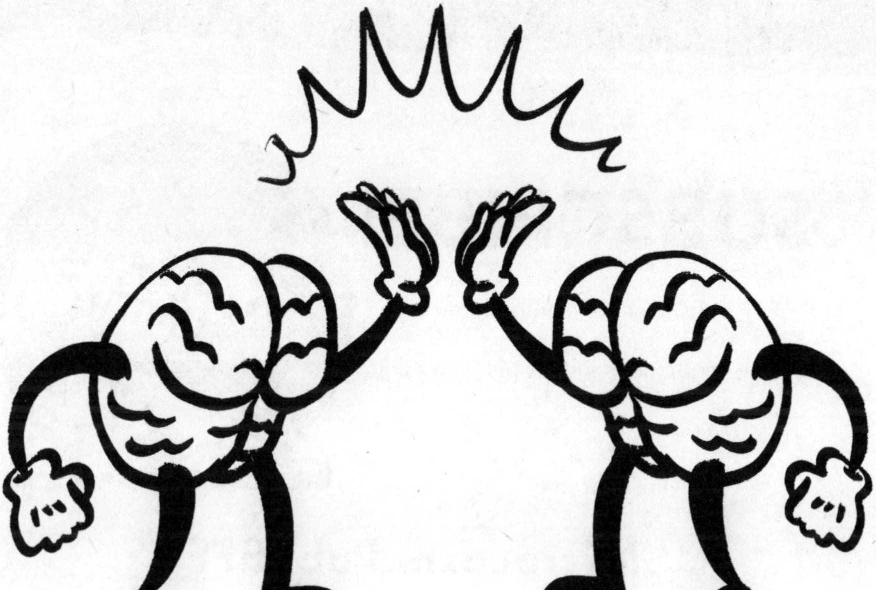